RURAL WATER SUPPLY AND SANITATION

RURAL WATER SUPPLY

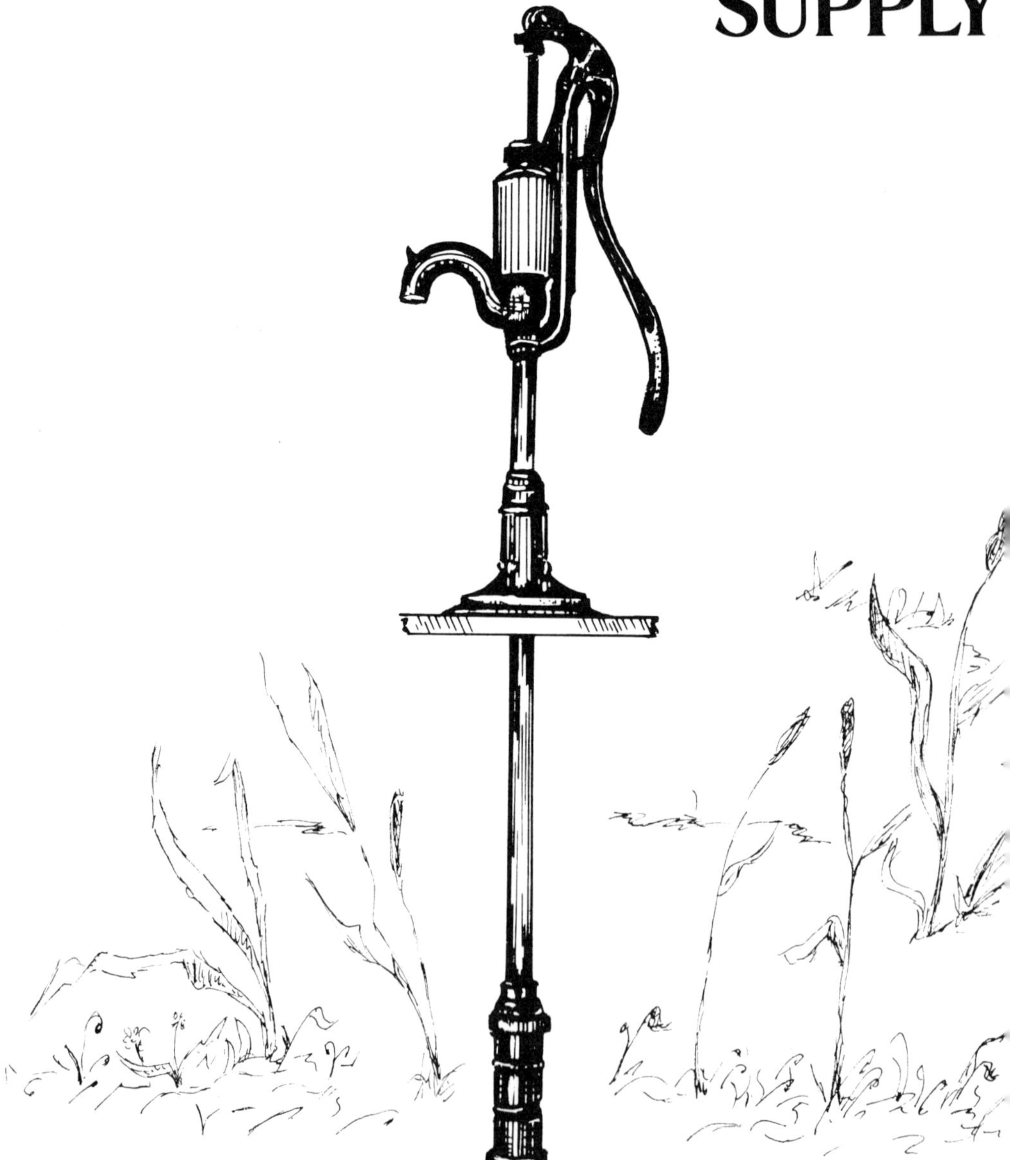

AND SANITATION

THIRD EDITION

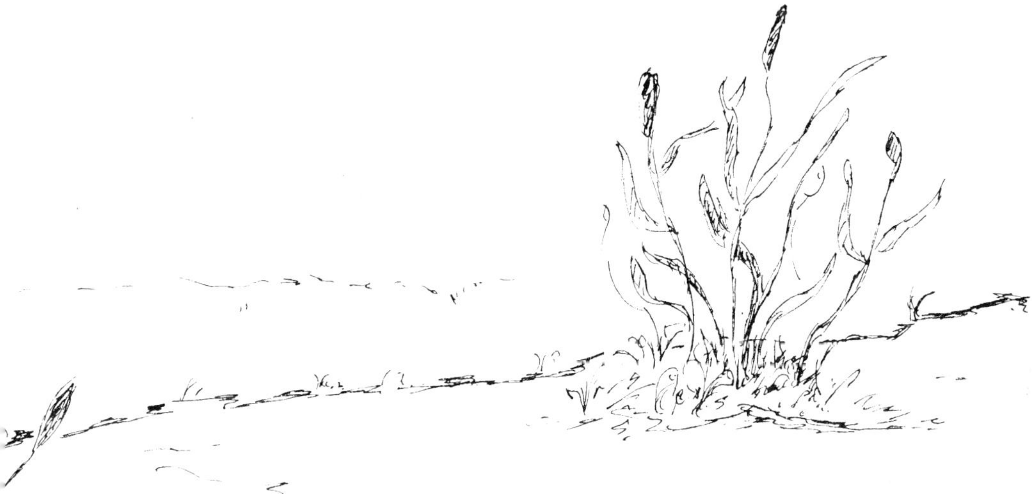

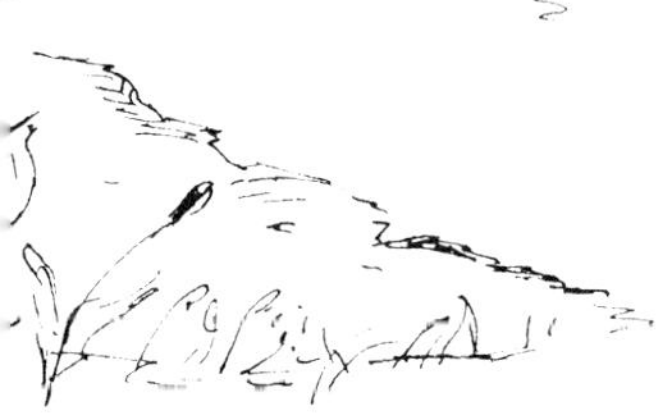

FORREST B. WRIGHT, Ph.D.

Professor Emeritus of Agricultural Engineering
New York State College of Agriculture
Cornell University, Ithaca, New York

ROBERT E. KRIEGER PUBLISHING COMPANY
HUNTINGTON, NEW YORK

Original edition 1939
Second edition 1956
Third edition 1977

Printed and Published by
ROBERT E. KRIEGER PUB. CO., INC.
645 NEW YORK AVENUE
HUNTINGTON, NEW YORK 11743

Library of Congress Cataloging in Publication Data

Wright, Forrest Blythe, 1896-
Rural water supply and sanitation.

Reprint of the 2d ed. published by Wiley, New York, in Wiley farm series.
1. Water-supply, Rural. 2. Plumbing. 3. Sewerage, Rural. I. Title.
[TD920.W75 1975] 628.7 75-14110
ISBN 0-88275-334-7

Printed in the United States of America.

DEDICATED

to the betterment of rural life

Preface to the Third Edition

For this edition of the book the author has endeavored to include all of the most important new developments in materials and techniques in the field of rural water supply and sewage disposal. Also, reference is made to the relation of the subject matter of the book to the over-all ecology of our times. New instruction material and new illustrations have been added where necessary.

Both metric and English units of measurement are indicated in most places where measurements are involved. A list of measurement conversion factors is included in the back of the book.

It has been the aim of the author to present the subject matter in such a way that one who masters the contents of the book should be able to take the fullest advantage of the possible water sources provided by nature, should be able to plan and construct a safe, convenient, and sanitary sewage disposal system, and should be able to service and keep in repair his plumbing and sewage-disposal systems at a minimum expense.

The book is divided into two parts. In the first part the important aspects of water supply and sewage disposal for the rural home and farmstead are discussed. Particular emphasis is placed upon methods of securing adequate sources of potable water, the selection and installation of pumping equipment, treatment of water where necessary, the design and installation of supply plumbing systems, and the design and installation of sanitary sewage and waste disposal systems. Important jobs connected with water supply and sewage disposal are presented in the second part of the book. These jobs are of a practical nature and will be helpful to anyone who wishes to plan or actually install water supply or sewage disposal equipment. References are given to the related subject matter in the first part of the book. These references should be read carefully before the jobs are started.

FORREST B. WRIGHT

Ithaca, N.Y.
March, 1976

Acknowledgments

For this revised edition the author gratefully acknowledges the valuable suggestions given by the following persons: Professor J.E. Kiker, Jr., College of Civil Engineering, University of Florida, Gainesville, Fla.; Professor W.C. Wheeler, Department of Agriculturing Engineering, University of Connecticut, Storrs, Conn.; Mr. G.E. Henderson, Co-ordinator, Southern Association of Agricultural Engineering and Vocational Agriculture, Athens, Ga.; and Mr. F.R. Ligouri, Tompkins County Health Department, Ithaca, N.Y.

The author is also indebted to the following for many of the illustrations and some text material: Morse Chain Co., Ithaca, N.Y.; U.S. Department of Agriculture, Washington, D.C.; Florida Power and Light Co., Sarasota, Fla.; Norfolk Port Authority, Norfolk, Va.; U.S. Weather Bureau, Washington, D.C.; Professor Harold Gray, Department of Agricultural Engineering, Cornell University, Ithaca, N.Y.; Sears Roebuck and Co., Philadelphia, Pa.; H.L.G. Co., Kalamazoo, Mich.; *Farm Journal,* Philadelphia, Pa.; Edward E. Johnson, Inc., St. Paul, Minn.; The Deming Co., Salem, Ohio; The F.E. Myers & Brothers Co., Ashland, Ohio; Goulds Pumps, Inc., Seneca Falls, N.Y.; National Association of Domestic and Farm Pump Manufacturers, Chicago, Ill.; Decatur Pump Co., Decatur, Ill.; William C. Popper and Co., New York, N.Y.; Mr. Clay Chadwick, Sarasota, Fla.; Orangeburg Manufacturing Co., New York, N.Y.; The Phillip Sitton Septic Tank Co., Dayton, Ohio; Portland Cement Association, Chicago, Ill.; San-Equip Inc., Syracuse, N.Y.; New York State Department of Health, Albany, N.Y.; Department of Poultry Husbandry, Cornell University, Ithaca, N.Y.; Copper and Brass Research Association, New York, N.Y.; Professors W.J. Riley, E.O. Eaton, C.N. Turner, and J.C. McCurdy, Cornell University, Ithaca, N.Y.; Mr. Paul Wright, Ithaca, N.Y.; Mr. F.R. Ligouri, Tompkins County Health Department, Ithaca, N.Y.; Professor J.E. Kiker, College of Civil Engineering, University of Florida, Gainesville, Fla.; Reinhold Publishing Corp., New

York, N.Y.; Mr. S.R. Weibel, Robert Taft Sanitary Engineering Center, Cincinnati, Ohio; Crane Company, Engineering and Research Division, Chicago, Ill.; Professor Arthur Schultz, Department of Agricultural Engineering, North Dakota Agriculture College, Fargo, N. Dak.; Rural Electrification Administration, Washington, D.C.; American Society of Agricultural Engineers, St. Joseph, Mich.; Lancaster Pump and Manufacturing Company, Lancaster, Pa.; Trend Manufacturing Company of America, Inc., Jacksonville, Fla.; Amco Chemicals Corporation, Industrial Products Division, Stow, Ohio; Delta Faucet Company, Greensberg, Indiana; Jet Areation Company, Cleveland, Ohio; and Borg-Warner Plumbing Products, Mansfield, Ohio; The Christian Science Monitor and Mr. Stewart Dill McBride.

For valuable assistance and understanding co-operation in the mechanical preparation of the manuscript the author is deeply indebted to his wife Mildred.

Contents

Part One

Part Two

List of Tables

PART ONE

Importance of Water 1

Water Is Essential for Life

The use of water by man, plants, and animals is universal. Without it there can be no life. *Every living thing requires water.* Man can live nearly two months without food, but can live only three or four days without water.

Water Is Essential for Health and Sanitation

In our homes, whether in the city or in the country, water is essential for cleanliness and health. The average American family uses from 65,000 to 75,000 U.S. gallons (54,166 to 62,500 Imp. gals.) of water per year for various household purposes.

Water Is a Principle Raw Material for Food Production

Water can be considered as the principal raw material and the lowest cost raw material from which most of our farm produce is made. It is essential for the growth of crops and animals and is a very important factor in the production of milk and eggs. Animals and poultry, if constantly supplied with good running water, will produce more meat, more milk, and more eggs per pound of feed and per hour of labor. If there is a shortage of water there will be a decline in farm production, just as a shortage of steel will cause a decrease in the production of automobiles. For these reasons it is good business for a farmer to carefully plan and install an *adequate* water system.

In addition to the direct use of water in our homes and on the fram, there are many indirect ways in which water affects our lives. In manufacturing, generation of electric power, transportation, recreation, and in many other ways water plays a very important role.

IMPORTANCE OF WATER IN OUR ECOLOGY

A subject which is now becoming of great importance to all of us is the matter of a balanced ecology, that is, a balance in the relationship between living things and the environment in which they live. Obviously water plays a critical role in this relationship. All living things depend upon it. For example, all animal life depends, directly or indirectly, upon vegetation for food, and vegetation will not grow without water. Vegetable matter, such as leaves and stems, can be converted to soil by bacterial action. Bacteria need water in order to thrive. New plants growing in this soil take up nutrients through their roots in the form of a solution in water. Any break in this ecological chain can mean a failure of the whole ecological system.

Water Conservation and Sanitation Are Important

Our use of water is increasing rapidly with our growing population. Already there are acute shortages of both surface and underground waters in many localities. We in the United States are pumping more than three times as much water out of the ground as we did 30 years ago. As a result, in some areas, the land is sinking, the water table has been lowered until the wells have to be deepened or abandoned. Along coastal areas the lowering of the fresh water table has allowed salt water to filter inland and ruin many wells.

Careless pollution and contamination of our streams, lakes, and underground sources has greatly impaired the quality of the water we do have available. It is, therefore, of utmost importance for our future that good water conservation and sanitary measures be practiced by everyone. Otherwise we may some day find that there is not enough good water to go around.

It has been estimated that, in the United States, the average daily consumption of water is 165 U.S. gallons (137 Imp. gals.) per person. If each of the 220 million persons saved, on the average, 5 U.S. gallons (4.17 Imp. gals.) per day the total saving would be 1.1 billion U.S. gallons (0.92 billion Imp. gals.) per day. In one year we would save 365 times that much, or 400 billion U.S. gallons (333 billion Imp. gals.).

Our ground water has been accumulating over the past centuries. If we remove it faster than precipitation can replace it, we will eventually deplete the supply. There are two ways in which we can prevent the depletion. One is to use less water, and the other is to provide better means of replenishing the supply.

The following suggestions will be helpful in reducing our use of water without sacrificing its full benefits. Some of the suggestions may seem trivial, but, as indicated above, if *everyone* saves a *little*, the overall savings will be very significant.

1. Repair all water leaks, including dripping faucets and leaking toilets. See Fig. J-4-1, pg. 264, for possible savings.

2. See that the hot water pipes are as short as possible, and are insulated so that less water will have to be drawn to get hot water.

3. Reduce shower time. Turn the water off while soaping the body. For tub baths draw one or two inches less water in the tub. Where septic tanks are used, suggestions 1, 2 and 3 will reduce the load on the disposal field.

4. Wash dishes and do laundry only when there are full loads for the machines. Automatic machines draw about the same amount of water per cycle regardless of the load.

5. When washing a car or farm machinery use the water sparingly and turn the hose off when not using it.

6. Use water saving toilets. (See Fig. J-5-4, page 273.) Install and use the type of toilet flush valve shown in Fig. J-5-3, page 273.

7. Water lawns and gardens adequately, but not wastefully. Don't leave hoses or sprinklers running overnight.

For replenishing the ground water supply such measures as reforestation, less drainage of wet lands, less paving of surface areas, soil erosion control to reduce run-off, or any other measures which will cause more water to soak into the ground will add significantly to our ground water supply.

Important Uses of Water

Figures 1-1 through 1-7 illustrate some of the important uses of water.

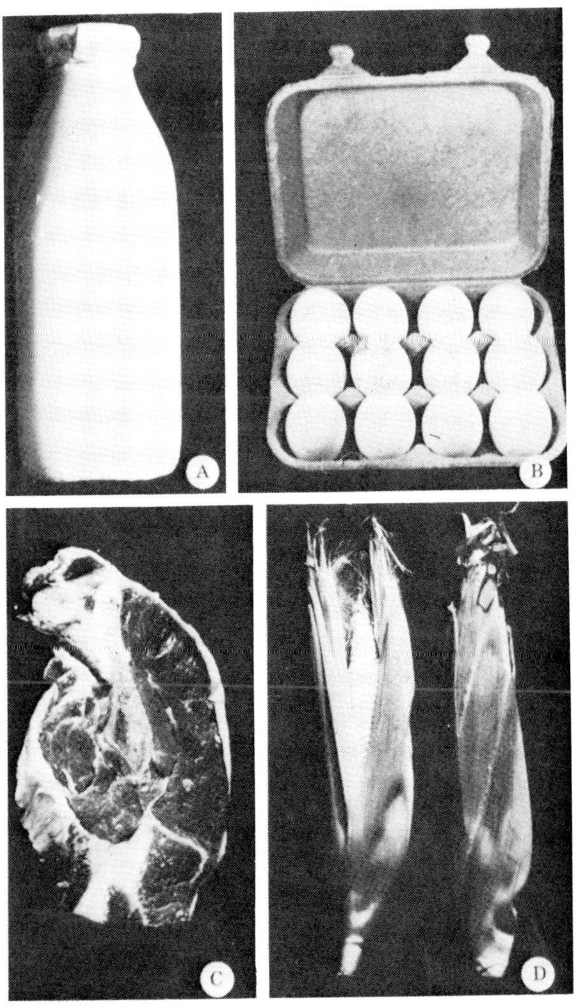

Fig. 1-1. A — Milk is 88% water. To produce one quart of milk a cow requires from 3½ to 5½ quarts (3.31 to 5.20 liters) of water. (From F.B. Morrison, Cornell University.)

B — Eggs are 66% water. To produce one dozen eggs hens require about 5 quarts (4.73 liters) of water. (From H.J. Bruckner, Cornell University.)

C — Beef is 77% water. To produce a pound of beef an animal must drink many times that much water.

D — It takes 365 pounds (164.56 kg.) of water to produce one pound (453.6 gms.) of dry matter in corn.

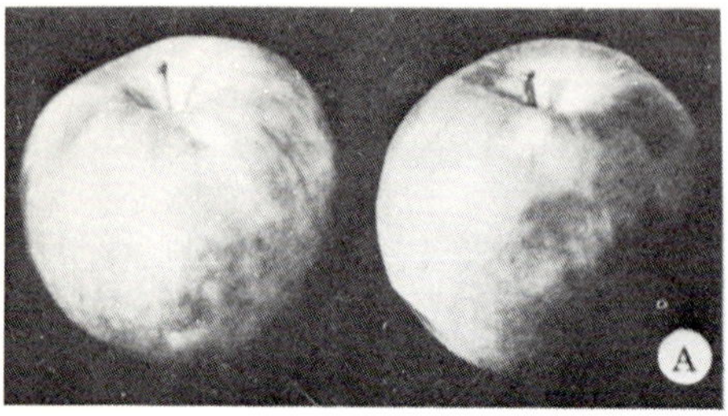

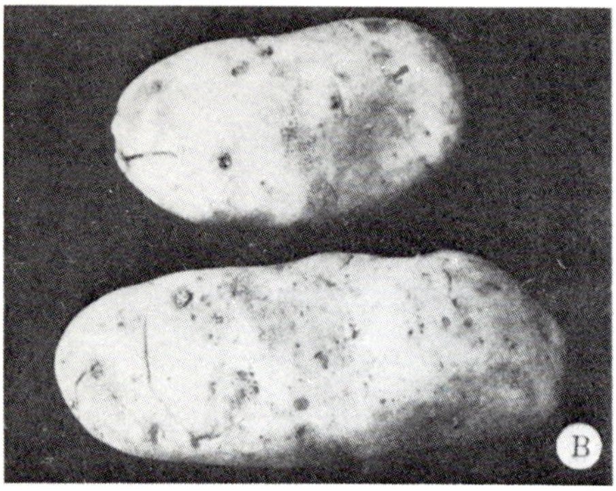

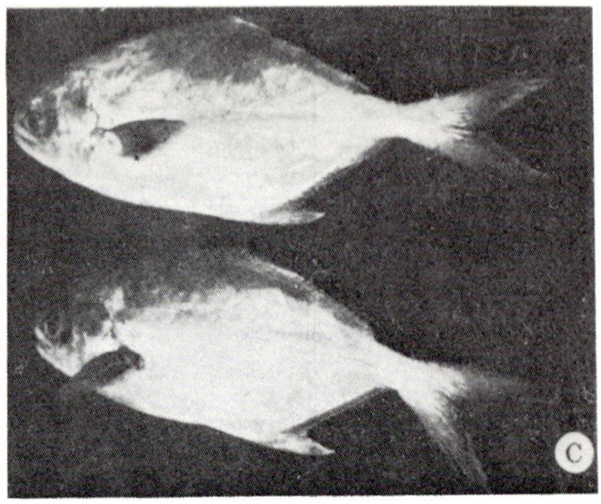

Fig. 1-2. A — Apples are 87% water. The tree on which they grow must have water many times the weight of the fruit.

B — Potatoes are 75% water. To grow an acre of potatoes tons of water are required.

C — Fish are 80% water. They not only consume water but must have large volumes of water in which to live.

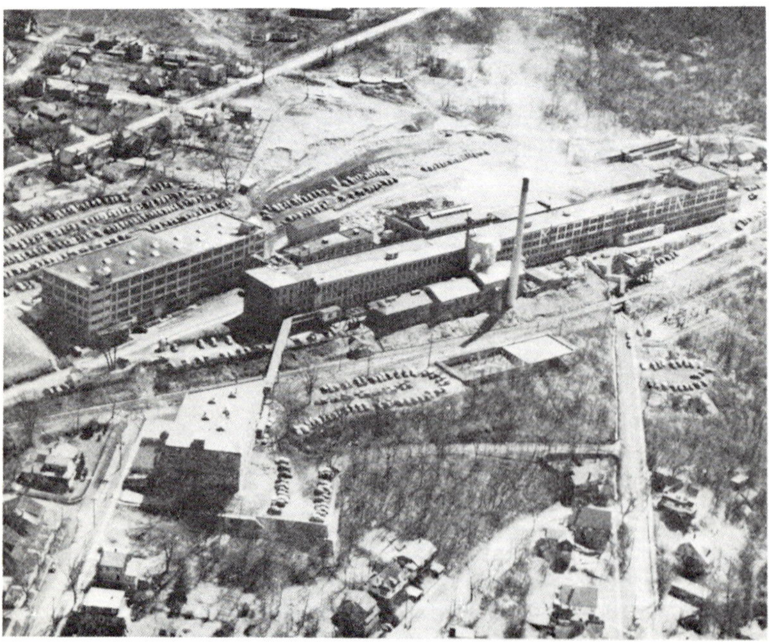

Courtesy Morse Chain Co., Ithica, N.Y.

Fig. 1-3. A manufacturing plant which produces power chains and sprockets. In 1974 this plant used 55 times as much water as steel in the manufacturing process.

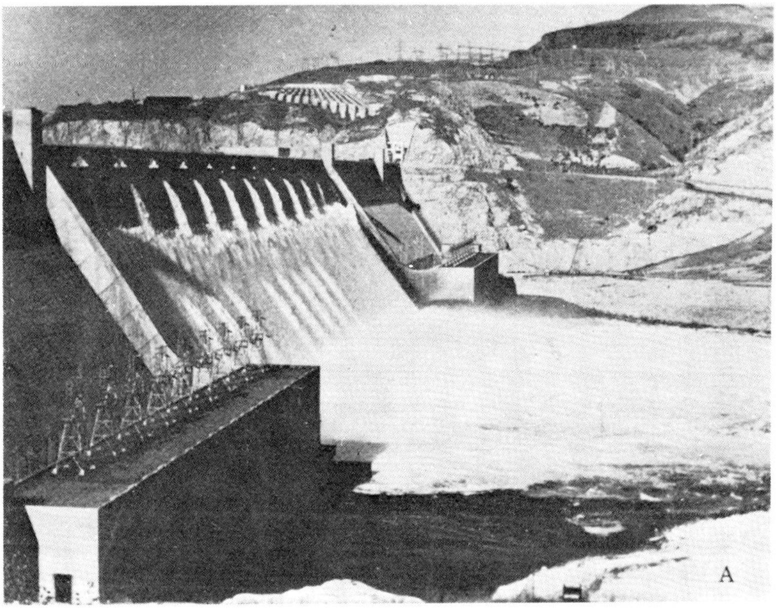

Courtesy U.S. Department of Agriculture

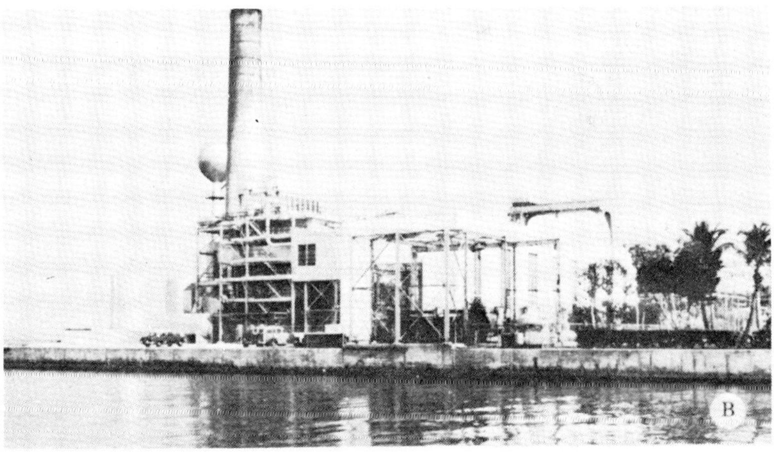

Courstey Florida Power and Light Co.

Fig. 1-4. Water is used for generating electric power. A — Grand Coulee Dam on the Columbia River in central Washington. The falling water provides power for one of the largest generating plants in the world. Also, part of the electric power is used to pump river water over the hills in the background for irrigation of thousands of square miles of fertile land.

B — A steam-generating plant at Sarasota, Fla. In such plants some water is used for steam and large quantities are used for cooling the condensers. Such plants use 500 to 700 tons of water for every ton of coal burned under the boilers. It is for this reason that steam-generating plants are always located at or near large bodies of water.

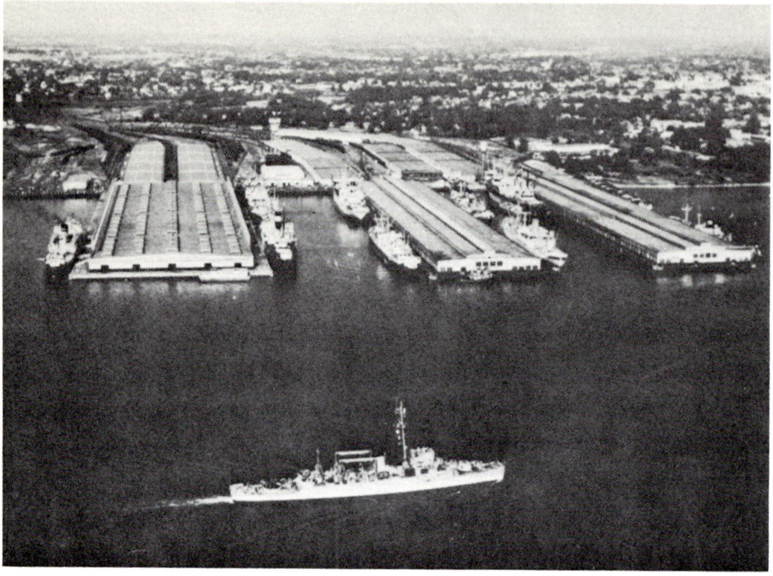

Courtesy Norfolk Port Authority

Fig. 1-5. The Lamberts Point Docks at Norfolk, Va., one of the largest shipping points in the world. Our rivers, lakes, and oceans provide cheap means of transportation.

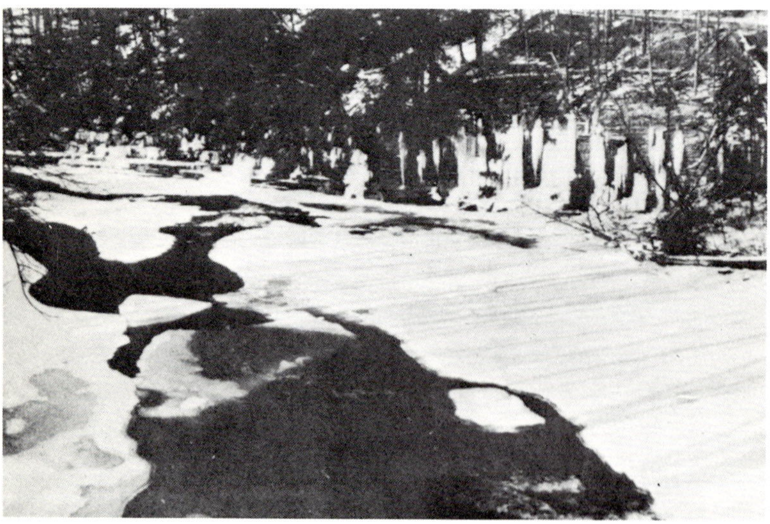

Fig. 1-6. Water plays an important part in the weather and climate. Water erosion is constantly changing the surface of the earth.

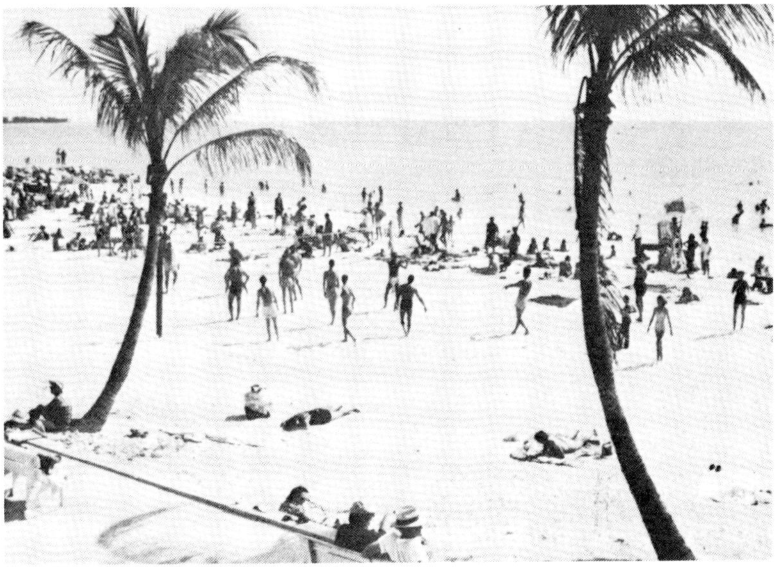

Fig. 1-7. Water plays an important part in the nation's recreational activities. This is Lido Beach, Fla.

The Nature and Sources of Water 2

NATURE OF WATER

Chemical Composition

Chemically pure water is a combination of two elements, hydrogen and oxygen. See Fig. 2-1. The chemical symbol is H^2O and the chemical name is hydrogen monoxide.

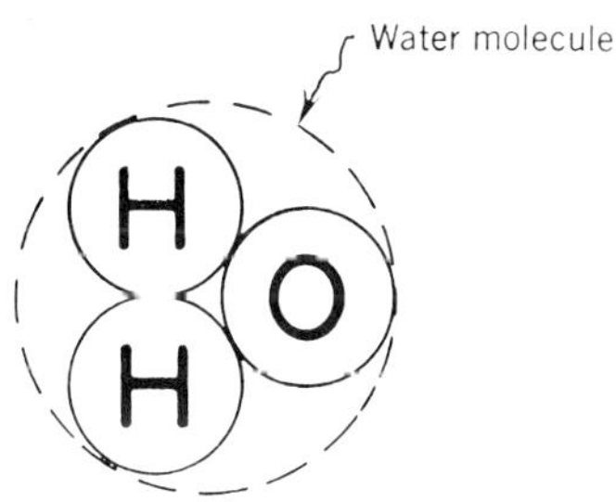

Fig. 2-1. Schematic drawing of a molecule of water consisting of two atoms of hydrogen and one of oxygen.

Physical Properties

Water exists in three states: 1. as a liquid; 2. as a solid (ice and snow); and 3. as a gas (water vapor).

Water in liquid form weighs approximately 62.5 pounds (28.41 kg.) per cubid foot or 8.3 pounds (3.77 kg.) per U.S. gallon. This is 830 times heavier than air. However, in the form of vapor, water is 133 times lighter than air, volume for volume, which partly explains why water vapor rises in the atmosphere to form clouds.

Water reaches its greatest density at 39.2°F (4°C), freezes at 32°F (0°C), and in open containers boils at 212°F (100°C) at sea level. Upon freezing to ice, water expands in volume by about one-tenth and exerts a pressure of 33,000 pounds (15,000 kg.) per square inch (6.45 sq. cm.). It is this pressure that bursts water pipes in freezing weather.

In the process of freezing and thawing of large bodies of water, there are exchanges of enormous amounts of heat energy between the water and the atmosphere. This in turn affects the climate in the vicinity of the water. Heat given off by the water in the fall may prevent an early frost and heat taken on by the water in the spring may so cool the air that buds and tender plants will be held back until all danger of frost is past. It is for these reasons that much of our fruit is grown near large bodies of water.

Water has the ability to dissolve solids and to absorb gases and other liquids, hence it is often referred to as the "universal solvent." Because of this solvent power all natural water contains minerals and other substances in solution which have been picked up from the air, the soil, and rocks through and over which it passes. Untreated sea water contains such quantities of mineral substances, particularly salts, that it is unfit for domestic use. Some ground water also contains such quantities of salt, sulphur, iron, sediment, acids, or mixtures of these that it is unfit for domestic purposes unless it is treated in some manner to remove, or neutralize these objectionable qualities.

Potable water.

Water which is clean and contains nothing injurious to health is called "potable water."

Water picks up, and sometimes nourishes, pathogenic (disease-producing) bacteria. Epidemics of typhoid and cholera have been caused by contaminated public water supplies. For this reason cities spend large sums of money to treat their water supplies to make them clean and safe to drink. In rural areas where people must depend upon private water supplies, it is just as essential to health to see that the water they use is potable. Various means of treating private water supplies are outlined in chapter 4.

THE WATER CYCLE

In nature, water is constantly changing from one state to another. See Fig. 2-2. The heat of the sun evaporates water from land and water surfaces. This water vapor (a gas), being lighter than air, rises until it reaches the cold upper air where it condenses into clouds. Clouds drift around according to the direction of the wind until they strike a colder atmosphere. At this point the water further condenses and falls to the earth as rain, sleet, or snow, thus completing the water cycle.

Growing plants take up water from the soil through their roots and give up great quantities of it through the foliage by evaporation and transpiration. It is claimed by some authorities that an averaged size oak tree will, during a five month growing season, give off through its leaves 28,000 U.S. gallons (23,324 Imp. gals.) of water. A large sunflower plant will give off one quart (0.94 liters) of water daily. Lawn grass will give off large quantities of water. Grass, therefore, growing over a sewage disposal area will dispose of considerable quantities of the liquid effluent from the septic tank.

Precipitation

Water in any form returning to the earth from clouds is referred to as *precipitation*. Precipitation is measured in terms of inches of liquid water. The annual precipitation (rain, sleet, and snow) in any locality is the total inches of water falling throughout the year. Fig. 2-2 illustrates the disposition of precipitation under average conditions.

The amount of water involved in the *water cycle* varies from place to place on the earth's surface. Figure 2-3 indicates the average annual precipitation in inches for different areas of the United States. An inch of rain on an acre of land constitutes 27,154 U.S. gallons (22,619 Imp. gals.) of water.

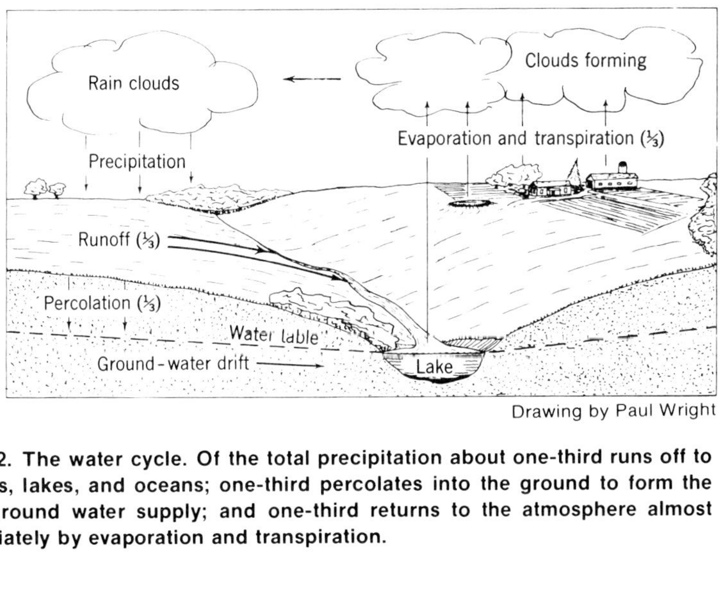

Drawing by Paul Wright

Fig. 2-2. The water cycle. Of the total precipitation about one-third runs off to streams, lakes, and oceans; one-third percolates into the ground to form the underground water supply; and one-third returns to the atmosphere almost immediately by evaporation and transpiration.

SOURCES OF WATER FOR DOMESTIC USE

There are three possible sources of water for our daily use. One is rain water collected from roofs or buildings or special water sheds and stored in cisterns or ponds. Another is natural surface water, in streams and lakes. The third and most important in rural areas is ground water stored in the earth's crust.

Rain Water

In regions where there is a fair amount of precipitation, water is often collected from building roofs or from outdoor water sheds, and

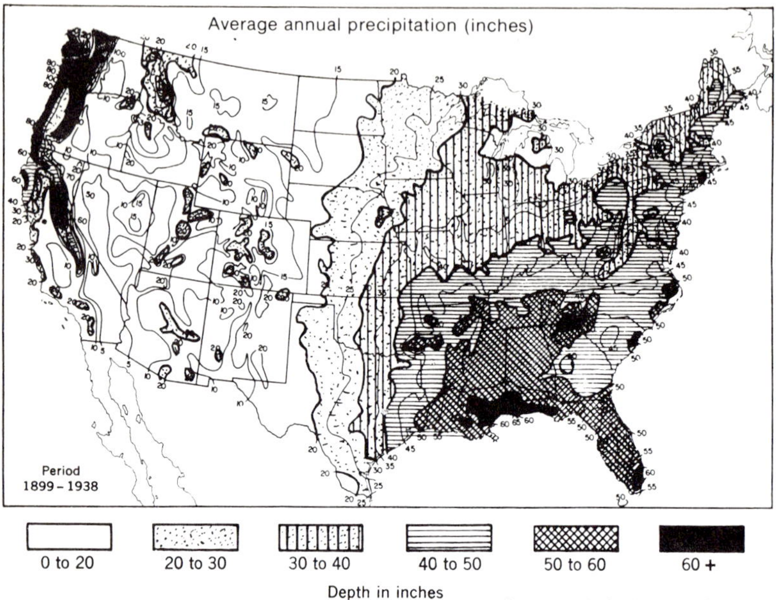

Courtesy U.S. Weather Bureau

Fig. 2-3. Average annual precipitation in different areas of the United States, in inchs.

stored in cisterns or ponds. In some rural sections of the country, cistern water is used for all domestic and farm purposes, including drinking. This is particularly true where ground water is difficult to obtain or, if obtainable, is for any reason unsatisfactory. When cistern water is used for drinking the cistern should be filled only with clean rain water and should be well protected from contamination. See Chapter 3 for the construction of cisterns. To be absolutely safe for drinking, cistern water should be boiled, chlorinated, or otherwise sterilized.

Cistern water is soft water; therefore, in regions where ground water is especially hard, cisterns are frequently used as a source of soft water for the hot-water supply in homes.

Farm ponds are an increasingly important source of water for livestock, irrigation, spraying, and fire fighting. When correctly constructed and properly managed they also provide an important source of food fish. They are useful for recreation such as fishing, swimming, boating, and skating. See Chapter 3, pages 49-52, for the development of ponds.

Natural Surface Waters

Natural surface waters from streams, lakes, and ponds are used extensively for irrigation (see Figs. 2-4 and 2-5), for industrial purposes, and for city water supplies. They are also used to some extent for domestic purposes in rural areas. When used for city water supplies or

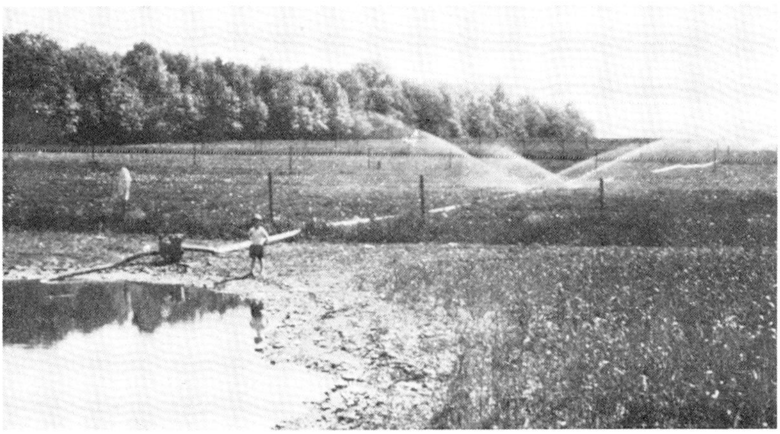

Courtesty Professor Harold Gray, Cornell University

Fig. 2-4. Pumping water from a pond for irrigation.

for domestic purposes, surface waters usually must be treated by filtration and chlorination to make them potable. Figure 7-5, page 110, illustrates a city water supply.

Ground Water

That portion of the total precipitation which soaks into the earth's crust (approximately one-third) percolates downward into the porous spaces in the soil and rock where it remains, or from which it finds its way out to the surface in some way. Figure 2-6 illustrates some of the characteristics of the earth's crust and how they affect the underground water supply.

Ground-water storage.

The principal source of water for domestic uses in rural areas is stored ground water from springs and wells. Some cities also use ground water from wells. In some regions irrigation water is pumped from wells. See Chapter 3, pages 22 - 45, for the development of springs and wells.

The character of ground water from springs and wells depends upon the nature and condition of the soil and rock through which it passes. If it contacts very little soluble material it will be soft water, and because of the filtering action of the soil it may be cleaner and purer than rain water.

WATER TABLE

The water table is that level in the earth's crust where all of the voids in the soil and rocks are filled with water and from which water will flow freely. In other words, it is the upper surface of free ground water within the saturated zone. Figures 2-7 through 2-10 illustrate water tables under various conditions.

Springs are often a result of outcroppings of the water table, as illustrated in Fig. 2-8.

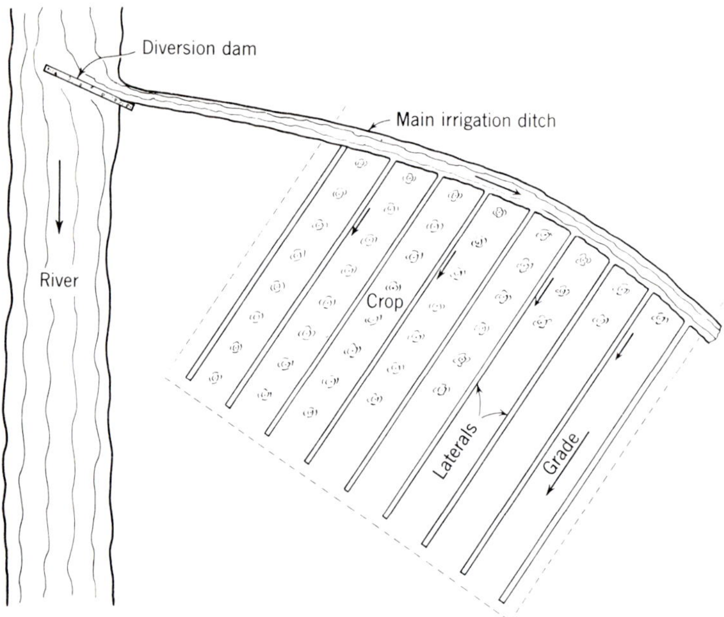

Fig. 2-5. Stream water diverted for flood irrigation.

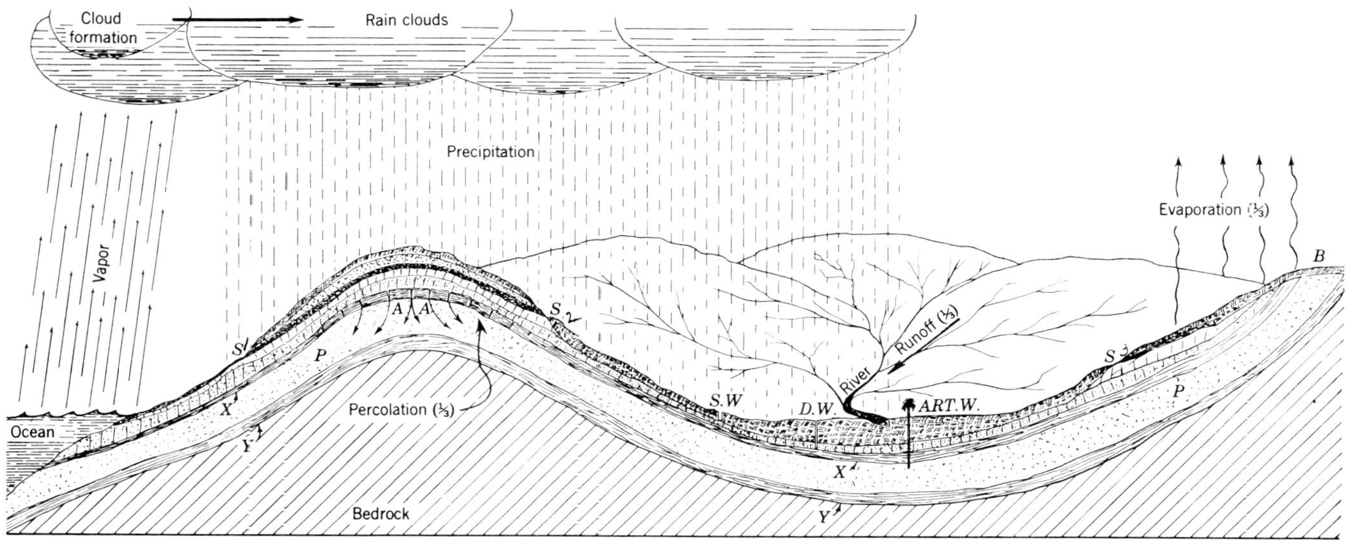

Fig. 2-6. A cross section of a possible arrangement of the earth's crust showing how water may be distributed over and through it. A part of the precipitation runs off at the surface forming creeks and rivers; a part may soak into the ground and return to the surface at springs, S, or wells, S.W. and D.W.; yet another portion may percolate deeper through cracks and faults, A.A. and B, into a porous strata, P, where it may be carried many miles to the ocean or to artesian wells, marked ART.W. on the drawing. Strata X and Y are impervious. The water at spring 3 will likely be hard because of the limestone through and over which it flows. Precipitation may pick up dust and gasses from the atmosphere.

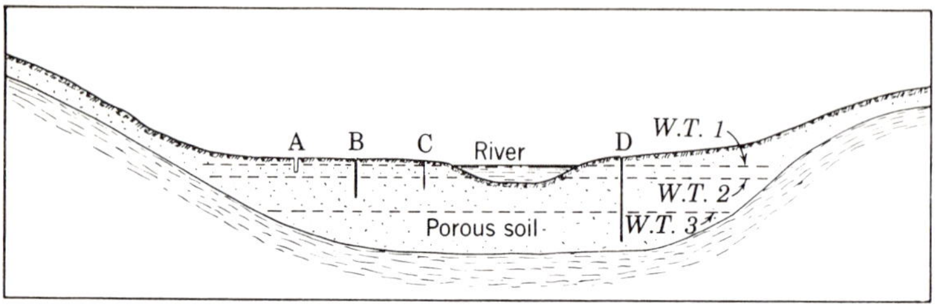

Fig. 2-7. Variations in water table in a river valley where the soil is very porous. The water table will rise and fall with the level of the stream as shown at W.T. 1 and W.T. 2. If the stream dries up in a dry season and the ground water is pumped out in quantity the water table may drop below the stream bed as indicated at W.T. 3. Such areas can sometimes be recharged by regulating stream flow with impounding dams. This is a good water conservation measure.

The shallow well at A would be dry except at high steam level. Wells B and C would flow except when the stream was dry, and well D would flow unless the water table dropped below the bottom of the well.

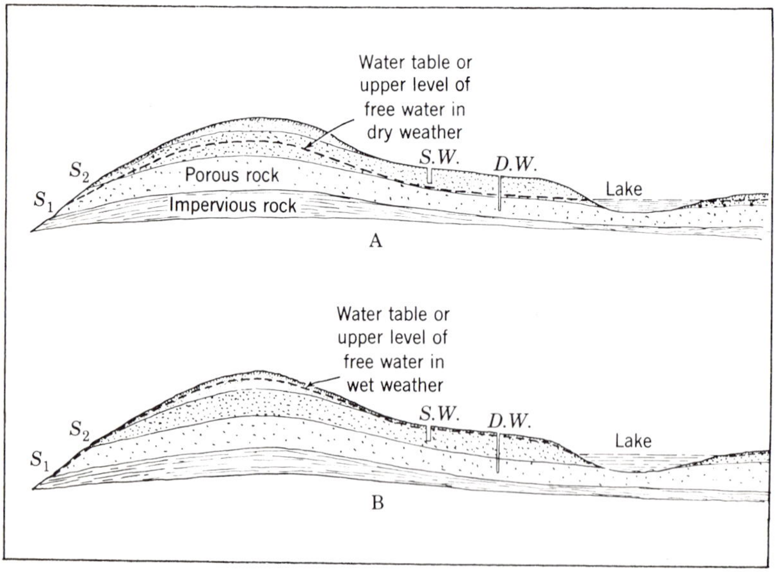

Fig. 2-8. A — Ground water in dry weather. The water table or free water is low because of lack of rainfall. Spring 2 (S^2) and the shallow well (S.W.) are dry.

B — Ground water in wet weather. The ground water is high owing to plentiful rainfall. During such periods spring 2 and the shallow well will flow, and spring 1 (S^1) and the deep well will have increased flow.

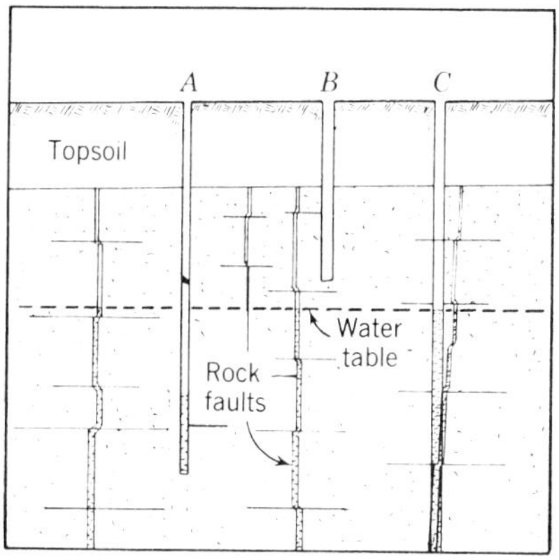

Fig. 2-9. Water table in bedrock. If the rock is faulted as shown, the water may collect in the faults and flow in quantity for long distances.

Wells drilled between faults as at A may have a very weak flow because the water moves slowly through the rock. A shallow well as at B may go dry in dry weather. A well which strikes faults with flowing water as at C may have a very strong flow, but is more likely to be contaminated than water which filters through soil or rock.

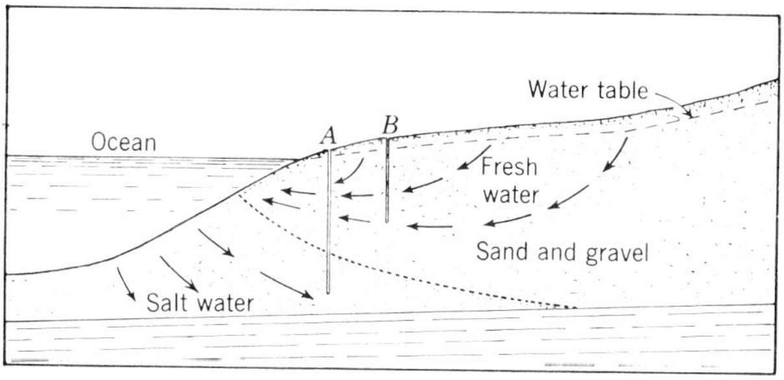

Fig. 2-10. Ground water near an ocean. If the soil is porous, sea water tends to drift in under the land. However, if precipitation is sufficient to maintain a water table of fresh water above the ocean level, as shown, the drift of fresh water toward the ocean will keep the salt water out.

Deep wells near the shore as at A may penetrate salt water, or if shallower wells as at B are pumped hard enough the salt water may rise to them.

Development of Sources of Water 3

Development of Sources of Water

The primary considerations in developing sources of water are:

1. To determine the amount and quality of water needed.
2. To find and develop a source or sources which will supply the needs.
3. The sanitary measures to be employed.

AMOUNT OF WATER NEEDED

Table 3-I indicates the average daily consumption of water for a number of household and farm uses. Water needed for irrigation spraying, fire fighting, etc., would be in addition to these demands. By employing Table 3-I the needs for water for farmstead uses under average conditions can be calculated as indicated by the following example. Rural family needs are as great or greater than city family needs.

TABLE 3-I.

AVERAGE DAILY CONSUMPTION OF WATER.

Use	**U.S. Gallons per 24 hours**	**Imperial Gallons per 24 hours**
For each person where there is running water in the kitchen, bathroom and laundry	40 to 70*	33.3 to 58.3*
Each horse	12	10
Each steer, heifer or dry cow	15	12.5
Each high producing cow (including barn and milkhouse sanitation)	35	29.2
Each hog	4	3.3
Each sheep	1½	1.25
Turkeys (per 100 birds)	18	15
Chickens (per 100 birds)	7	5.8
Washing dairy utensils	30 to 50	25 to 42
Lawn and garden sprinkling	625 per 1000 sq. ft. per inch of water	521 per 930 m² per 2.5 cm of water

*With automatic dishwasher, garbage disposal, and automatic laundry equipment use the higher figure.

Example

Assuming a farm situation where there are four people living in the house. Running water is to be supplied in the kitchen, bathroom and to automatic laundry equipment. There are 30 head of high producing milch-cows, 10 head of steer, heifers, and dry cows, 2,000 chickens, and 6 hogs. How much water will be needed per 24 hours?

Solution	**U.S. Gallons**	**Imperial Gallons**
4 people at 70 gals. per person	280	230
30 milch cows at 35 gals. per head	1050	875
10 steers, heifers, and dry cows at 12 gals. per head	120	100
2,000 chickens at 7 gals. per 100	140	117
6 hogs at 4 gals. per head	24	20
Washing dairy utensils	50	42
Total daily demand	1664	1384

Water needed for irrigation can be calculated on the basis of acre inches or acre centimeters. One acre-inch of water equals approximately 17,000 U.S. gallons. The acre-inches to be applied times the number of acres will give the total amount of water needed.

In addition to the routine daily demands as illustrated above there may be periodic additional demands for such purposes as hosing down floors in animal shelters, washing cars, trucks and tractors, and fire fighting. If these additinal demands are to be met by the same water system that supplies the routine demands then the needs for water may be considerably increased.

For hosing down floors, washing vehicles, etc. allow a minimum of 5 U.S. gallons (4.2 Imp. gals.) per minute. For fire fighting allow 10 U.S. gallons (8.3 Imp. gals.) per minute.

QUALITY OF WATER

Any new or untried source of water should be examined for quality *before* expensive development is undertaken. Good-quality water for household purposes must be free of harmful bacteria, sediment, objectionable minerals, tastes, odors, etc. For watering animals, spraying, and irrigation it should at least be clear and free of any minerals, tastes, or odors which would be harmful or objectionable to plants or animals.

Contamination and Pollution

Although the terms contamination and pollution are often used synonymously, health authorities make the following distinction:

Contamination is the presence in water of bacteria from the intestinal tract of warm-blooded animals including man. The presence of such bacteria means that the water may carry human disease germs. The fact that water looks clear and sparkling is no assurance of its purity. Disease germs are invisible to the unaided eye.

Pollution is any undesirable quality of water other than contamination. Dirt, silt, organic matter, objectionable minerals, colors, odors, or tastes, acidity, and alkalinity are causes of pollution.

Although pollution is not necessarily a health hazard, it is often accompanied by contamination which *is* a health hazard. Contamination is most likely to accompany pollution by dirt, silt, and organic matter picked up by the water from the ground surface.

Deep underground waters are seldom dangerously contaminated if surface waters are excluded. This is due to the filtering action of the soil and rock through which underground water percolates. Exceptions occur where ground water follows cracks, faults, or channels in the bedrock as indicated in Fig. 2-9 at *C*.

Testing for contamination.

Tests for contamination should be made by qualified persons. Local county or municipal health officers usually co-operate in making these tests. In many communities there are health laboratories where health officers can have the tests made. Otherwise a State laboratory or a private laboratory may have to be used.

In any case it is essential that the samples be collected in an approved manner and in sterile containers. Most states have regulations covering the necessary procedures and copies of the regulations can usually be obtained from the State Health Departments.

In case a source of water is found to be contaminated and no other satisfactory source is obtainable, it is possible to sterilize the water by chlorination or boiling to make it safe for domestic use. Procedures for chlorination are discussed in Chapter 4. A health office should be consulted on the type of chlorinator to use and the method of installing it.

Testing for minerals.

If there is evidence of objectionable mineral content it may be advisable to have a chemical analysis made to determine the kind of treatment needed. Most manufacturers of water-treating equipment will make such an analysis free of charge for prospective customers. County, municipal, and state health departments usually make both bacteriological and chemical tests free of charge, or for a nominal fee.

Measurement of hardness.

Hardness of water is expressed in terms of calcium carbonate equivalent ($CaCO^3$). There are two numerical units in common use in the United States. They are: (1) parts per million (ppm), and (2) grains per U.S. gallon (gpg). Parts per million is the number of parts of calcium carbonate equivalent per million parts of water. Grains per U.S. gallon is the number of grains of calcium carbonate equivalent per U.S. gallon of water. In other English-speaking countries the unit, grains per Imperial gallon is widely used.

One gpg is the equivalent of 17.14 ppm. One ppm is equal to 0.0583 gpg.

Although water hardness resulting from dissolved calcium is not a health hazard, it does require excessive amounts of soap for washing purposes and often fills pipes and water heaters with a hard precipitate which interferes with the flow of water. Removal of excessive minerals by means of softeners is discussed in Chapter 4. If the hardness exceeds 6 gpg or 100 ppm it is considered good economy to use a water softener. Table 4-II on page 55 indicates the amount of soap wasted by hardness. Additional soap must be used for the washing action.

Sediment, color, taste, and odor.

Sediment in water is clearly visible. Every precaution should be taken to eliminate it, particularly if the source is surface water. Such water is very likely to be contaminated. If the source of sediment is underground or is of such a nature that it cannot be avoided, then filters and or chlorinators may have to be used. The use of filters is discussed in Chapter 4, pages 59-67.

Color in the water can of course be detected by eye, and tastes or odor can be detected by sampling. See Chapter 4 for treatment.

Acidity

Excessive acidity makes the water corrosive and may cause it to pick up lead in solution from the ground or from any contact with lead in the plumbing system. The maximum tolerance for lead in drinking water is 0.1 ppm. Page 62 of Chapter 4 describes methods of removing acidity.

LOCATING AND DEVELOPING ADEQUATE SOURCES

Development of Springs

A good spring is a sure source of water, whereas the drilling of a well is always a gamble. Good springs are not common but where they do exist they should be seriously considered as a source of water.

The following factors should be considered before an investment is made in the development of a spring:

1. Is the flow adequate for the needs, even in dry weather?
2. Is the water of satisfactory quality?
3. Is the spring located favorably for natural gravity flow? If not, would it be economically practical to pump the water?
4. Can the spring be adequately protected from pollution and contamination?

5. Would it be easier, cheaper, and surer to develop the spring than to drill a well?

Measuring the flow of a spring.

The rate of flow of a spring may be determined by bailing from the spring pool or by erecting a temporary dam below the spring as shown in Fig. 3-1 and catching the water in a measuring pail below the dam. This should be done in the driest season of the year in order to determine the minimum flow.

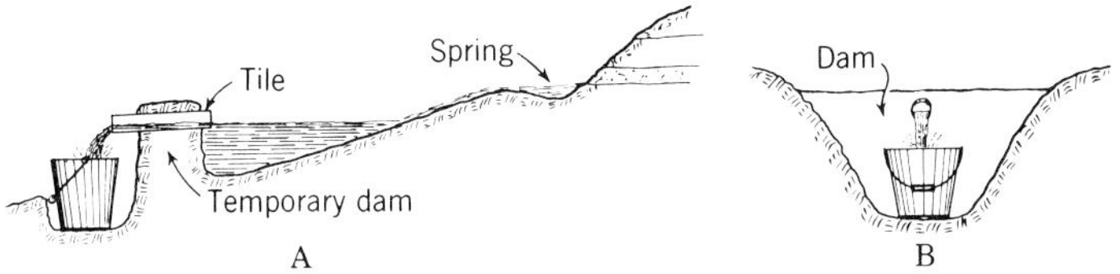

From Cornell Extension Bulletin No. 145

Fig. 3-1. Method of measuring spring flow. A — Cross-section view. B — Front view.

Quality of spring water.

If a spring supplies an adequate quantity of water the next step is to examine its quality as suggested on pages 20-21.

Location of spring with respect to the buildings.

A spring high enough above the buildings and not too far away can be made to supply water by gravity flow. This eliminates the cost of

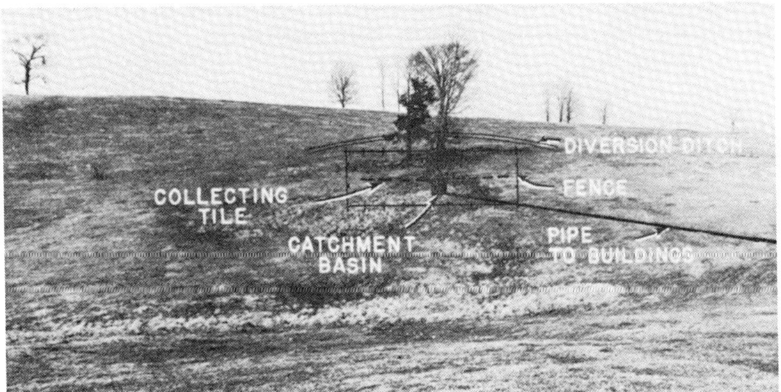

Fig. 3-2. A spring in a seepage area. The spring is just below the trees and supplies a fair amount of water. However, much of the available water escapes into the seepage area below the spring. Drainage tile installed as indicated by broken line would collect most of the water and lead it to a catchment basin. A sodded diversion ditch and a fence placed as shown would protect the spring area from surface water and animals.

installing and running a pump. The elevation of a spring should be measured and not judged by eye. Differences in elevations on land surfaces are very deceiving to the unaided eye. An elevation of at least 20 feet is desirable for satisfactory gravity flow. Job 8 gives instructions on methods of leveling for such purposes.

If the elevation is not sufficient for satisfactory pressure at the faucets, it may be possible to pipe the water to a storage tank and then pump it to the outlets, as indicated in Figs. 3-3 and 3-4.

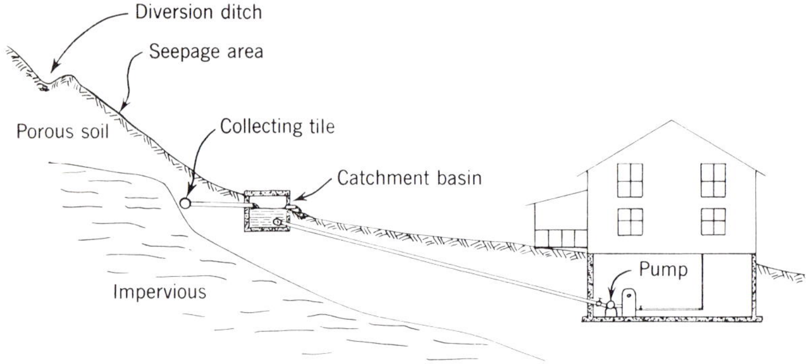

Fig. 3-3. An elevation view of an installation similar to that of Fig. 3-2, except in this case the spring is not high enough for gravity flow to the faucets. The tile is laid along the lower edge of the seepage with a slight grade toward the catchment basin. A pressure water system for boosting the pressure is shown in the basement. The suction pipe to the pump would need to be throttled with a valve or small-sized pipe in order to make an air-volume control work. See Fig. 7-20; page 123.

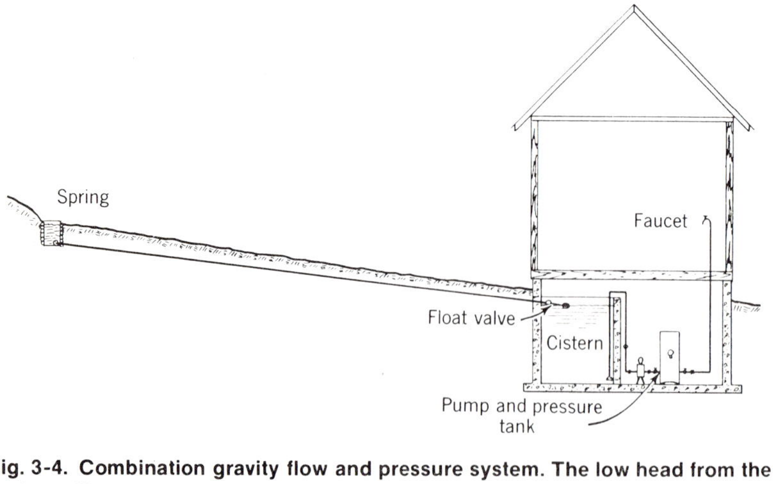

Fig. 3-4. Combination gravity flow and pressure system. The low head from the spring will not give the desired pressure at the faucets but will deliver water to a cistern 24 hours a day. A small pipe can be used from the spring. The pump will take water from the cistern and deliver it to the faucets at a satisfactory volume and pressure.

If the spring is lower than the buildings it will be necessary to pump the water all the way from the spring. It is very important in such an installation to be sure that the pipe lines are large enough.

Cost of developing a spring.

The cost of developing springs varies widely with the type of spring, the elevation, type and size of catchment basin needed, the amount and size of pipe, and the extent of fencing, ditching, tiling, and frost protection. Figures 3-2 through 3-6 illustrate spring developments.

As a rule, the catchment basin should be built below the spring, as indicated in Fig. 3-6, to allow a free flow of water. This is especially important with a weak-flowing or seepage type of spring. See Fig. 8-2, pg. 132.

Size of storage reservoir or catchment basin.

A rule of thumb for determining the size of storage is to build it large enough to hold at least one-half day's supply of water. The daily needs can be calculated from Table 3-I. The storage capacity in U.S. gallons is equal to the cubic feet of storage space times 7.48. For Imp. gals. divide U.S. gals. by 1.2.

Installing the pipe.

The three types of piping materials commonly used on gravity systems are: (1) galvanized steel pipe; (2) copper tubing; and (3) plastic tubing. These materials are described in Chapter 10, pages 164-168. The procedure for determining pipe sizes is outlined in Chapter 8 and Job 6. The size of pipe used can make the difference between a satisfactory installation and a complete failure.

In most cases it is best to lay the piping underground because there it is protected from frost, the heat of the sun, and mechanical damage. In warm climates the pipe need be only deep enough to shade it and to prevent damage.

Table 3-II indicates the recommended depths for frost protection for pipes in the various states. The higher values should be used at high altitudes, where the soil is wet, or where the pipeline runs under roads, driveways, or walks where snow is packed or kept cleaned off.

Flowing water does not freeze as readily as still water; therefore, if there is enough water available so that a faucet or valve can be left open in cold weather to keep the water in the pipe moving, the pipes can be laid at shallower depths than shown in Table 3-II. Water run to waste for this purpose should not be discharged into a septic tank as it might flood the disposal field.

Shallow trenches can be made with a plow. In some areas small trenching machines are available for deep trenches. These machines are fast and inexpensive compared to hand labor.

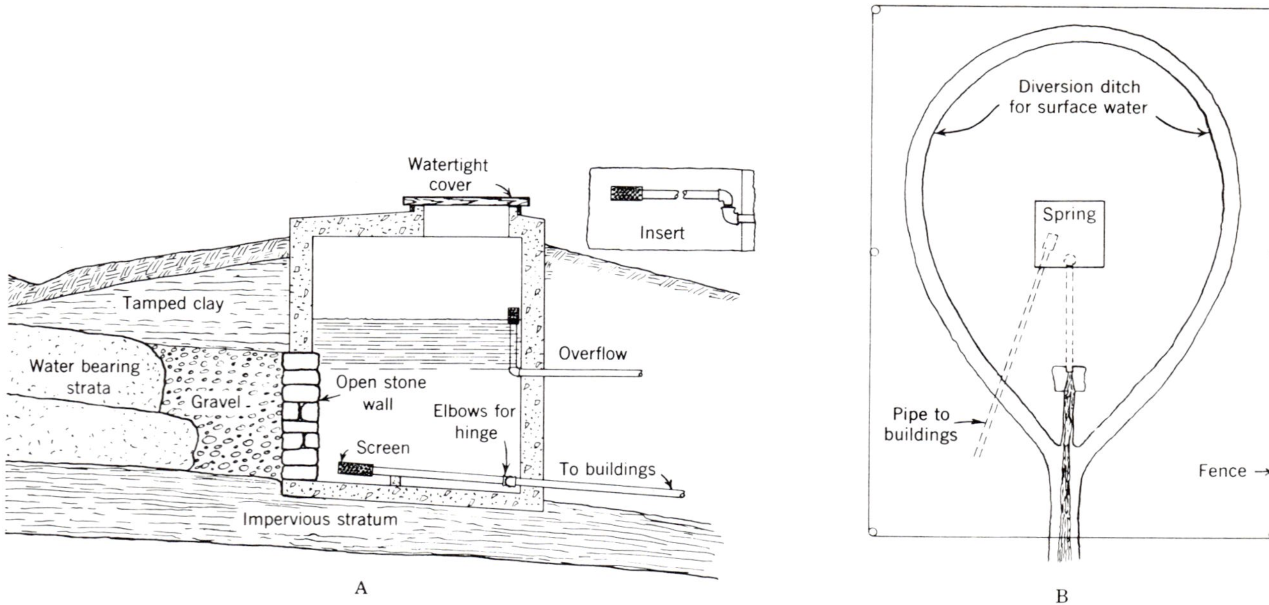

Fig. 3-5. A — A suitable catchment basin for a strong spring. For a weak spring the arrangement shown in Fig. 3-6 should be used. The insert shows the assembly for the discharge pipe which permits the screen to be lifted above the water for cleaning. B — Plan view showing a diversion ditch for surface water and a fence to keep animals away.

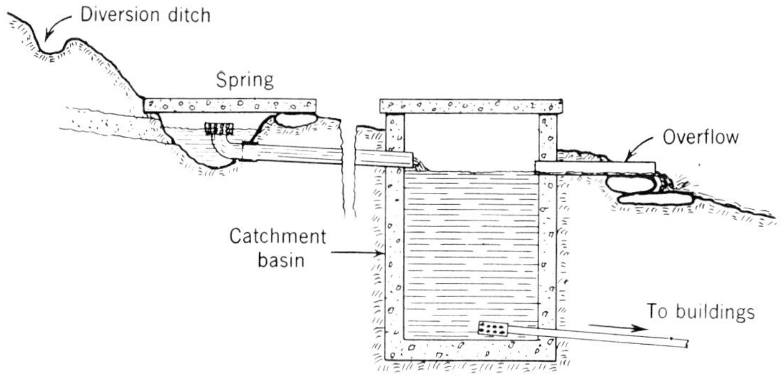

A

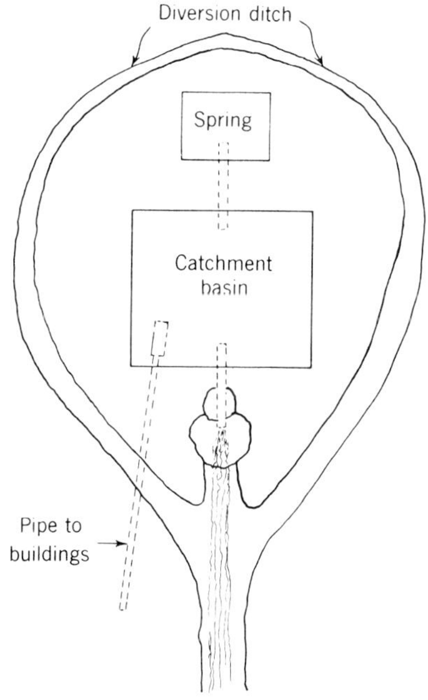

B

Fig. 3-6. A suitable storage basin for a weak spring. The storage basin can be located at any distance from the spring as indicated at A. At B is a plan view of such an installation. The storage basin should be built *below* the spring so that the water will have a free flow from the spring.

Sanitary precautions.

Like any other source of water a spring should be protected from surface water, animals, manured fields, sewage disposal systems, or any other source of pollution or contamination. This often means at least trenching above the spring and fencing in the area.

If the cost of developing a spring as outlined here compares favorably with the cost of a well and pumping equipment, the spring would be a logical choice, particularly in areas where good wells are difficult to obtain.

TABLE 3-II.
DEPTH AT WHICH TO LAY SMALL WATER PIPES FOR FROST PROTECTION IN DIFFERENT STATES.*

State	Depth, Feet	Depth, Meters	State	Depth, Feet	Depth, Meters
Alabama	1½ to 2	0.45 to 0.61	Mississippi	1½ to 2½	0.45 to 0.77
Arkansas	1½ to 3	0.45 to 0.91	Missouri	1½ to 2½	0.45 to 0.77
California	2 to 4	0.61 to 1.22	Montana	5 to 7	1.52 to 2.13
Colorado	3 to 5	0.91 to 1.52	Nebraska	4 to 5½	1.22 to 1.68
Connecticut	4 to 5	1.22 to 1.52	New Hampshire	4 to 6	1.22 to 1.83
Florida	1 to 2	0.30 to 0.61	New Jersey	3½ to 4½	1.07 to 1.37
Georgia	1½ to 2	0.45 to 0.61	New Mexico	2 to 3	0.61 to 0.91
Idaho	4 to 6	1.22 to 1.83	New York	4 to 6	1.22 to 1.83
Illinois	3½ to 6	1.07 to 1.83	North Carolina	2 to 3	0.61 to 0.91
Indiana	3½ to 5½	1.07 to 1.68	North Dakota	5 to 9	1.52 to 2.74
Iowa	5 to 6	1.52 to 1.83	Ohio	3½ to 5½	1.07 to 1.68
Kansas	2½ to 4½	0.77 to 1.37	Pennsylvania	3½ to 5½	1.07 to 1.68
Kentucky	2 to 3½	0.61 to 1.07	Tennessee	2 to 3	0.61 to 0.91
Louisiana	1½ to 2	0.45 to 0.61	Texas	1½ to 3	0.45 to 0.91
Maine	4½ to 6	1.37 to 1.83	Virginia	2 to 3½	0.61 to 1.07
Massachusetts	4 to 6	1.22 to 1.83	Wisconsin	5 to 7	1.52 to 2.13
Michigan	4 to 7	1.22 to 2.13	Wyoming	5 to 6	1.52 to 1.83
Minnesota	5 to 9	1.52 to 2.74	District of Columbia	4	1.22

*English Units Courtesy U.S. Department of Agriculture.

Development of Wells

By far the most common source of water for farms and rural homes is wells of one type or another. A water well may be defined as a hole or shaft sunk into the earth's crust to a depth below the free-water level or into deep-water-bearing strata for the purpose of obtaining ground water.

The following are important considerations in the development of a well for a water system:

1. Is there an existing well which can be made to serve?
2. If a new well must be developed: Where should it be located? What type of well should be constructed? What diameter well should be constructed?
3. What measures must be taken to protect a well, old or new, from contamination and pollution?
4. What pumping equipment, frost protection, housing, and power facilities will be needed?

Types of well construction.

There are five common types of well construction: dug wells, driven wells, jetted wells, bored wells, and drilled wells. To some extent, where soil and water conditions are favorable, well holes are "jetted" in with a high velocity stream of water. See Fig. 3-13.

Dug wells. The oldest type of well construction is the dug well as illustrated in Figs. 3-7 and 3-8. A hole 3 to 10 feet (0.91 to 3.05m) in diameter is dug into the earth, usually by hand, until a flow of water is obtained. The hole is then walled up and covered to protect it from surface water. Nearly all wells of pioneer days were of this type. In some areas dug well are 50 ft (15m) deep, or more.

Driven wells. In regions where there is water in porous strata at shallow depths the driven well is common. Figures 3-9 and 3-10 illustrate such wells. A specially designed well point such as illustrated in Fig. 3-11 is driven into the ground on the end of a pipe. See Fig. 3-12. Naturally such a well is not feasible where the soil is full of stones or where the water-bearing strata are below bedrock.

Jetted wells. Where soil conditions are favorable jetted wells can be constructed very economically. For example, in the sandy soils of parts of Florida jetted wells are very common. Fig. 3-13 illustrates one method of "jetting" a well. A high velocity stream of water pumped down the drill pipe dislodges the sand and soil and flushes them to the surface. A casing and, or, a screen can be driven down the hole following the jetting head.

Bored wells. In regions where the soil down to a water-bearing stratum is soft and free from stones, wells can be bored with special boring equipment as illustrated in Fig. 3-14. The hole can then be lined with tile or other suitable material, as shown, to support the walls.

Drilled wells. Drilled wells, when cased into bedrock and correctly sealed at the surface, afford maximum protection from contamination and pollution. Deep water-bearing strata are less likely to be contaminated from sewage systems, barnyards, outdoor privies, etc., than are shallow sources. Deep wells frequently penetrate more than one water-bearing stratum, therefore they may provide a stronger flow. Also, deep sources are less affected by droughts as the water-bearing formations are more likely to be extensive in area. In most regions a satisfactory source of water can be obtained at depth of 100 feet (30 + m) or less. Deep wells are more likely to provide high concentrations of minerals than are shallow wells. In some areas deposits of salt, sulphur, or other objectionable minerals make it impractical to drill deep for water. Such conditions can usually be determined by a survey of existing well conditions in the area. Drilled wells are made with special well-drilling rigs. Fig. 3-15 illustrates a percussion type of drilling rig. A heavy drilling bit is raised and dropped in the hole to deepen it. The cuttings are bailed or pumped out. Fig. 3-16 illustrates a rotary drilling rig. Here the drilling bit is rotated in the hole and the cutters on the under side of the bit cut through the various formations to deepen the hole. Cuttings are flushed or pumped out. The rotary drill is commonly used for drilling large diameter wells (8 inches (20.3 cm) or larger) to supply large volumes of water for irrigation, city water systems, etc.

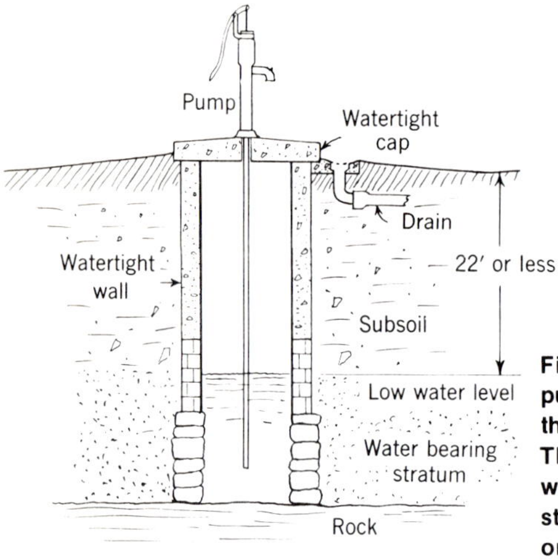

Fig. 3-7. A shallow dug well with pump on the top. The bottom part of the well wall is laid up without mortar. The top 6 to 8 feet should be made watertight with mortar between the stones and sand and cement plaster, or by use of concrete. If the well is large in diameter and therefore requires a heavy cover, a manhole should be constructed in the top.

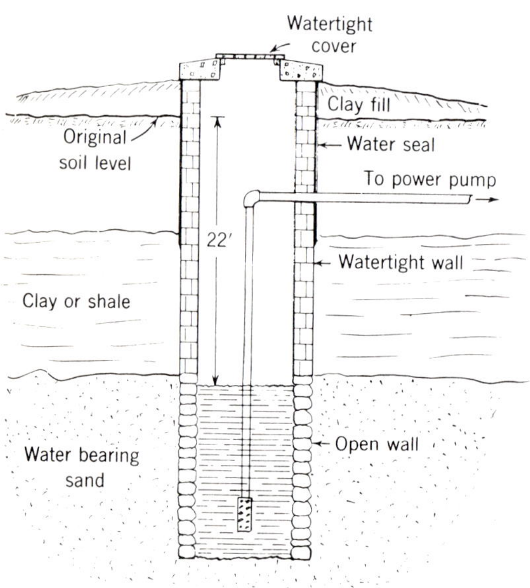

Fig. 3-8. A shallow dug well with pump located at a distance from the well. The level of the water is within 22 feet (6.71 m.) of the pump. The top part of this well wall is laid up with stone and mortar and is plastered and tarred on the outside near the top to keep out surface water. A clay fill also protects from surface water.

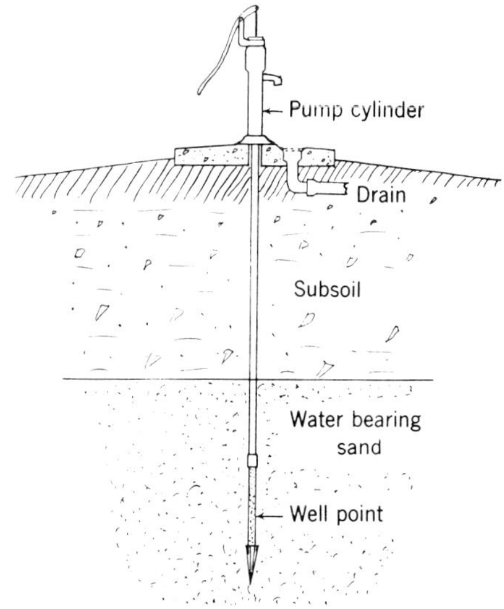

Fig. 3-9. A driven shallow well with the pump at the top of the well.

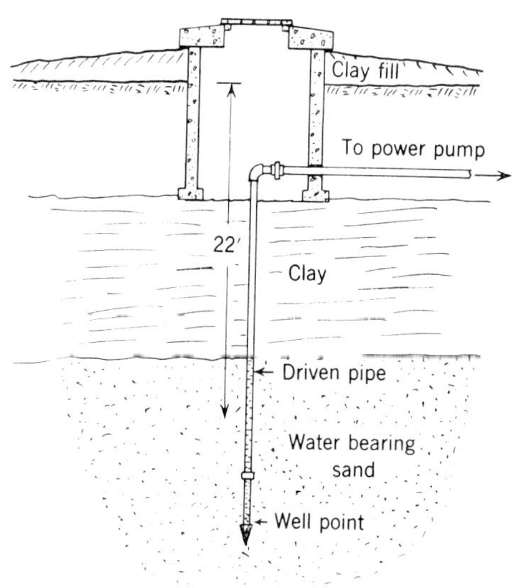

Fig. 3-10. A driven well with the pump located at a distance from the well. The driven well is inexpensive, but usually has a limited capacity. However, when used in multiple as shown in Figs. 3-26 and 3-27 can deliver high capacity.

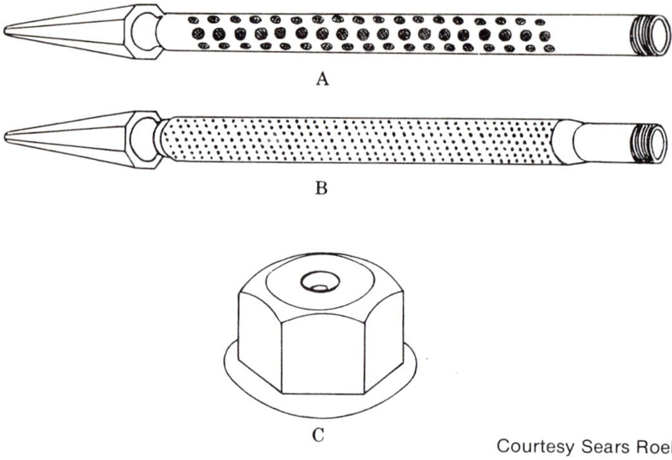

Courtesy Sears Roebuck and Co.

Fig. 3-11. Two types of wéll points at A and B. They are usually made of forged steel, stainless steel, or hard brass. At C is a drive cap.

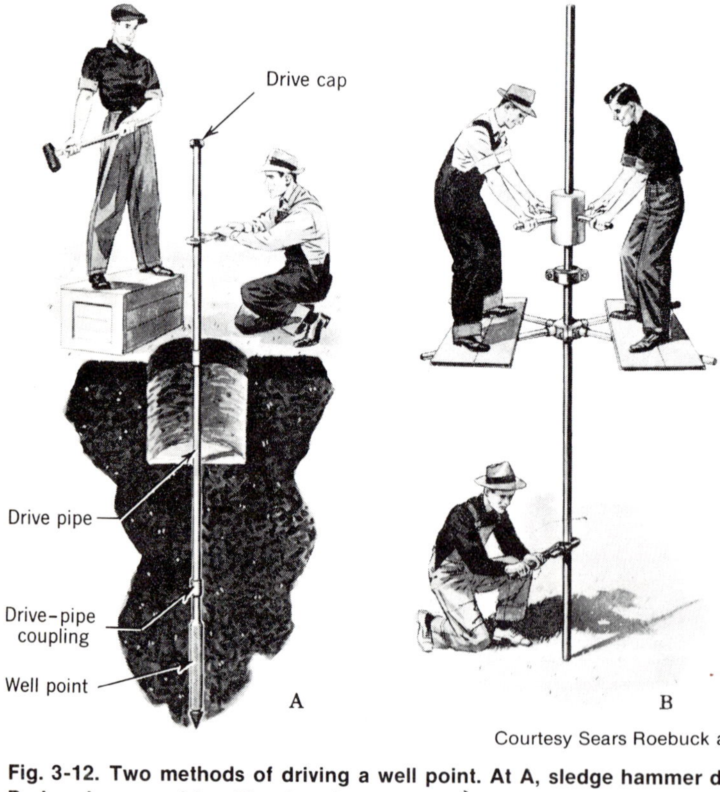

Courtesy Sears Roebuck and Co.

Fig. 3-12. Two methods of driving a well point. At A, sledge hammer drive. At B, drop hammer drive. The drop hammer can be operated by a percussion type of drilling rig.

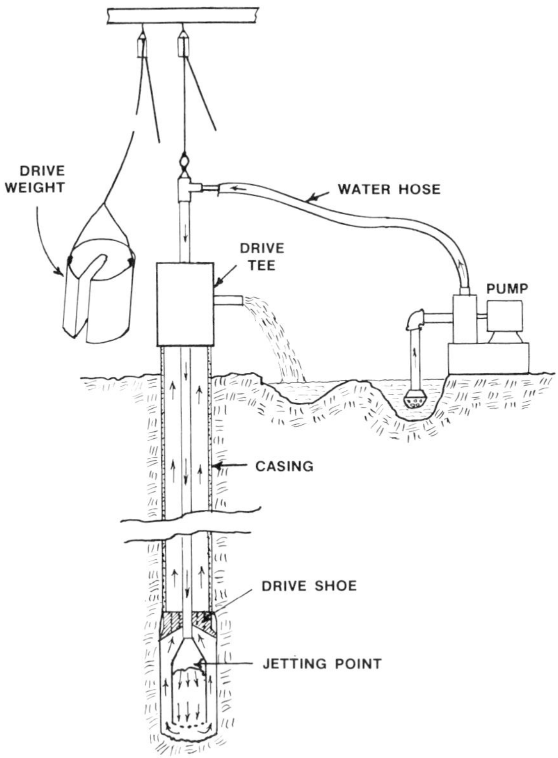

Fig. 3-13. A jetting rig for constructing a well. A high velocity stream of water is pumped down to the jetting point where it loosens the soil and flushes it out through the drive tee. The sediment settles out in the first pool and the water flows over into the sump at the pump to be recirculated into the well hole.

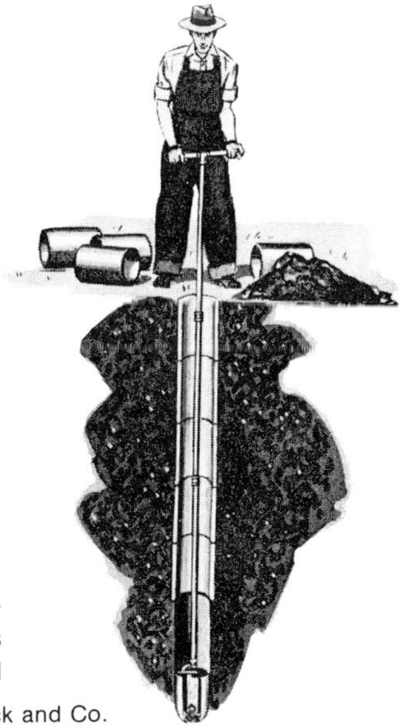

Fig. 3-14. Boring a well. The tile is used to prevent cave-in of the wall. Tractor-powered augers are frequently used instead of the hand tool shown here.

Courtesy Sears Roebuck and Co.

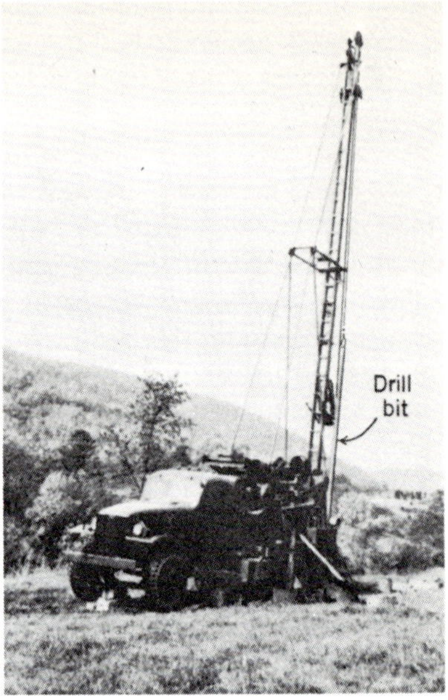

Fig. 3-15. A percussion type of well-drilling rig in position for drilling. The heavy drill with a cutting bit on the lower end is lifted and dropped by the rig so that a hole the size of the bit is drilled down into the earth's crust to a water-bearing stratum. Periodically the drill is pulled from the hole; the hole is flushed with water and then bailed with the bailer to remove the cuttings of the drill. Using this same rig the driller drives a casing down into the hole at least to bedrock to prevent cave-ins and to seal out surface water.

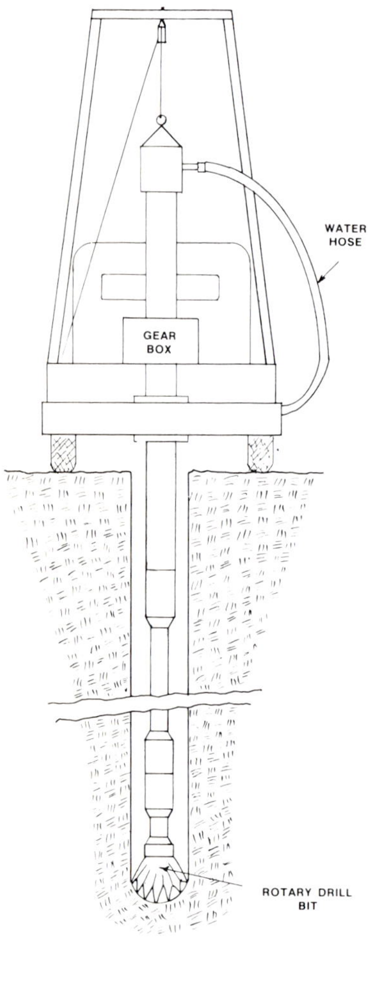

Fig. 3-16. A rotary drill rig. Works best in alluvial soils. Can drill through soft rock. Can drill well holes 3″ to 36″ in diameter and to depths of 6,000 feet (1828.8 m.) A casing is usually driven into the hole following the drill.

Developing Old Existing Wells

If often happens that an existing well on a property is adequate for modern needs if correctly developed, i.e., if cleaned and enclosed for protection from contamination and pollution. Old wells are often of the dug type and frequently are walled all the way up with stones laid without mortar. The cover is often badly deteriorated and does not exclude surface waters.

The first step in development of an old well is to measure its flow to see if it will meet the needs for water. A well which has the reputation of never going dry when pumped or bailed by hand may soon

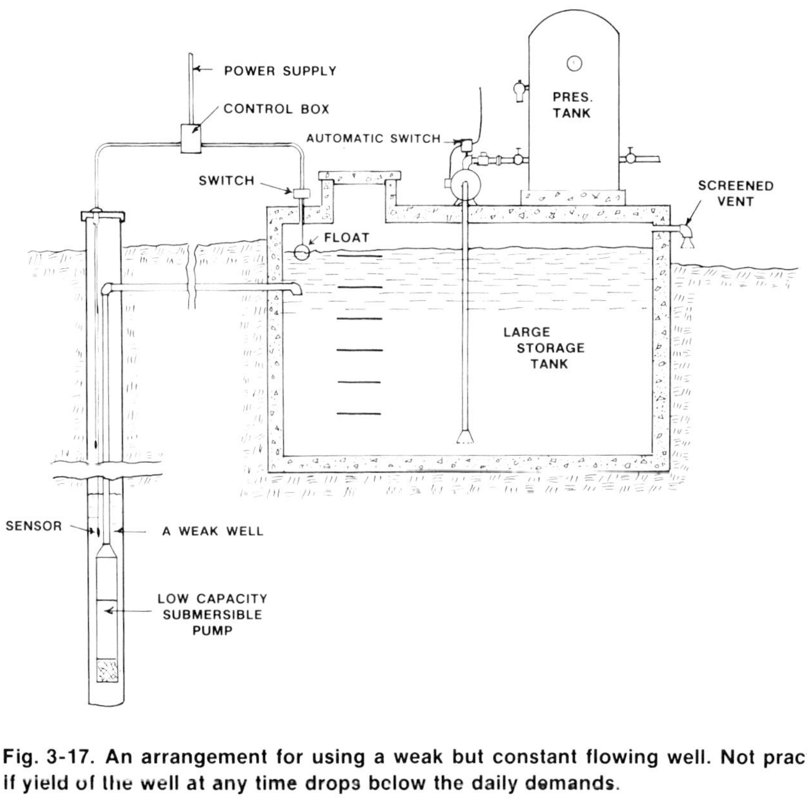

Fig. 3-17. An arrangement for using a weak but constant flowing well. Not practical if yield of the well at any time drops below the daily demands.

Although a small capacity submersible pump is indicated in the well, other types of pumps can be used and can be controlled by sensors. Sensors may also be used in the large storage tank in place of the float switch.

The operation of the system is as follows: When the water in the well rises to the upper sensor the well pump starts and pumps water into the large storage tank. When the water level in the well drops to the lower sensor the pump is shut off and remains shut off until the well fills again to the upper sensor at which time the well pump starts again. This perodic pumping continues automatically twenty-four hours a day, or until the water level in the large tank raises the float and turns the power off at the float switch.

When the pump at the pressure tank draws the level of the stored water down the float drops and closes the float switch thus returning the well pump to automatic operation.

go dry when pumped with modern equipment for supplying indoor plumbling. The flow can be determined by pumping or bailing. If there is evidence of considerable sediment in the bottom of the well it should be cleaned before final measurement of the flow is made. To obtain the minimum flow, measurement should be made during a dry season.

The rate of flow in a dug well having considerable storage capacity need not be as large as for a small-diameter drilled, bored, or driven well. In any case the minimum daily flow should at least equal the daily demands for water as calculated from Table 3-I.

A weak flowing well with a daily flow equal to the daily demand can sometimes be made adequate by providing an extra pump and extra storage capacity. A small capacity pump installed on the well together with an automatic float or electrode switch in the well can be used to pump water from the well whenever the water rises to a certain level in the well. This small capacity pump delivers the water to an extra storage tank from which a larger capacity pump can pump the water into a pressure tank to supply the outlets. Fig. 3-17 illustrates such an installation.

If the flow of an old well is adequate the next step is to have the water tested for quality as suggested on pages 20-22.

If the quantity and quality of water are satisfactory, the well construction should be checked and repaired if necessary. The well wall should be watertight down 6 to 8 feet (1.83 to 2.44 m) below the surface. There should be a good top placed high enough to permit grading of the ground surface downward from the cover. See Figs. 3-7 and 3-8. New piping into the well should be installed at the time of these repairs.

Developing New Wells

The development of a new well may involve considerable expense. It is important, therefore, that the matter be given careful consideration beforehand.

Generally speaking, ground water is found in porous strata which underlie extensive areas, very much like large underground streams, ponds, or lakes. Under such conditions a good well is just as likely to be found at one spot around a yard or a farmstead as at another.

In regions where the bedrock is faulted, in limestone areas where underground water has cut channels, or in glacial till where there are streaks of sand, water may collect in and flow along these "easy flow" channels to form *true veins* of water. A well hole which strikes such a vein is likely to have good flow. On the other hand, if the hole is drilled, perhaps only a few feet away, it may be a dry hole. See Fig. 2-9 at *A* and *B*. In such areas the location of a successful well is very much of a gamble.

There is no infallible method of locating a successful well previous to drilling. All methods fail at times to produce satisfactory results.

Water witching.

One of the ancient methods for locating underground water which has persisted to the present time is that of "water witching" or "dowsing" with a forked twig or some other type of divining instrument. Various kinds of wood and even metals are advocated by practitioners of this method.

Some hold the instrument in one way and some in another. All claim to have some rare, if not supernatural, power, which is imparted to the instrument to make it dip or otherwise indicate the presence of underground water. Figure 3-18 illustrates one method of grasping a forked twig for divining purposes.

In the author's opinion the practice of water witching, whatever its form, is based upon a false premise, namely, that ground water is to be found only in veins or in concentrated underground pools. All scientific data indicate that this is the exception rather than the rule. As stated previously, water is usually found in strata which underlie rather large areas. Although it is recognized that some people are firm believers in the practice, one with technical training finds it difficult to credit the practice until there is at least *some* scientific evidence that it has value.

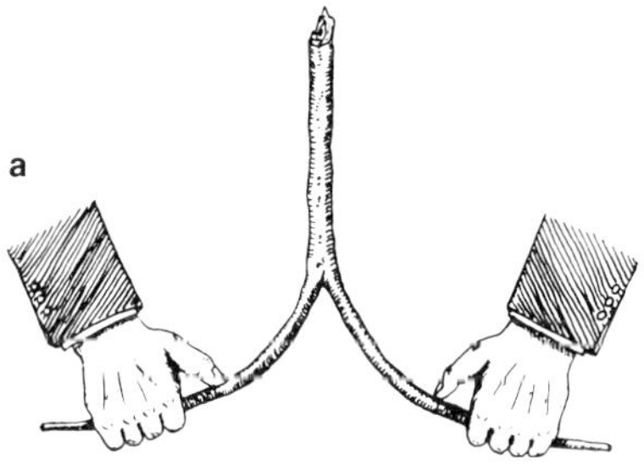

Fig. 3-18. One method of holding a water-witching stick.

Drawing by Paul Wright

Survey method.

The most reliable method of locating underground water is to have a qualified geologist make a preliminary survey and then put down some test holes to check the geological data. All of this is too expensive for the average farmer or householder, although it is common practise when expensive wells for city water supplies, for large industries, or for irrigation are anticipated. A reasonably good forecast of results can be had at little expense by a survey of existing neighboring wells. This, and the good judgment of a competent driller, will in most cases produce the desired results. It is wise to keep in mind the fact that if ground water is available anywhere within the general area of a set of buildings it probably will be available at the most convenient place that is safe from sources of pollution and contamination.

In general the most convenient location for a well is near the building or buildings where the most water is used. A location next to the foundation of a house provides easy access for servicing and repairs and keeps piping, wiring, and frost-proofing costs to a minimum.

Type of well to construct.

The great majority of new wells are now made by drilling. However, if it is known that driven, jetted or bored wells are generally successful in the area these may be tried. Dug wells are now seldom constructed because of labor costs.

Depth of wells.

The depth of wells is as variable as the distance to water-bearing strata. The deeper the well has to be the more expensive the construction and, as a rule, the more expensive the pumping equipment. Also the energy costs for pumping from great depths are more than for pumping from shallow sources.

Shallow wells.

For convenience in selecting pumps, wells are classified into two groups, namely, *shallow wells* and *deep wells*. A shallow well is one in which the water level always stands within "sucking" distance of a pump located at or near the top of the well. The sucking distance varies with the type of pump and the altitude of the well above sea level. At sea level the sucking distance is 15 to 28 feet (4.57 to 8.53 m), depending upon the type of pump used. For any type of pump, the sucking distance decreases about 1 foot for every 1000 feet (305m) of elevation above sea level. See Table 5-I, page 76. Figures 3-7 through 3-10 illustrate shallow wells. Pumps which can be used for pumping from such wells are called shallow-well pumps.

Deep wells.

A deep well is one in which the water level is, or at times may be, below sucking distance of the pump located at or near the top of the well. To pump water from such a well the pumping unit (cylinder, turbine, or jet) must be lowered into the well until it is within sucking distance of the water. In practise the pumping unit is usually placed down *in* the water to avoid the loss of priming. Figures 8-7, and 8-11 illustrate a deep well. Pumps used on deep wells are called deep-well pumps.

Well diameter.

The greater the diameter of a well the greater its water storage capacity per foot of depth. See Table 3-III. Also large-diameter wells are likely to have a higher rate of flow. Large-diameter wells should be considered where there are high peak demands or where the nature of the water-bearing strata is such that small wells will not have a satisfactory flow. Because of the extra cost of large-diameter wells 4- and 6-inch diameter wells are generally used for domestic water supplies, but in many cases better supplies could be had from larger diameter wells.

TABLE 3-III.
STORAGE CAPACITY OF WELL, IN GALLONS PER UNIT OF DEPTH*.

Diameter of Well		Capacity in U.S. Gals. per Ft. Depth	Capacity in Imp. Gals. per Unit Depth	Diameter of Well		Capacity in U.S. Gals. per Ft. Depth	Capacity in Imp. Gals. per Unit Depth
2"	5.08 cm.	0.163	0.14	1'	30.48 cm.	5.89	4.91
3"	7.62 cm.	0.368	0.31	2'	60.96 cm.	23.66	19.72
4"	10.16 cm.	0.654	0.55	3'	91.44 cm.	53.02	44.18
5"	12.70 cm.	1.020	0.85	4'	1.22 m.	94.27	78.56
6"	15.24 cm.	1.470	1.22	5'	1.52 m.	147.22	122.68
7"	17.78 cm.	2.000	1.67	6'	1.83 m.	212.02	176.68
8"	20.30 cm.	2.620	2.18	7'	2.13 m.	288.60	240.50
9"	22.86 cm.	3.310	2.76	8'	2.44 m.	377.02	314.18
10"	25.40 cm.	4.090	3.41	9'	2.74 m.	477.15	397.63
11"	27.94 cm.	4.950	4.12	10'	3.05 m.	589.05	490.88

*English Units Courtesy Sears Roebuck and Co.

Artesian wells.

Artesian wells are those in which water rises to a considerable distance above the water-bearing stratum from which the water is obtained. Occasionally such wells flow out the top, as illustrated in Fig. 3-19.

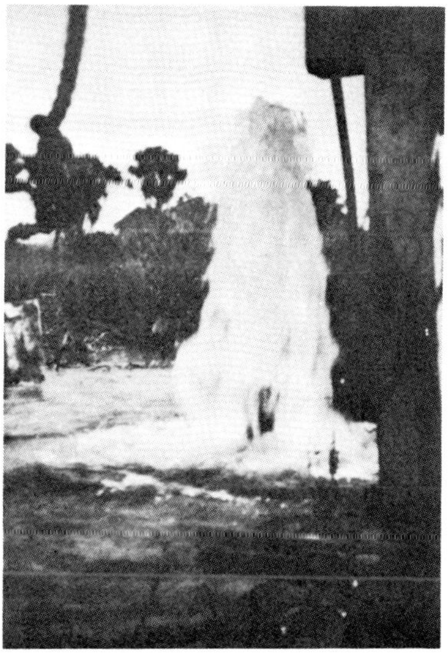

Fig. 3-19. A gushing artesian well. Figure 8-14 illustrates how such a well can be capped.

Courtesy Edward E. Johnson, Inc., St. Paul, Minn.

Contract for drilling.

It is good business to have a complete understanding with the well driller in regard to what he is to do for the price quoted. A written contract is the best. Read the contract carefully before signing.

Measuring the flow of new wells.

Well drillers have bailing equipment for measuring the flow of small drilled wells. The flow of other types of wells can be measured by bailing or pumping. The daily flow of a well should at least equal the daily demands for water.

Pumping equipment.

The selection and installation of pumping equipment are discussed in Chapters 6, 7, and 8.

Protection of wells.

A new well should always be chlorinated to sterilize it. Then the water should be tested as indicated on pages 20-22 before it is used for drinking purposes. Local health authorities should be consulted on this procedure.

The fact that a new well proves to be safe does not necessarily mean that it will always remain so. Seepage from sewage disposal areas, entrance of surface waters, drainage from barnyards, graveyards, and even manured fields can, in time, so contaminate a well as to make it unsafe for human consumption. See Figs. 3-20 and 3-21. Every precaution should be taken to safeguard the well from any and all such sources of contamination. Good housing is important in this respect. See Chapter 8, pages 140, 142-144.

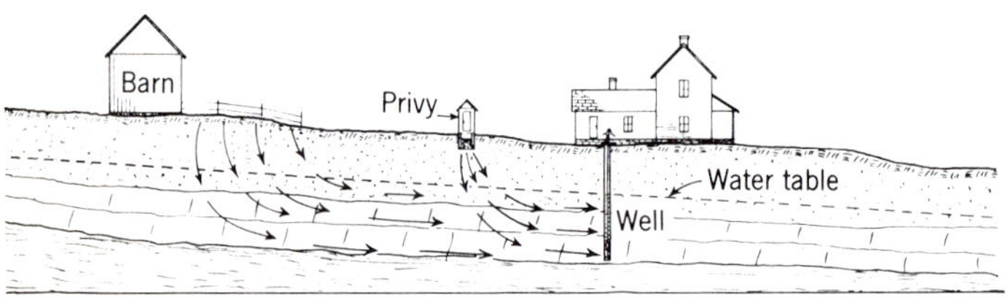

Fig. 3-20. A very poor well location. In such a case the well is likely to be badly contaminated from the privy and barnyard.

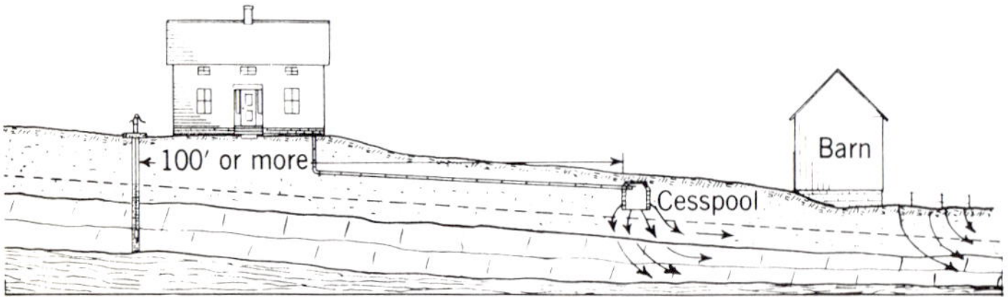

Fig. 3-21. A satisfactory location of the well with respect to the cesspool and barn.

Suggestions for Maintaining the Flow of Springs and Wells

The amount of water obtainable from springs and wells depends upon two factors: the amount of natural ground water available at the location and the capacity of the well or spring to draw that water from the ground.

A shortage of natural ground water in any particular location is something which cannot always be remedied. However, the following suggestions may be helpful. Ground water comes from precipitation soaking down into the earth's crust from the surface; therefore any measure which will increase absorption at the surface is likely to increase the supply of ground water. Any water that runs off and into a stream may not find its way into a well or spring. Wooded areas, grass lands, swampy areas, terracing, contour farming, or any other conservation measure which will hold surface water until it soaks into the ground is likely to improve the flow of water to a well or a spring in the same vicinity.

In localities where there are large demands for water for industrial purposes, air conditioning, city water supplies, or even for irrigation purposes, it is sometimes practical to recharge the ground-water storage area by diverting stream flow into absorption areas or by returning at least a portion of the water, after use, to the ground through recharging wells. This, however, is seldom practised on farms or for rural home water supplies.

The flow of water in both springs and wells can be appreciably diminished by the accumulation of sediment. See Figs. 3-22, 3-23, and 3-24. In such cases a good cleaning may restore the normal flow. The flow of wells can often be improved by the use of screens at the bottom of the well, by the use of explosives, or by acid treatment.

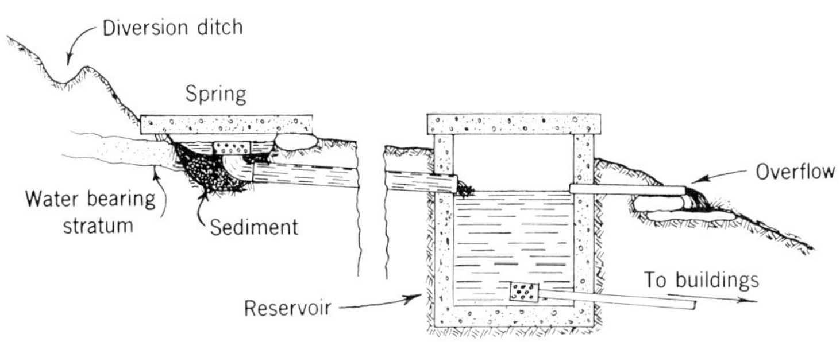

Fig. 3-22. Sediment in the bottom of a spring can greatly reduce the flow of water.

In some types of water-bearing formations there is a tendency for the well hole to fill up with a cave-in or fine sand. This is especially true on large-diameter wells which have a strong flow and are pumped hard. Well screens are often used to prevent this. Also, in some formations the finer particles of soil and sand are so tightly packed that

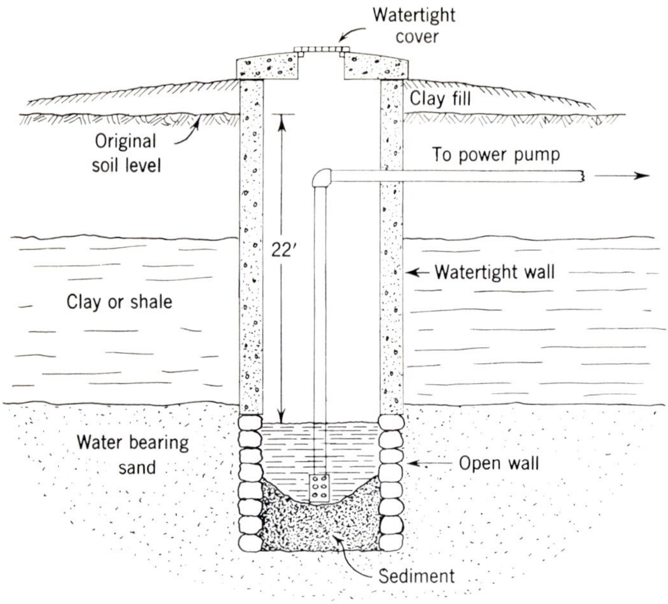

Fig. 3-23. The accumulation of sediment in the bottom of a dug well may restrict the flow of water.

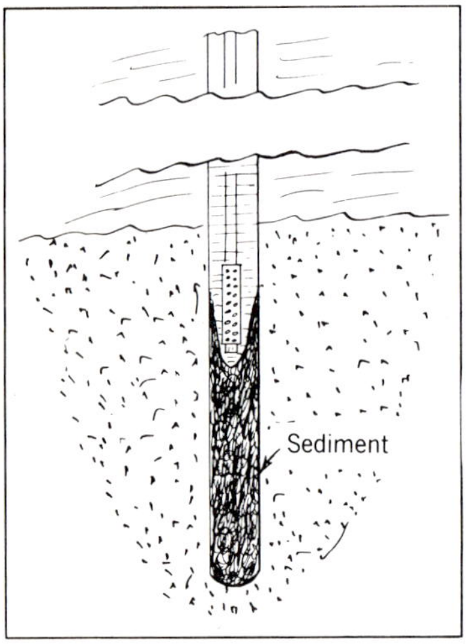

Fig. 3-24. Sediment in the bottom of a drilled well may restrict the flow.

the flow of water is retarded. With the proper equipment a well driller can enlarge the hole in the formation, install a well screen, and pack gravel around the outside of it as indicated in Fig. 3-25. This greatly increases the flow area around the screen and therefore the flow of water. Large wells used by industry, municipalities, and for irrigation are often equipped with such screens.

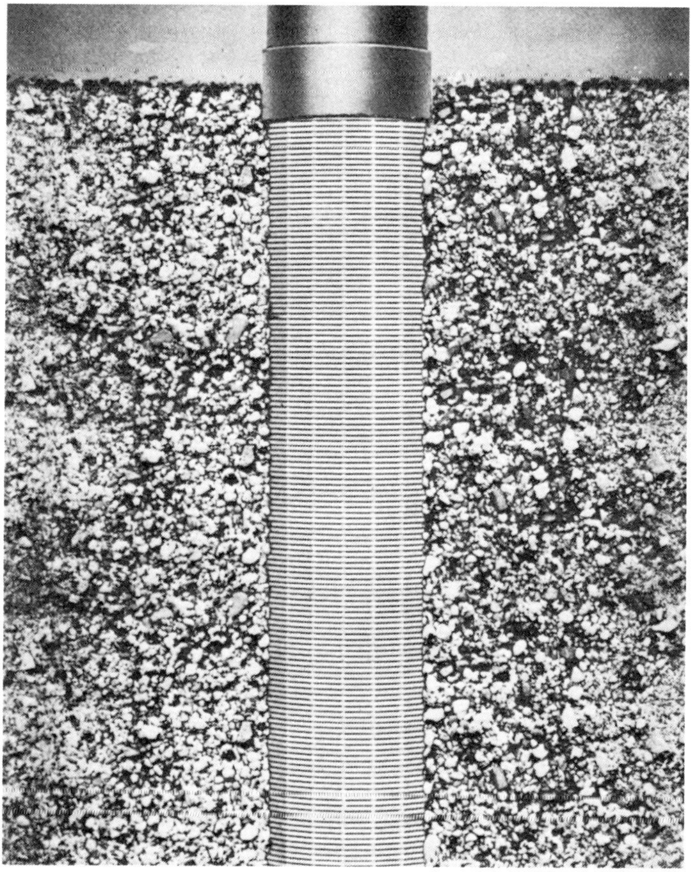

Courtesy Edward E. Johnson, Inc., St. Paul, Minn.

Fig. 3-25. A well screen packed with gravel to increase and maintain the flow. This same graveling effect can be produced in gravel beds by surging water through the screen to flush out the sand for a distance back from the screen. Many well drillers have equipment for doing this kind of work.

Explosives should be used with caution and only as a last resort. Under favorable conditions an explosive charge will open the porous strata and increase the normal flow of water. Under other conditions explosives may further compact the formations and decrease the flow or even open cracks in rock and let what water there is escape, thus destroying the well. Such treatment should be undertaken only by experienced persons.

In some regions, particularly in limestone areas, there is a tendency for the well screen and even the soil or rock to become clogged with

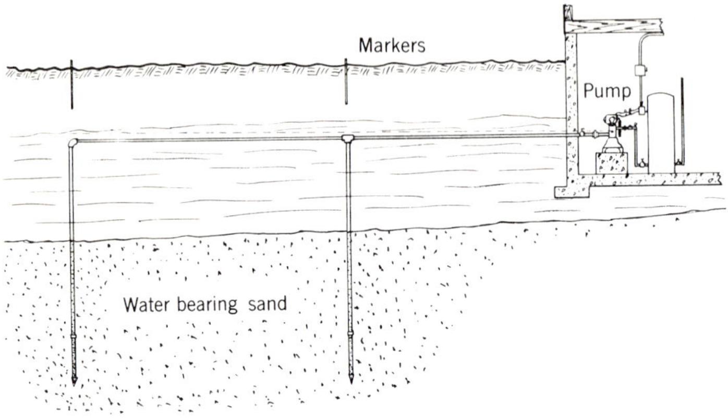

Fig. 3-26. An arrangement for increasing the water supply from driven wells. Water must be within sucking distance of the pump.

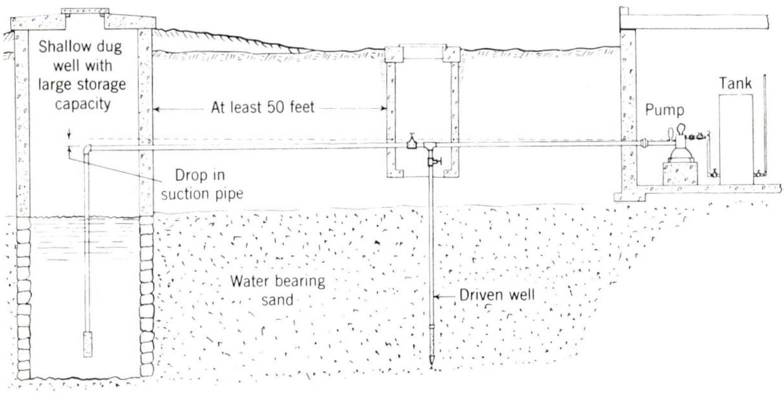

Fig. 3-27. A driven well and a dug well connected to the same pump. The valve arrangement enables one to pump from either or both wells. The valves should be of the gate type and should be made accessible as shown. The packing around the valve stems must be kept tight. The union should have a rubber gasket.

lime deposits to such an extent that the flow of water is reduced. An acid treatment consisting of surging an acid solution through the screen and the surrounding soil will sometimes clear the well of the obstructing deposits. However, this too is a treatment which should be undertaken only by trained personnel. It can be dangerous if done incorrectly.

In some cases the flow of wells can be increased by deepening the well.

Where the nature of the water-bearing stratum is such that the movement of water through it is too slow, two or more wells can be used, as shown in Figs. 3-26, 3-27 and 3-28.

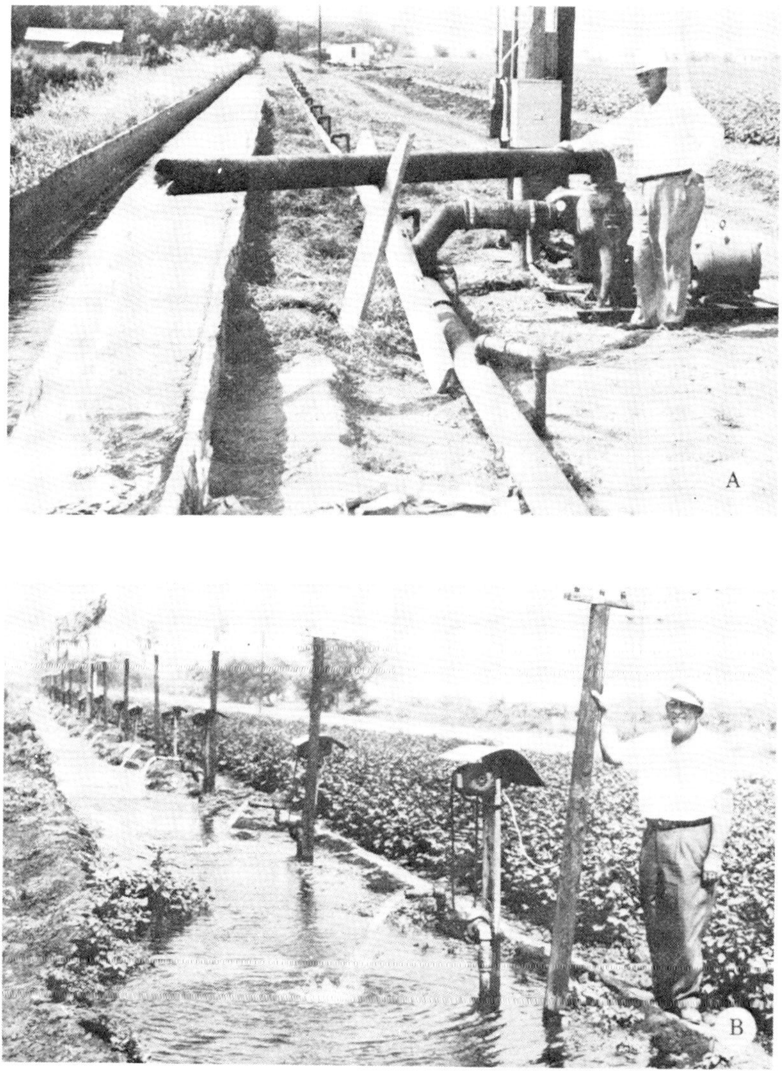

Courtesy Farm Journal

Fig. 3-28. Two methods of pumping from multiple wells. At A one pump of large capacity pumps from a number of driven wells all on about the same level. At B each well has an individual pump. The discharges could be connected to a manifold pipe to lead all of the water off to one place if desired. The arrangement at B is best where it is necessary to pump from various levels. Either system is practical for situations where there is plenty of ground water at shallow depths yet the movement of ground water is too slow to supply adequate flow at one well.

Construction of Cisterns

Cisterns are most generally used as supplementary sources of water, usually where ground water is in short supply or is for any reason unsuited for the needs. Where ground water is quite hard cisterns are often used to supply the hot water side of the plumbing system. The following are important considerations in the planning and construction of cisterns:

1. Is there enough rainfall to make cisterns worth while with the available collecting area?
2. What size cistern should be built?
3. How and of what materials should the cistern be constructed?
4. Where should it be located?
5. What treatment should the water have to maintain the desired quality?

Rainfall.

The average annual precipitation together with the available collecting area (roofs or water sheds) will determine the amount of water which can be collected. One inch of precipitation on 100 square feet of horizontal surface is equal to 62.3 U.S. gallons. (2½ cm of rain on 9.29 sq. m. of horizontal surface is equal to 51.92 Imp. gallons). Thus, if there is an annual precipitation of 24 inches (60.96 cm) and the available collecting area is 500 square feet (46.45 sq. m.) the maximum amount of water which can be collected is equal to 62.3 U.S. gallons × 24 inches × 5 or 7476 U.S. gallons. (6230 Imp. gallons).

Size of cistern to build.

The size of cistern to build is determined by: 1. the amount of water needed; 2. the amount of collecting area available, usually building roofs; and 3. the amount and distribution of rainfall.

The total demands for water for a home or a farmstead can be calculated from Table 3-I. An estimation of that portion of the total demand to be supplied by cisterns can be used as the starting point in calculating the size needed. The storage capacity of cisterns, in U.S. gallons, is equal to the cubic feet of storage space times 7.48. (For Imp. gals. divide U.S. gals. by 1.2).

There is no point in building a cistern that is too large for the collecting area or the available rainfall. The collecting area and the amount and distribution of rainfall should be considered together if the cistern is to hold all of the water available.

If the total annual precipitation is well distributed throughout the year, then the cistern need be only large enough to hold 1 months' or 6 weeks' supply. On the other hand, where most of the precipitation occurs in a short season of 2 or 3 months the cistern would need to be large enough to store the dry season supply.

If there are several separate buildings on a property with sizeable roofs it is of course possible to build cistern capacity for all of them. If they are widely separated and if water is to be used at each, then a cistern at each building of a size suitable for its roof may be the best arrangement.

The effective building roof area for collecting water is not the roof area, but is the *ground area covered by the roof*. For example, in Fig. 3-29 the effective collecting area would be determined by the measurements at ground level, or 35′ × 28′ which equals 980 sq. ft. If measurements on the roof were used the area would be 35′ × 20′ × 2 or 1400 sq. ft. The difference is 420 sq. ft.

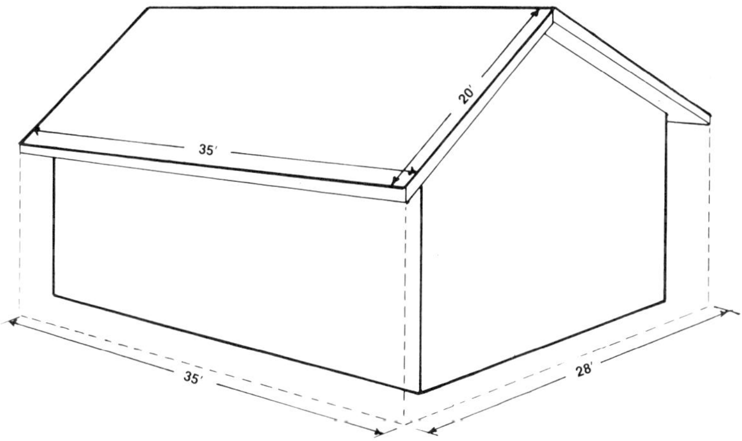

Fig. 3-29. The effective water collecting area of a roof is the *ground area* covered by the roof. For the above building it would be 35′ × 28′ and *not* 35′ × 40′.

Materials for construction.

The best type of construction is cast-in-place reinforced concrete. However, bricks, masonry blocks, or stones laid up in mortar and plastered on the inside and tarred on the outside toward the top are used especially for round underground cisterns. Wooden or metal tanks are also used aboveground where there is no danger of freezing.

Location.

Cisterns are usually located in or near the building from which the water is collected. Underground locations keep the water in better condition and give frost protection. Indoor locations are usually cheaper if the cistern can be made an integral part of the building foundation. However, indoor cisterns are more difficult to protect from dirt and rodents. Figures 3-30, 3-31, and 3-32 illustrate typical forms of cistern construction.

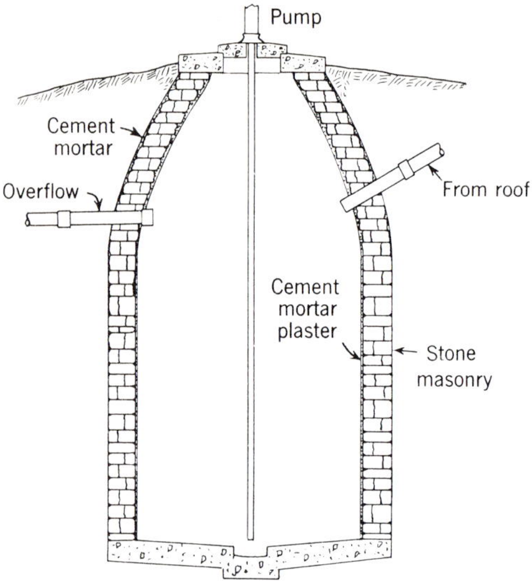

Fig. 3-30. An underground round cistern walled up with stone, bricks and mortar and plastered with cement mortar. It is good practice to coat the outside of the wall near the top with tar to help keep out surface water. This type of cistern is suitable for use at a barn, or to supply soft water for the hot-water side of a plumbing system, provided it is filled only with clean water.

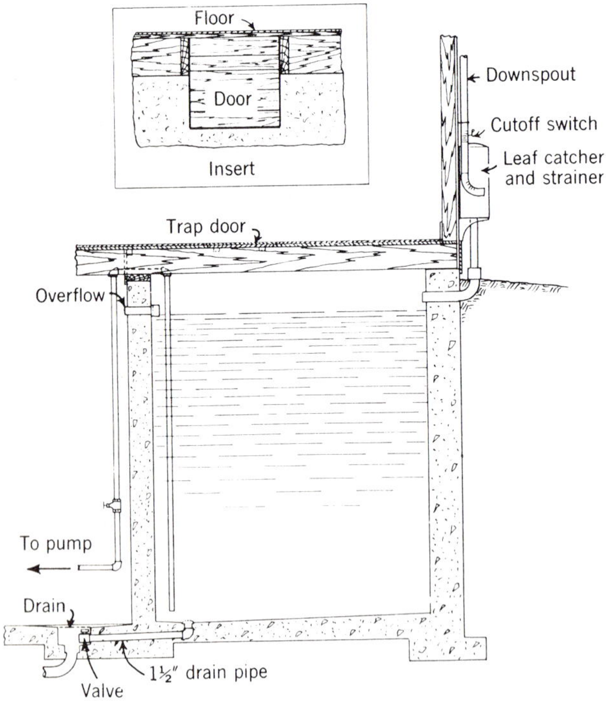

Fig. 3-31. A cistern suitable for a basement. The foundation wall serves as one or more sides of the cistern, the other walls being constructed of concrete. Note that the cistern is entirely enclosed to keep out dust and rodents and that a leaf catcher and strainer is provided on the down spout. Entrance to the cistern for cleaning and repairs may be through a trap door, as shown, or through a special door in the side between two floor sills as shown in the insert.

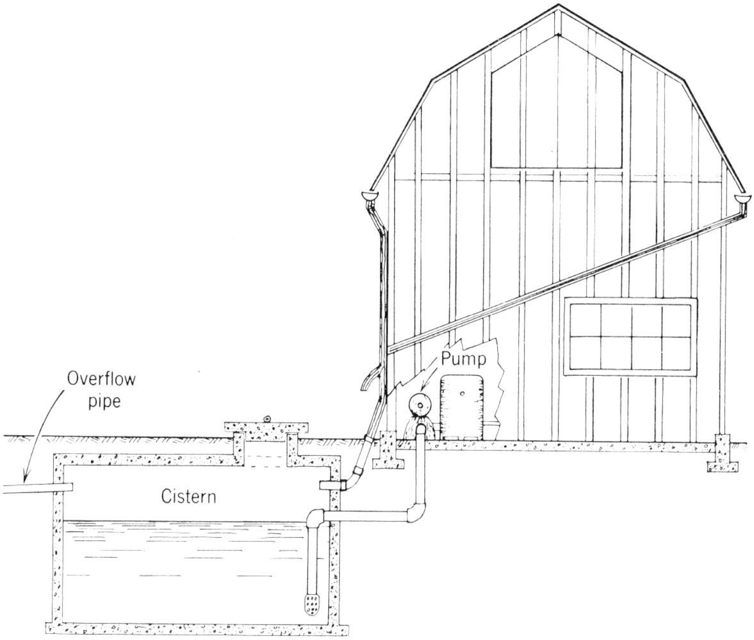

Fig. 3-32. A large-capacity underground concrete cistern. A large-capacity pump installed on such a cistern will provide water for fire fighting. The manhole provides access for the suction hose of fire-fighting apparatus and for cleaning. For fire protection the cistern should be located at least 25 feet (8 m.) from buildings.

Treatment of cistern water.

Where cistern water is dirty or contaminated it should be filtered and chlorinated if the water is to be used for drinking or cooking purposes. Details of water treatment are covered in Chapter. 4.

Construction of Farm Ponds

The following are important considerations in the construction of farm ponds: 1. size to build; 2. location; 3. type to build; and 4. costs.

Size to build.

If a pond is to be used only for a limited purpose, such as watering livestock or as a reserve for fire fighting, it can be relatively small if at least 8 feet deep, and should be located near the point of use. If large volumes of water are needed, as for irrigation or to supply water for many different purposes, then the size must be larger and the location may have to be chosen on the basis of available watershed rather than convenience to buildings. For best results a pond should be at least 8 feet (2.5 m.) deep and the drainage area should be several times the surface area of the pond depending upon the amount and distribution of rainfall.

Allowing for evaporation and leakage losses in dry weather, the capacity of a pond should be about double the estimated demands for water. The capacity of a pond in U.S. gallons can be calculated as follows:

1. Measure the average depth in feet.
2. Measure the average width and average length in feet, or if the pond is round, measure the diameter.
3. Multiply average depth by average width by average length by 7.48. For round ponds multiply average depth by diameter squared by 7.48.

Example

Average depth 6 feet, average width 100 feet, average length 200 feet.

6′ × 100′ × 200′ = 120,000 cubic feet of water
1 cubic foot of water = 7.48 gallons
Therefore, 120,000 × 7.48 = 897,600 gallons*

This volume of water (neglecting losses by evaporation and leakage) would supply 1 acre-inch of water for 33.5 acres of land or over 2 inches for 14 acres.

*For Imperial gallons divide U.S. gallons by 1.2.

Location of pond.

A pond must be located where the soil is of such a nature that it will hold water. Borings or test holes should be made in a proposed location to determine the nature of the soil. Heavy clays are best, but silt clays and clay loams are suitable. Sandy or gravelly soils are unsuited. Clay soils underlain by porous soils are unsuited unless the pond is lined with 2 or 3 feet of heavy clay or sheets of plastic. Faulted or porous rock close to the surface should be avoided. The earth fill, or dam if any should be as watertight as the bottom.

In order to fill a pond with water it must be located where there is sufficient watershed or flowing water as from a spring or brook. A natural saucer-shaped area, a shallow ravine with a small flowing stream, or a fairly level area near a large stream where water can be diverted to the pond are ideal locations and often can be constructed at the lowest cost. For example, a relatively small dam across a deep ravine can impound large volumes of water.

In general a pond should be located as near to the buildings as the foregoing conditions will permit.

Type to build.

There are four types of construction for ponds: 1. surface or "watershed" ponds; 2. spring-fed ponds; 3. dugout ponds; and 4. diversion ponds.

Surface or watershed ponds derive their water from surface runoff of rain water from nearby sloping land. A fill across a low point in a field is a good example. See Fig. 3-33. Such a pond must have a watertight fill with a spillway to take care of excess water. The watershed should be in sod to prevent silting and should be clean. Barnyard drainage should not be used.

Spring-fed ponds are built near to and below continuously flowing springs. The usual construction is to build a dam across the spring brook. The dam should be far enough below the spring so that the pond will not flood the spring. If the spring flow is strong enough to supply all water needed, surface water should be diverted. This provides better quality water and avoids pond damage by flooding. Spring-fed ponds are excellent for growing fish.

Dugout ponds are simply holes dug into fairly level soil where surface water can flow in or where underground seepage can fill the pond. The latter is common in Florida and other areas where there is a high water table. There is no fill to construct. As, in the case of the watershed pond, the drainage area, if any, should be in sod to prevent silting and should be clean. This type of pond is very common because there are more places where it can be built.

Diversion ponds are possible only where there is a stream of water available. Such ponds are usually constructed near the stream at such a level that at least a portion of the stream flow can be diverted to the pond by ditch or pipe. The pond should be located where the stream will not overflow it in flood season. The flow of water to the pond can be regulated by suitable controls on the feed pipe or ditch. All flood waters should be diverted to avoid silting. This and the spring-fed pond usually provide the best water as the flow through them keeps the water fresh.

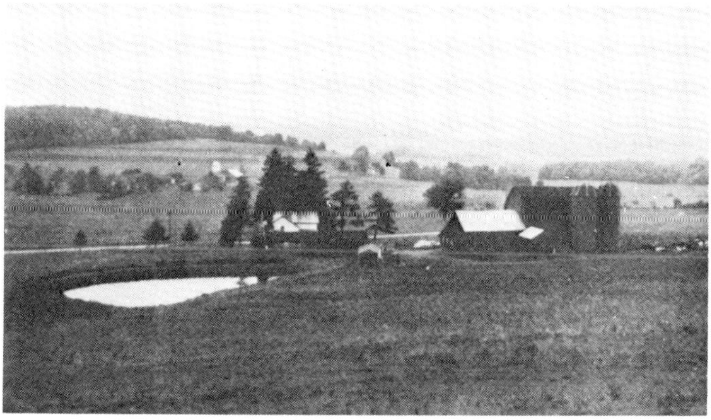

Fig. 3-33. A small farm pond in eastern United States. Rain water flows to this pond from the sodded watershed above it. It is used for watering livestock; for fire fighting; for swimming, boating, and skating; and as a source of food fish.

Any constructed fill for a pond dam should be made of clay or other watertight material. The fill should be well tamped and planted with sod and shrubbery to hold it in place. See Fig. 3-33. Spillways should be of concrete or masonry and large enough to take care of maximum flood waters.

If food fish are to be grown, the pond depth should be 8 to 12 feet (2.5 to 3.7 m.) with minimum area at least ¼ acre. (0.2 ha). Careful planting and fertilization are essential in most cases to insure an adequate food supply for the fish. For best results animals should be fenced away. If animals are to be watered from a pond, the water should be piped to a watering trough if possible. If the pond water is to be used for household purposes, animals should be fenced from the entire watershed area. Treatment of pond water for domestic use is described in Chapter 4.

Some states have laws regulating farm pond construction. These laws apply to such features as depth, volume, area of watershed, etc. Any one contemplating the construction of a pond should make sure that such laws are understood and complied with.

Development of Natural Lakes and Streams

Natural lakes and streams must be taken as nature provides them. Obtaining water from them is principally a matter of selecting and installing the necessary pump, treatment equipment, and piping. These problems are discussed in Chapters 4 to 7.

Water Treatment 4

The treatment of water to improve its quality involves additions to, subtractions from, or chemical changes in the raw water. The subject is broad enough to justify a whole book. Space will not permit a lengthy discussion here; therefore only the usual minimum treatments of water used for domestic purposes will be presented.

Water used for domestic purposes in rural areas is, in the majority of cases, satisfactory as it comes from the well or spring. However, in some localities, for one reason or another, the water is not satisfactory unless treated. The most common treatments are: 1. for excessive mineral content, hardness in particular; 2. for acidity; 3. for objectionable odors or flavors; 4. for removal of sediment; and 5. for contamination.

REMOVAL OF MINERALS

Practically all natural ground water contains minerals. The kind and extent of mineral content varies widely with the exposure of the water to various sources of soluble minerals as it flows over and through the earth's crust. Table 4-I indicates the most troublesome minerals found in domestic water supplies, the reasons why they are troublesome, and the tolerance range below which treatment is seldom necessary.

In rare instances other minerals are found in such concentrations that the water needs treatment or is unsuitable for use. For example, near an ocean, sea water may find its way into wells which are pumped hard, and sea water contains many objectionable minerals. Some waters contain so much silica in solution that excess scale formation occurs. However, this is rare with domestic water supplies.

Treatment for Hardness

Hardness in water results from the presence of calcium salts and/or magnesium salts in solution. *Total hardness is equal to the sum of the two.* Calcium hardness is sometimes referred to as "temporary

TABLE 4-I.

MINERALS COMMONLY FOUND IN DOMESTIC WATER SUPPLIES FOR WHICH TREATMENT IS SOMETIMES NECESSARY.*

Mineral	Reasons for Treatment	Tolerance Range Below Which Treatment Is Seldom Necessary
Calcium	Produces hardness	5 gpg or 85 ppm**
Magnesium	Produces hardness	5 gpg or 85 ppm Calcium and magnesium together should not exceed 5 to 6 gpg or 85-103 ppm
Sulphur (hydrogen sulphide)	Bad tase and odor. Highly corrosive to plumbing, stains clothing, etc.	Trace
Salt	Bad taste. Highly corrosive.	Trace
Iron	Stains clothing and plumbing fixtures. In excess give water bad taste and color. Interferes with water softener. May cause growth of iron bacteria which clogs screens, strainers, and pipes.	0.3 ppm

*From Nordell's *Water Treatment*, Reinhold Publishing Corporation, New York, 1951. Reproduced courtesy of the publisher.

**gpg = grains per gallon. ppm = parts per million.

hardness" while magnesium hardness is called "permanent hardness." This distinction is due to the fact that calcium salts are much less soluble in water than are magnesium salts; therefore the calcium salts precipitate more readily and are deposited as lime scale when the water is heated. With high concentrations of calcium salts there is often precipitation even in cold-water pipes.

Hardness in water is objectionable for the following reasons:

1. It requires excessive amounts of soap for washing. See Table 4-II.

2. Soap reacts to calcium and magnesium salts, forming an insoluble precipitate which lodges in the fabric of clothing, making it gray in color, harsh, hard to clean, and less durable. There is also a harsh effect on human skin and hair.

3. The precipitate soils plumbing fixtures, plugs drain pipes, and in extreme cases may interfere with the operation of a septic tank.

4. When hard water evaporates from dishes, glassware, car bodies, fruit, milk containers, and other objects washed or rinsed in it, a cloudy film or dusty looking spots are left on the surfaces. In the case of milk containers this residue may harbor bacteria and cause a high bacterial count in the milk.

5. Some foods cooked in hard water, particularly beans and peas, become tough and rubbery. Baking soda added to the cooking water tends to counteract this.

6. When the water is heated, calcium hardness readily precipitates and forms scale on the container in which it is heated. Thus water heaters, hot-water pipes (see Fig. 4-1), teakettles, and cooking pots and pans may soon become heavily coated with lime scale. It has been estimated that heavy lime deposits on water heaters, furnaces, etc., can increase the fuel costs by one-third. Also, such water used in engine cooling systems will form scale on the inside of the cooling jackets and radiators, reducing the effectiveness of the cooling systems.

TABLE 4-II.
SOAP WASTED BY HARD WATER*.

Hardness: Grains per Gallon	Hardness: Ppm	Pounds of Soap Wasted per 1000 Gallons of Water
5	86	7½
7	120	10½
10	171	15
15	257	22½
20	343	30
25	428	37½
30	514	45
40	686	60
50	856	75
60	1027	90

*From Nordell's *Water Treatment*, Reinhold Publishing Corporation, New York, 1951, p. 52. Reproduced courtesy of the publisher.

Water softners

It is estimated that 80% of the farms and rural homes in the United States have hard-water problems. The best solution for these problems is water softeners. Water softeners used for domestic purposes are of the zeolite type.

Zeolite softeners consist of a tank containing a bed of granular synthetic zeolite chemicals (sometimes referred to as "white sand") resting on a bed of quartz gravel, as indicated in Fig. 4-2. Another type of softener using a natural "green sand" is used primarily for iron removal. Green-sand softeners have much less capacity for removal of carbonates.

Principles of operation. When hard water is passed through an active bed of granulated zeolite the calcium and magnesium are taken up by the zeolite, thus leaving the water soft. At the same time the zeolite gives up to the water an equal amount of sodium. The process is known as a *sodium-cation exchange*, i.e., the zeolite takes up the hardness and adds sodium to the water.

In service the zeolite gradually loses its sodium and therefore its capacity to soften the water, with the result that eventually unsoftened water will flow through. Before this point is reached the softener should be backwashed, regenerated, and rinsed.

Following the backwash a measured quantity of salt brine is flushed through. The chlorine of the salt combines with the calcium and magnesium to form soluble chlorides of calcium and magnesium. These soluble chlorides are taken up by the water and can then be flushed to waste. The sodium of the salt restores the sodium to the zeolite.

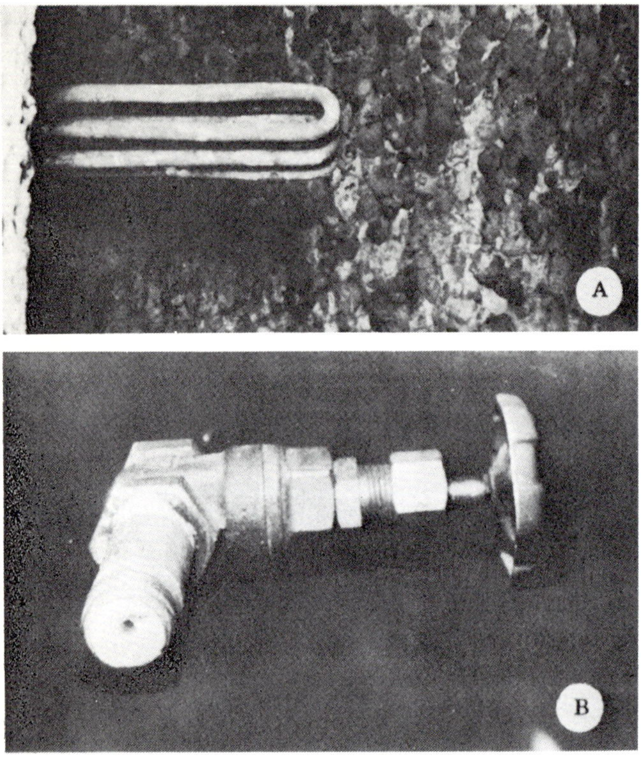

Fig. 4-1. A — Scale on inside surface of a hot-water tank. B — Calcium deposit on inside of hot-water pipe.

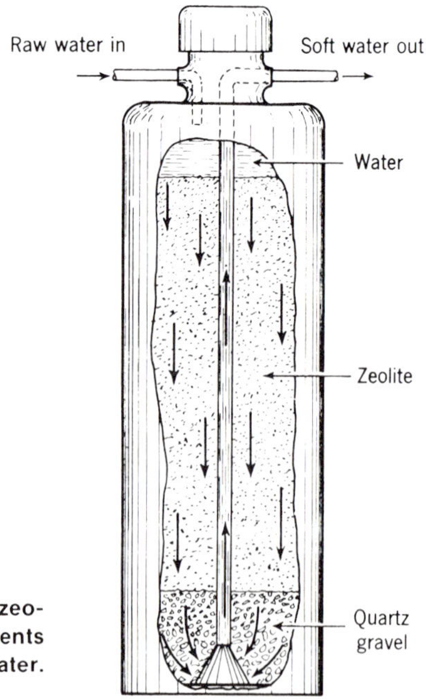

Fig. 4-2. A mannal regeneration zeolite water softener showing contents and direction of circulation of water.

This is the regeneration process. In regenerating any softener the manufacturer's directions should be followed explicitly.

Types of softeners. Many different brands of softeners are on the market. Most of the manufactures offer a line of five or six models at a rather wide price range depending upon the size, the degree of automatic operation, and the quality of materials. For example, one manufacturer offers six different models ranging from a simple all-manual regeneration model to a completely automatic regeneration model.

Selecting the size of softener. The size of softener to install is dependent upon three factors: 1. the total hardness of the water; 2. the amount of water to be softened; and 3. with manual regeneration, the frequency of regeneration desired.

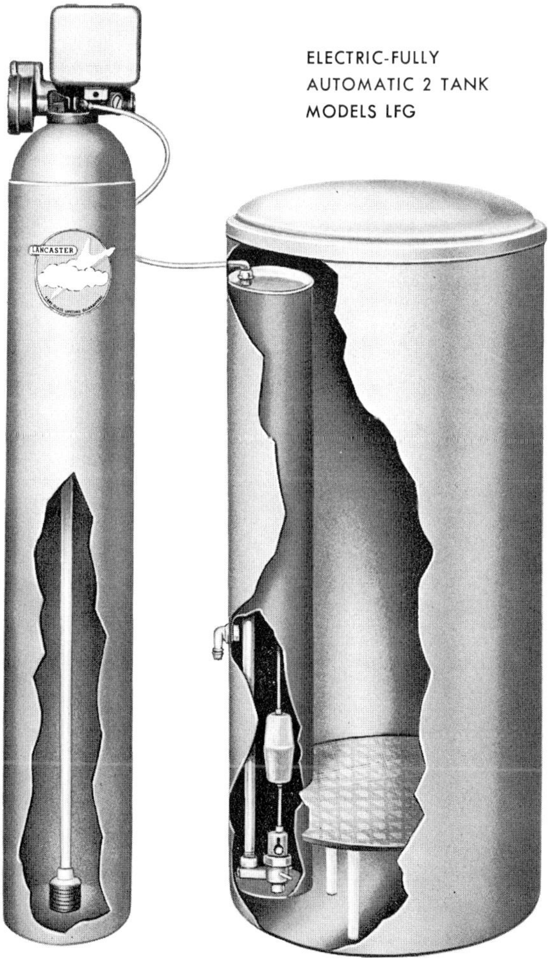

Fig. 4-3. A fully automatic, 2-tank, water softener. Electrically operated. The tank on the left contains the softening material and the tank on the right contains the salt brine. Softener tank is rust and corrosion resistant. Brine tank is constructed of heavy gague fiber-glass. Removes disolved iron as well as hardness.

Courtesy Lancaster Pump & Mfg. Co., Lancaster, Pa.

In shallow wells, springs, and other surface supplies the hardness of the water may vary greatly from season to season. The size of the softener should be based upon the highest degree of hardness. Deep wells and large bodies of surface water are likely to have a remarkably uniform degree of hardness throughout the year.

For domestic use it is common practice, where the total hardness of the water does not exceed 170 ppm (10 gpg), to soften only the hot-water supply. For harder water some of the cold water is also softened, especially for laundry purposes. For extremely hard water, 500 to 1200 ppm (30 to 70 gpg), it is highly desirable to soften the entire supply. Water with a hardness over 1200 ppm (70 gpg) is ordinarily considered unfit for domestic purposes. Table 4-III gives estimated average demands per person per week for soft water under four types of plumbing installations. Figure 4-4 illustrates plumbing connections for the most usual types of installations, namely, items 3 and 4 in Table 4-III.

TABLE 4-III.
DEMANDS FOR SOFT WATER. GALLONS PER PERSON PER WEEK.

Types of Installation	U.S. Gallons per Person per Week	Imperial Gallons per Person per Week
1. All water softened	250 to 500	208 to 417
2. All water softened except for toilets and for sprinkling	150 to 300	125 to 250
3. All hot water and the cold water for laundry softened	125 to 150	104 to 125
4. Only hot water softened	90 to 100	75 to 83

The frequency of regeneration is a matter of choice. With automatic regeneration models the regeneration periods can conveniently be set for almost any frequency. However, with the manually operated models the time required for each regeneration may make it desirable to install a larger softener in order to reduce the frequency of this time-consuming chore. In most cases it is desirable to regenerate not more than twice per month.

Ratings for softeners. Softeners are rated as to the maximum flow rate per minute, and the total softening capacity in grains of hardness and in gallons of soft water delivered per regeneration. See Table 4-IV. A flow rate of 10 U.S. gallons (8 Imp. gals.) per minute is adequate for a small family with a kitchen, laundry, and one bath. A faucet will flow 3 to 5 U.S. gallons (2.5 to 4.2 Imp. gals.) per minute on the average; therefore the 10 U.S. gallon-per-minute flow rate would provide adequate flow for two faucets simultaneously. In general, the desired flow rate can be determined by estimating the number of soft-water faucets which are likely to be in use at one time and multiplying that number by 5.

Water-softening service.

In some communities a water-softening service is available through business firms which make a specialty of this. A common procedure is for the firm to install and maintain the softeners on customers' premises for a monthly, quarterly, or annual fee. Some of the larger firms will also provide additional treatments, as for iron or sulphur, when necessary.

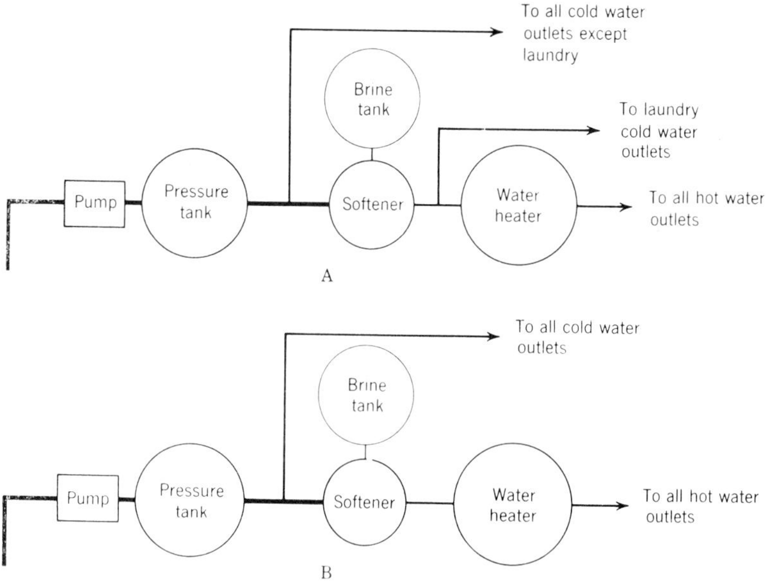

Fig. 4-4. Two plumbing installations for water softeners. A — To soften all hot water and the cold water for the laundry. B — To soften hot water only.

Softeners as filters.

The zeolite type of softener does afford some degree of filtration. However, softeners are not designed for that specific purpose; therefore, if there is any appreciable amount of sediment in the water a filter should be installed ahead of the softener, as indicated in Fig. 4-5. An appreciable amount of sediment in the zeolite bed greatly reduces the capacity of the softener. Also, waters with a high iron concentration will form a precipitate which will interfere with the softener. In the latter case an iron trap or a green sand softener should be installed ahead of the zeolite softener where the filter is in Fig. 4-5.

Treatment for Iron, Sulphur, and Salt

Forms of Iron in Water

Iron may be present in water in several forms. By far the most common form found in springs and well water is ferrous bicarbonate. This is a colorless salt which exists in solution. It is this form of iron which the water also picks up from rusting pipes.

Although iron-bearing water may be clear when first drawn, upon standing exposed to the air for a time it will become cloudy and eventually will show a reddish-brown precipitate. It is this precipitate which produces the stain from the water. Manufacturers of iron re-

TABLE 4-IV.
CAPACITY OF SOFTENERS*.

Model No.	Max. Flow Rate per Minute, Gallons	Total Capacity, Grains†	Hardness of Water, Grains‡ 6	10	15	20	30	40	50	60	70	Salt Tank Capacity, Pounds	Pounds of Salt per Complete Regeneration
			U.S. Gallons of Soft Water per Regeneration**										
1	8	15,000	2500	1500	1000	750	500					200	8
2	10	20,000	3333	2000	1333	1000	700	450				300	12
3	14	30,000	5000	3000	2000	1500	1000	675	480			300	17
4	18	40,000	6666	4000	2666	2000	1300	900	640	466		500	22
5	24	50,000	8333	5000	3333	2500	1650	1100	800	580	430	500	27
6	30	60,000	10,000	6000	4000	3000	2000	1300	1000	700	514	700	32
7	36	80,000	13,333	8000	5333	4000	2700	1800	1300	930	686	1000	42

*Based on data from H.L.G. Co.
**For Imperial gallons divide U.S. gallons by 1.2.
†To obtain capacities in gallons per regeneration not shown in this table, divide the total capacity in grains (column 3) by the hardness of the water to be softened.
‡Figures for capacities of 40, 50, 60, and 70 grains of hardness represent a 10%, 20%, 30%, and 40% reduction respectively from the normal capacity to allow for loss of softening capacities during regeneration and rinsing.

moval equipment usually make water analyses free of charge for a prospective customer. The type of iron removal unit to use should be determined on the basis of the water analysis.

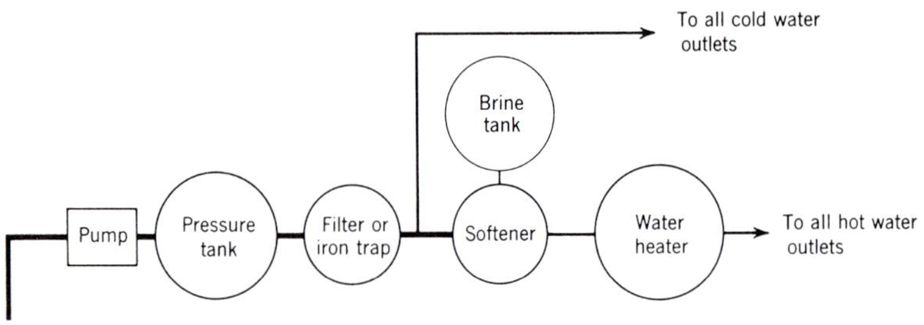

Fig. 4-5. Plumbing installation for a filter or an iron trap in conjunction with a softener.

Iron removal.

Iron in the form of ferrous bicarbonate can be removed from water in a number of ways, but for domestic water supplies from private sources such as springs or wells the best methods are by means of "iron traps" or by areation. A natural green-sand softener is often used for this purpose. White-sand zeolite softeners can also be used for iron removal but they are more expensive if used only for iron removal.

For iron water which is clear when first drawn, polyphosphates can be fed into the water by special feeding devices.

Figure 4-7 illustrates the external appearance of one type of filter which can be used for iron, sulphur, or sediment, depending upon the chemicals used in the tank.

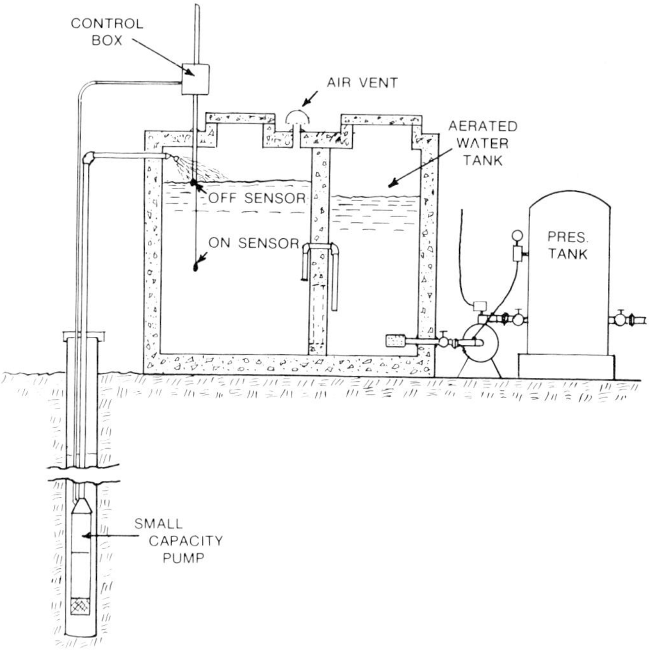

Fig. 4-6. An aerating tank for reducing sulphur and iron in water. Spraying the water into the tank at the left releases the disolved sulphur gasses in the water. The finer the spray the better. The sulphur gasses escape through the vent. The lower sensor turns the pump on when the water in the spray tank reaches a low level and the higher sensor turns the pump off when the water level rises to the desired level.

Areation also tends to oxidize iron in the water. The oxidized iron particles will settle to the bottom of the tank and should be cleaned out occasionally. If the water has a high concentration of iron it will be necessary to have a filter between the two tanks as indicated by the dashed lines in center wall. Otherwise a pipe connection as shown will be satisfactory.

Removal of sulphur.

Hydrogen sulphides, in concentrations up to 6 ppm, can be removed by special filters of the type illustrated in Fig. 4-7. For concentrations above 6 ppm the water must be aerated before filtering.

Aeration can be accomplished by spraying the raw water into a catchment basin as indicated in Fig. 4-6. The aerated water can then be pumped into the plumbing system. Commercial aerating devices are on the market which will do a better job. See Fig. 4-8.

Traces of sulphur can be removed economically by chlorination. The standard chlorinators used for bacterial treatment can be used for this purpose. See Fig. 4-14.

Removal of salts.

It is possible to remove salts from water, even from sea water, but the process is tedious and expensive. For these reasons the process is little used except on a small scale for emergency purposes such as supplying potable water for shipwrecked sailors and fliers.

If the salt concentration in a domestic water supply is high enough to make the water unfit for use the usual practice is to abandon the supply.

Treatment for Acid

Waters containing carbon dioxide in quantity are acid waters. Cistern and pond waters containing decaying vegetation are likely to be acid. The acid concentration usually found in domestic water supplies has little effect upon the washing qualities. It does, however, cause corrosion of piping and may pick up lead in solution. With iron pipe the water will be a rusty red and with copper a bluish green. Both will stain clothing.

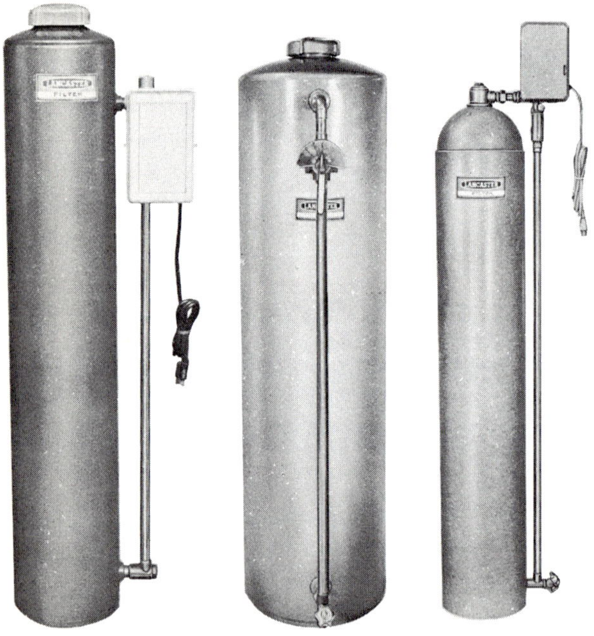

METAL AUTOMATIC

METAL MANUAL

FIBRE GLASS MANUAL OR AUTOMATIC

Courtesy Lancaster Pump and Mfg. Co., Inc., Lancaster, Pa.

Fig. 4-7. The external appearance of one type of filter and neutrelizer now on the market. Depending upon the contents of the containers, these devices can be used, (1) As filters for sediment and turbidity, (2) As iron filters, (3) For neutralizing acid water, and (4) For removing color taste and odors caused by chlorine, sulphur, mold, fishy taste, muddy taste and swampy taste.

Small cartridge type of filters are available for installing ahead of a faucet to remove sediment, taste and odor from the water at that one faucet. Practical for use where it is desirable to improve the quality of water for drinking and cooking only.

Acidity can be neutralized by passing the water through a bed of crushed marble or limestone. Alkaline feeders are also available which automatically feed an acid neutralizer into the water.

A commercial unit similar in appearance to that shown in Fig. 4-7 but containing a bed of crushed marble can be used, or a home-made acid neutralizer can be installed. The latter should be approved by health authorities before being put into operation.

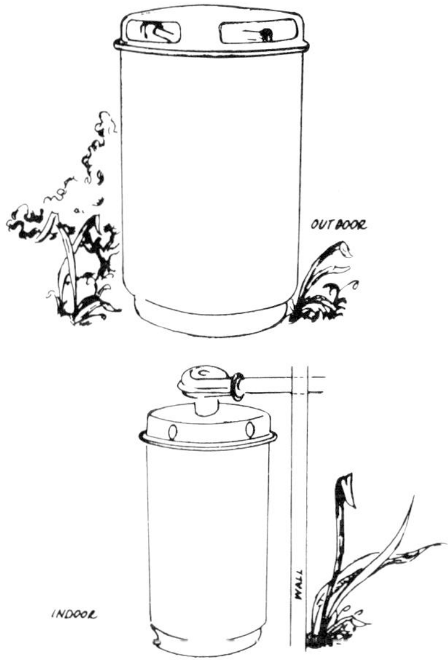

Fig. 4-8. Two models of commercial areators for removing sulphur, gas and iron from water. Upper tank is for outdoor installation and lower tank is for indoor installation where freezing temperatures prevail. Note the vent on the indoor model to lead the sulphur and gas odors to the outside. Both tanks are constructed of fiberglass.

Aeration of stagnant flat tasting water will improve its quality. The manufactures of this equipment claim that areation of waters with oxygen content under 12 parts per million can increase dairy herd production, probably because the cows will drink more of it, and water is the principle raw material from which milk is made.

REMOVAL OF OBJECTIONABLE TASTE, ODOR, AND COLOR

A common cause of objectionable taste and odor is the presence of algae in the water. Also, decaying vegetation in the water source, such as a pond, lake or stream may cause objectionable taste and odor. Algae are microscopic green plants, flourishing in ponds, lakes, and sometimes in streams. The algae take up free oxygen from the water and thus produce a flat taste. High concentrations give the water a distinct greenish color.

Algae can be removed from water by treatment with copper sulphate. About 0.5 ppm or 4½ pounds per million gallons of water applied in solution over the surface of the water in April, May, or June is usually effective. In some cases two treatments about 1 month apart are necessary. Concentrations of copper sulfate higher than those mentioned will be harmful to fish living in the water.

Other organic compounds, odors, and tastes can be removed by passing the water through activated charcoal filters. A commercial unit similar in appearance to Fig. 4-7, but filled with activated charcoal, is effective, easy to install, and inexpensive to operate.

Color resulting from organic compounds is difficult to remove. A chemical analysis of the water may be required to determine the method of removal, if any.

TREATMENT FOR SEDIMENT

Sediment can be removed from water by settling and filtering. The type and size of filter to install depends upon the amount and kind of sediment in the water and the use to be made of the water.

For filtering iron precipitate and small amounts of other kinds of sediment which might be found in wells and springs, commercial types of filters such as shown in Fig. 4-7 can be used. For large amounts of water or where the water is loaded with sediment as might be the case with stream or pond water, larger filters are necessary.

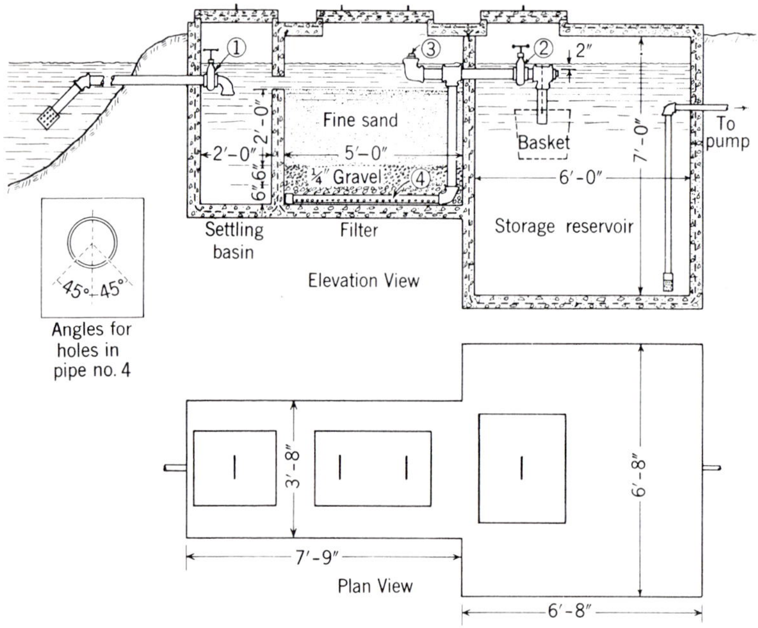

Partly from Farm Journal

Fig. 4-9. Plan of a slow sand filter for installation near the shore of a lake, pond, or stream. If installed near a stream it must be protected from flooding. Dimensions are for a capacity of 750 U.S. gallons (625 Imp. gals.) per day based upon 50 gallons (42 Imp. gals.) per day per square foot of filter surface. Settling basin removes heavier sediment when the water is exceptionally roily. The reservoir should have a capacity for at least a 2-day supply of water.

If the water has an objectionable taste, a charcoal filter similar to that of Fig. 4-7 can be installed in the pumping system, or activated charcoal can be hung in a wire basket over the inlet pipe in the reservoir as indicated by the dash lines.

1 Inlet valve. 2 Filter outlet valve. 3 Plug-in connection for backwashing. 4 Perforated collecting pipe at bottom of filter. The selling basin should be cleaned out occasionally.

For extreme turbidity it may be advisable to add alum to the water before filtering. Alum dispensers are available commercially for installation on domestic systems. Figures 4-9 through 4-12 illustrate home-built filters. Filters should be located where they will not be flooded and the intake should be out in the water far enough and high enough so that bottom mud will not be drawn into the filter. Figure 4-10 to 4-13 illustrate types of intake arrangements.

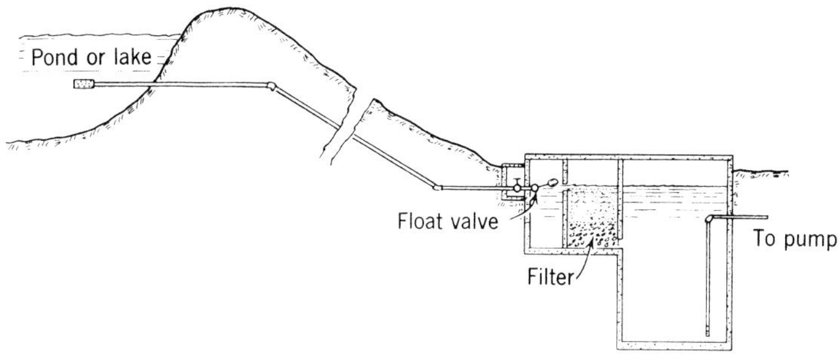

Fig. 4-10. A filter fed by gravity flow. A float valve must be installed at the filter intake as shown to regulate the flow of water from the source.

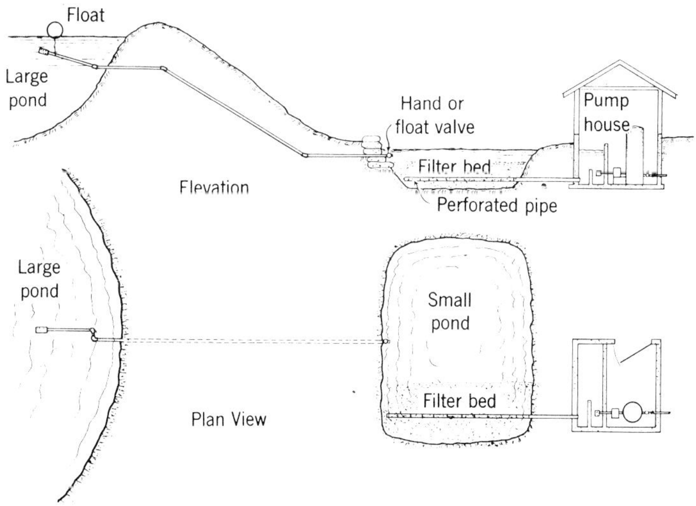

Fig. 4 11. A plan for filtering pond water. The small pond serves as a settling basin and as a place for the sand filter. It should be large enough to hold at least 3 or 4 weeks' supply of water. If the water is quite muddy, settling can be accelerated by treatment with chemicals as follows: 1. Mix 1 part lime to 2 parts of alum. 2. Sprinkle this mixture uniformly over the surface of the small pond at the rate of ½ pound for each 1000 U.S. gallson (833 Imp. gals.) of water in the pond. An alternate method is to dissolve the lime-alum in water and spray it over the surface at the same rate. The chemicals will form a "flock" in the water which will settle to the bottom and take the mud with it.

If the water is to be used for household purposes it will need chlorination. If the water has a bad taste it can be improved by aeration or by filtering through a bed of activated charcoal. The filter bed must be cleaned occasionally.

The water must move slowly through the filter or the filter bed will not be effective. The flow rate should not exceed 50 gallons per square foot (42 Imp. gals. per sq. m.) of surface per day. The filter shown in Fig. 4-9 has a surface area of 3 by 5, or 15 square feet (1.39 sq. m.). This multiplied by 50 U.S. gallons per square foot (42 Imp. gals./sq. m.) equals 750 gallons (625 Imp. gals.) per day.

All filters need cleaning periodically to keep them sanitary and to avoid a reduction in the flow of water. The commercial type of filter can be cleaned and sterilized by backwashing. The types illustrated in Figs. 4-9 through 4-11 can be cleaned by draining and scraping off the top surface. After cleaning any removed sand should be replaced by fresh sand and the filter should be sterilized by chlorination.

Chlorination is for disinfecting the filter only and is not effective after a few hours. If the water at the source is contaminated, a chlorinator should be installed on the pump as for any contaminated water. See Fig. 4-14. A health officer should be consulted on chlorination procedures.

TREATMENT FOR CONTAMINATION

The cheapest and most effective method of treatment of large volumes of water for contamination is by means of chlorination. For small quantities of water such as the requirements for drinking purposes, the water can be treated by boiling for 20 minutes, or by adding chlorine pellets usually available at drugstores.

A number of chlorinating devices for domestic water systems are on the market. Local health authorities should be consulted before selecting a chlorinator for any particular location. Figure 4-14 illustrates one type installed on a pressure water system.

Although approved chlorinators are somewhat expensive, the operating cost is negligible and the total cost may be less than that of establishing a new uncontaminated source of water. In fact, in densely populated areas it may be impossible to obtain uncontaminated ground water.

The chlorinators used for contamination treatment can also be used for removing slight traces of sulphur.

MULTIPLE TREATMENT OF WATER

Treatment of water for only one purpose such as softening is a relatively simple matter and in most cases an owner, with the aid of a health officer and a local dealer for the specific equipment, can obtain good results. However, if the water must be treated for multiple purposes such as softening, filtering, and removal of sulphur and iron, then advice should be sought from a person or a firm well qualified to make a complete water analysis and recommendations for combinations of conditioning equipment. Manufacturers of conditioning equipment usually provide this service free of charge to prospective customers. Any multiple treatment installation should conform to local health department regulations.

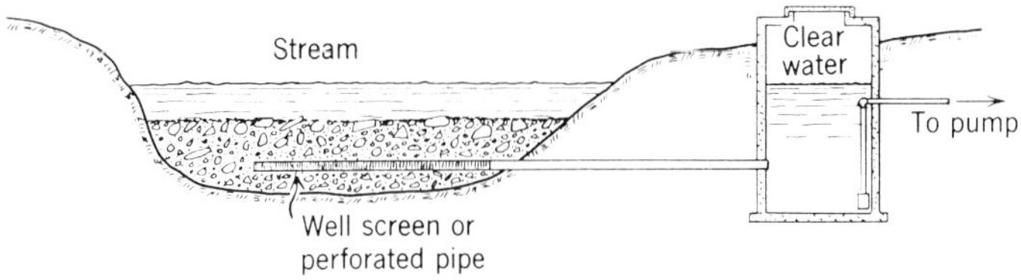

Fig. 4-12. Plan for understream filter. A well screen or a perforated pipe buried in a gravel bed in the bottom of a stream and connected to a clear water well can furnish an abundance of water for irrigation, livestock, or fire fighting. It is of doubtful value in a stream which carries a heavy load of silt or has a deep mud bottom.

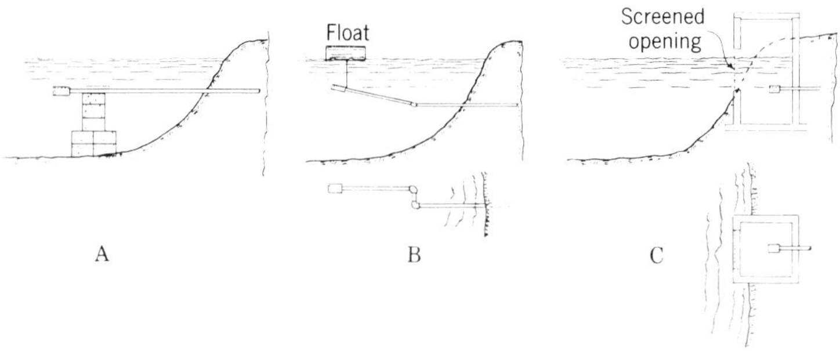

Fig. 4-13. Optional intake arrangements for filters. Can also be used for pumps.
A — For use where water level is constant and the bottom is sand, gravel, or rock.
B — For use where the water level fluctuates. A small steel drum will serve as a float. Flexible plastic pipe can be used without the elbow hinge.
C — For use in a stream where flood water might damage an installation such as A or B.
If the water tends to be stagnant and has a flat taste, the inlet screen should be supported near the surface as shown at B where there is more oxygen in the water.

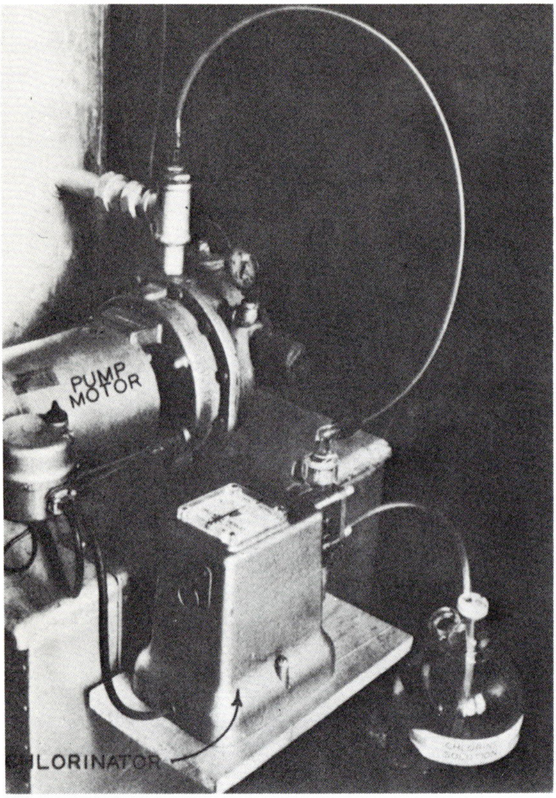

Fig. 4-14. A chlorinator for a domestic water system. Has capacity for chlorinating up to 1200 U.S. gallons (1000 Imp gals.) per hour at pressures as high as 100 pounds per square inch. Rate of feed is adjustable by means of the knob on the end and is indicated on a dial under the plastic plate. The rate of feed should be such that there is residual chlorine in the water at the faucets. This can be determined by a simple test with the "residual chlorine test kit" obtainable with the chlorinator. The chlorine solution can be made from bleaching agents available at grocery stores. This type of chlorinator has a positive feed and is operated by a self-contained motor. It should be connected to the pump motor side of the automatic switch so that the chlorinator operates only when the pump is running.

Problems of Head and Pressure 5

DEFINITIONS AS APPLIED TO WATER

When used in connection with handling water, head refers to the vertical height of a column of water above a certain point, and is considered as causing or counteracting the flow of water. For example, if water stands at a height of 20 feet in a pipe, as shown in Fig. 5-1, there will be 20 feet of head on the bottom end of the pipe. This 20 feet of head will exert a total pressure on the bottom of the pipe equal to the weight of the column of water. This pressure may be expressed in terms of pounds per square inch (psi) or grams/sq. cm. A column

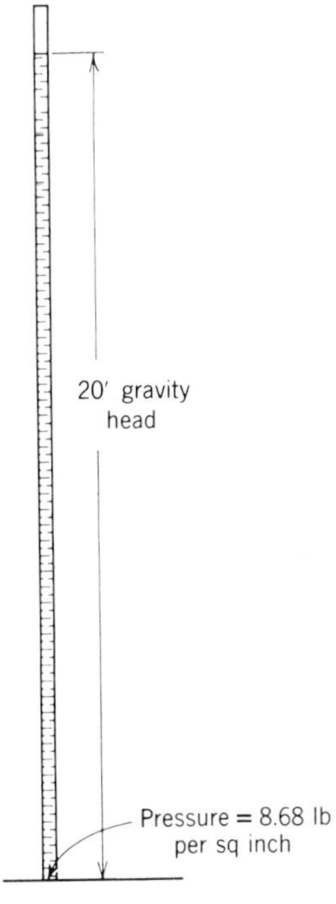

Fig. 5-1. Gravity head.

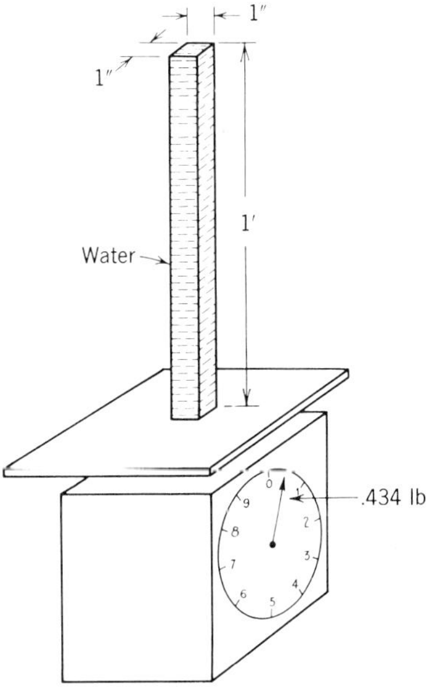

Fig. 5-2. A column of water 1 inch square and 1 foot high weighs 0.434 pound. The scales were set for the tare of the container.

of water 1 inch square and 1 foot high weighs 0.434 pound. See Fig. 5-2. Therefore, the pressure per square inch on the bottom of the pipe equals 20 feet × 0.434 pound, or 8.68 pounds. If the bottom of the pipe were opened this head would cause water to flow out.

Pressure is a force created in some manner to make the water flow. It may be created by the weight of the atmosphere (atmospheric pressure), by the weight of a column of water, by means of pumps, compressed air, etc.

KINDS OF HEAD

In handling water we speak of four kinds of hea, namely: gravity head, pressure head, suction head, and friction head.

Gravity

Gravity head is the actual vertical height of a column of water above a reference point. The head shown in Fig. 5-1 is gravity head.

Pressure

Pressure head is the vertical height in feet to which any given pressure will force water. One pound of pressure will force water to a height of 2.3 feet. The pressure head in feet, then is equal to the pounds pressure × 2.3. For example, in Fig. 5-3, with a pressure of 10 psi in the tank, the water will rise in the pipe to a height of 23 feet (10 pounds × 2.3).

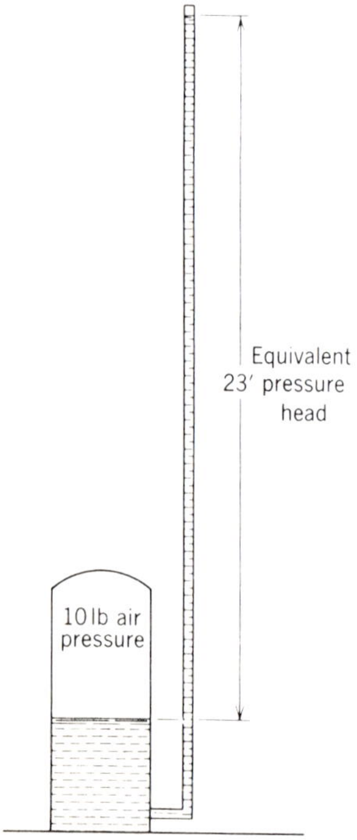

Fig.5-3. If the pressure of the air on the water is 10 psi, the pressure head is the equivalent of 10 pounds × 2.3, or 23 feet of gravity head.

Suction

Suction head, a term applied to pumps, is considered as the total equivalent head in feet on the suction side of the pump against which the pump must work in order to get water. The equivalent suction head is made up of (1) gravity head and (2) friction head. For example, if a pump is "sucking" water through a vertical distance of 15 feet as shown in Fig. 5-4, the suction head on the pump will be the vertical distance plus the friction head, whatever that may be.

Where the pump is located at some distance from the well as shown in Fig. 8-7, the amount of friction head may be very considerable.

Many pumps are guaranteed to work against at least 22 feet (6.7m) of total suction head at sea level. One has a guaranteed suction lift of as much as 28 feet (8.5 m) at sea level. Straight centrifugal pumps may be limited to about 15 feet (4.5 m) at sea level.

Friction

Friction head is the head required to overcome friction between flowing water and pipes. Water is caused to flow through pipes by gravity head, pressure head, or "suction" head.

Any portion of such heads used up in overcoming friction is called "friction head." Thus, friction head may be considered as lost head or obstructing head. To have any flow of water the gravity, pressure, or suction head must first overcome the friction head.

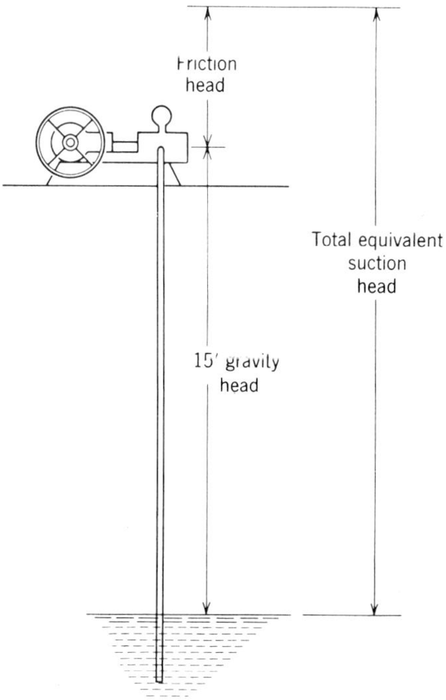

Fig. 5-4. Suction head on a pump is made up of gravity head plus friction head.

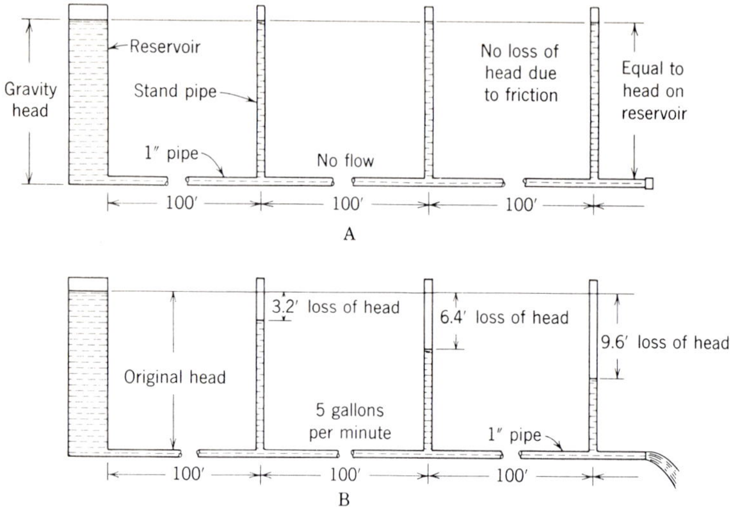

Fig. 5-5. Loss of head due to friction. If standpipes are erected on a pipeline as shown at A and the system filled with water, and if there is no flow through the pipe, the water will stand at the same level in all the standpipes. If the water is allowed to flow at the rate of 5 gallons per minute as indicated at B, the level of the water in each successive standpipe will be lower because of the loss of head by friction along the pipeline.

The amount of head lost due to friction depends upon several factors such as (1) the length of pipe, (2) the diameter of the pipe, (3) the smoothness of the inside of the pipe, (4) the number and kind of fittings, valves, and faucets in the pipe line, and (5) the rate of flow. For example:

1. *The longer the pipe, the greater the loss of head due to friction for any given diameter of pipe and rate of flow.* Thus with a 1-inch pipe and a rate of flow of 5 gallons per minute, as shown in Fig. 5-5B, the loss of head through 100 feet is 3.2 feet; through 200 feet is 6.4 feet; through 300 feet is 9.6 feet, etc.

2. *The smaller the diameter of any given length of pipe, the greater the friction losses for any given rate of flow.* Thus with a rate of flow of 5 gallons per minute through 100 feet of ¾-inch pipe, as shown in Fig. 6-6A, the loss of head due to friction is 10.5 feet. Through 1-inch pipe for the same rate of flow, the loss is only 3.2 feet, as shown in Fig. 5-6B.

3. *The smoother the inner surface of any given pipe, the less the friction losses for any given rate of flow.* Thus the losses in pipe A, Fig. 5-7, are less than in pipe B.

4. *The fewer the fittings and valves on a pipe line, the less the friction losses for any given rate of flow.* Thus the losses in pipe A, Fig. 5-8, are less than in pipe B.

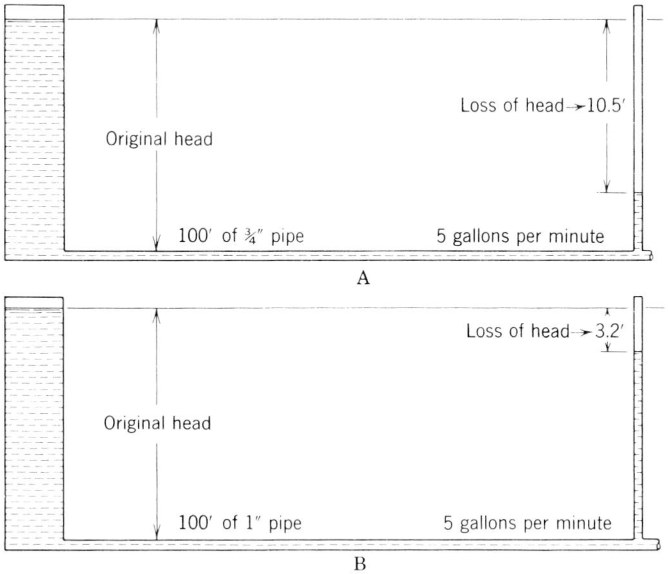

Fig. 5-6. Other things being equal, the loss of head due to friction is greater in a small pipe than in a large pipe.

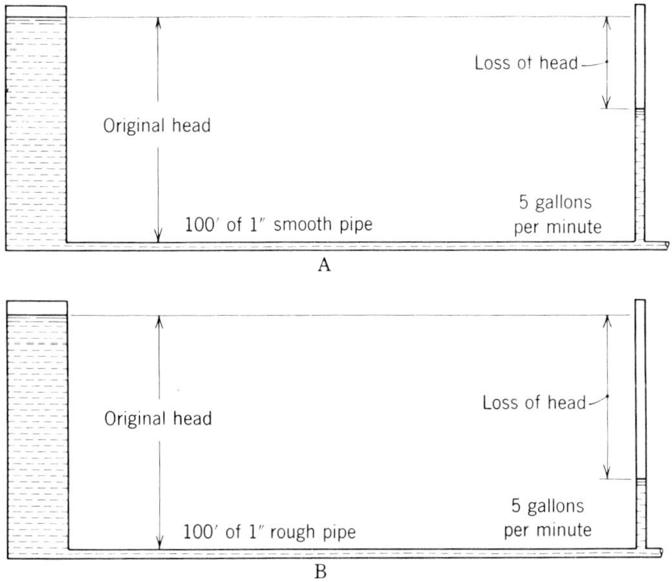

Fig. 5-7. Other things being equal, the loss of head due to friction is greater in a rough pipe than in a smooth pipe.

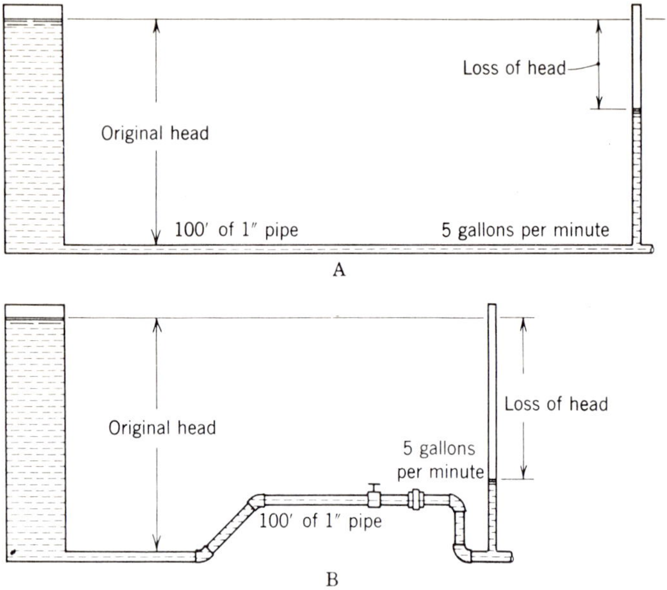

Fig. 5-8. Other things being equal, the loss of head due to friction is greater in crooked pipe or pipe with many fittings than it is in a straight pipe with few fittings.

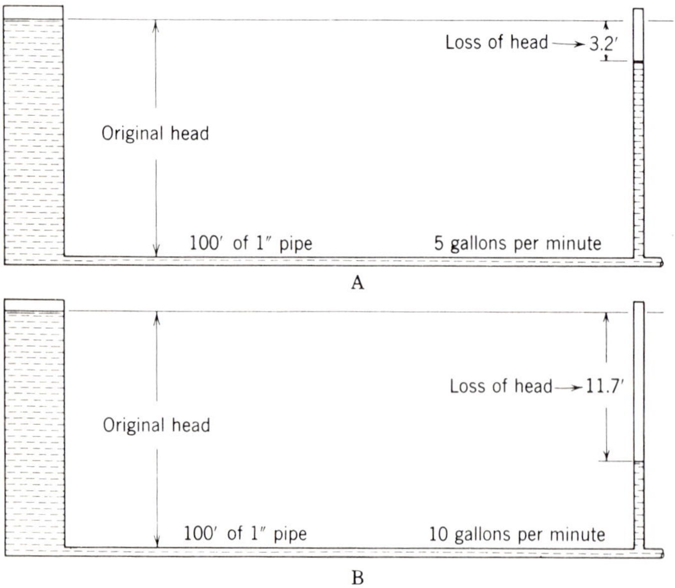

Fig. 5-9. The loss of head due to friction varies with the rate of flow of water.

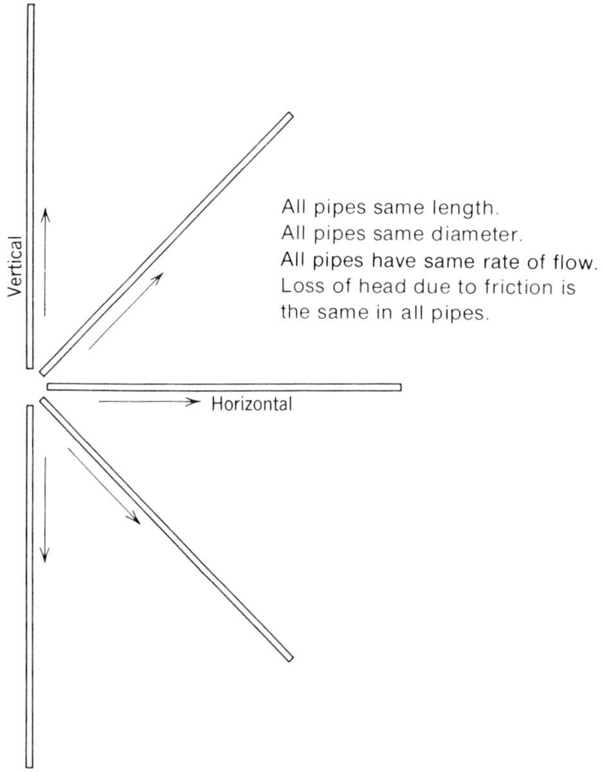

Fig. 5-10. The loss of head due to friction is not affected by the angular position of the pipe.

5. *The higher the rate of flow through any given pipe, the greater the friction losses.* Thus with a rate of flow of 5 gallons per minute through 100 feet of 1-inch pipe, as shown in Fig. 5-9, at A, the loss of head due to friction is 3.2 feet. If the rate of flow were increased to 10 gallons per minute, as shown at B, the loss of head due to friction would be 11.7 feet. Friction increases as the square of the velocity.

6. *Friction losses are not affected by the angular position of the pipe.* The friction losses under similar pipe and rate of flow conditions will be the same whether the water flows uphill or downhill. In Fig. 5-10 the losses due to friction are the same in each pipe.

7. *Friction losses are not affected by the pressure on the water in the pipes.*

Use of friction tables.

The losses of head due to friction in various sizes of pipe and with various rates of flow are presented in Table J-6-II, page 279. By use of this friction table, one may readily determine the friction losses or rate of flow under various conditions. See Job 6.

TABLE 5-I

BAROMETRIC PRESSURES AT DIFFERENT ALTITUDES*
WITH EQUIVALENT HEAD OF WATER AND THE VERTICAL SUCTION LIFT OF PUMPS

	Barometric Pressure, psi	Equivalent Head of Water, Feet	Practical Suction Lift of Pumps,† Feet
Sea level	14.70	33.95	22
¼ mile (1,320 feet) above sea level	14.02	32.38	21
½ mile (2,640 feet) above sea level	13.33	30.79	20
¾ mile (3,960 feet) above sea level	12.66	29.24	18
1 mile (5,280 feet) above sea level	12.02	27.76	17
1¼ mile (6,600 feet above sea level	11.42	26.38	16
1½ mile (7,920 feet) above sea level	10.88	25.13	15
2 mile (10,560 feet) above sea level	9.88	22.82	14

*Courtesy Goulds Pumps, Inc.

†Practical suction lift of pumps is equal to the vertical distance to which water is to be lifted plus the head of friction and other losses, if any.

METRIC EQUIVALENT OF ABOVE TABLE

	Grams per sq. cm.	Equivalent Head in Meters	Practical Suction Lift in Meters
Sea level	1034	10.35	6.70
¼ mile	948	9.87	6.40
½ mile	940	9.38	6.10
¾ mile	894	8.91	5.49
1 mile	844	8.46	5.18
1¼ mile	803	8.04	4.88
1½ mile	784	7.66	4.57
2 mile	694	6.96	4.26

KINDS OF AIR PRESSURE

In handling water with domestic equipment there are two kinds of air pressure to be considered: atmospheric and pneumatic.

Atmospheric

Atmospheric pressure results from the weight of the atmosphere extending above the earth's surface. At sea level the weight of the atmosphere is 14.7 psi (1.03 kg./sq. cm.). At higher levels, the pressure is less as shown in Table 5-I.

If we assume that the water in a well is at sea level, on each square inch of surface of water the atmosphere will exert a pressure of 14.7 psi as shown in Fig. 5-11A. This uniform pressure levels the surface of the water so that it stands at the same level inside and outside the pipe. "Water seeks its own level."

Now if an airtight plunger is placed in the pipe at water level and the plunger is raised as shown at B. the atmospheric pressure on the water in the pipe is reduced. This causes an unbalanced condition along the surface of the water, and the water will rise in the pipe. The water rises, not because the plunger is pulling up on it, but because there is greater pressure on the water outside the pipe than there is on the inside of the pipe. If a long pipe is used, as shown at C, and the plunger is drawn continuously upward, water will be forced up the pipe by the atmospheric pressure on the surface of the water in the well until the weight per square inch of the column of water in the pipe equals the weight per square inch of the atmosphere, or 14.7 psi. A column of water approximately 34 feet high is required to exert a pressure of 14.7 psi.

Ordinary water pumps are not capable of creating perfect vacuums. This, together with the fact that there are likely to be small leaks in the pipe and vapors from the water, reduces the practical "suction lift" of ordinary pumps to about 22 to 25 feet at sea level. Pumps in poor repair will have less suction lift than pumps in good repair.

If the location of the water is higher than sea level, both the theoretical and practical suction lifts are decreased, as may be seen in Table 5-I. At an elevation of 5000 feet, which is equivalent to that of the plains immediately east of the Rocky Mountains, the practical suction lift is only about 17 feet (5.2 m).

Pneumatic

Pneumatic pressure is air pressure over and above atmospheric pressure. It is this pressure which is registered on the pressure gauge and which makes water flow from hydropneumatic or "pressure" tanks. It also functions in air chambers on reciprocating pumps to even out the flow.

Pneumatic pressure may be expressed in psi. Each pound of pressure per square inch will force water up an open pipe a distance of 2.3

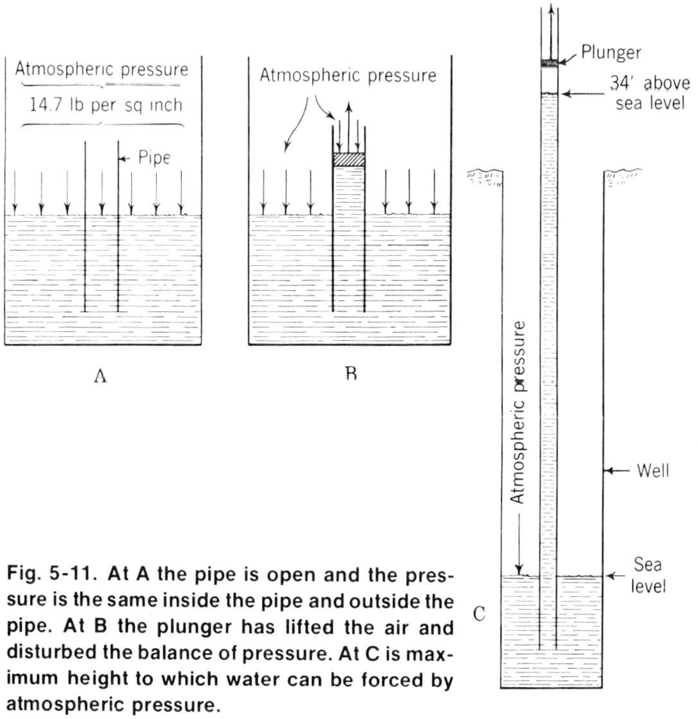

Fig. 5-11. At A the pipe is open and the pressure is the same inside the pipe and outside the pipe. At B the plunger has lifted the air and disturbed the balance of pressure. At C is maximum height to which water can be forced by atmospheric pressure.

feet. Therefore 1 pound of pressure is equal to 2.3 feet of head. If the pneumatic pressure in a water tank is 20 pounds then the water can be forced to an elevation of 20 × 2.3 or 46 feet. Twenty pounds of pneumatic pressure is then equal to 46 feet of gravity head.

From the foregoing discussion it can be seen that head and pressure can be converted, one to the other. Head in feet divided by 2.3 equals pounds of pressure. Pressure in pounds multiplied by 2.3 equals head in feet. Job 6, page 277, illustrates how to use head and pressure in calculations for pumps and water systems.

Pumps
Types and Principles of Operation 6

GENERAL CLASSIFICATION OF PUMPS FOR DOMESTIC AND FARM USE

Domestic and farm water pumps in general can be classed in two main groups, namely *"lift" pumps* and *force pumps*. Lift pumps and force pumps can, in turn be classified as *shallow-well* and *deep-well* pumps. See Table 6-I.

Lift Pumps

Lift pumps are designed to pump water from the source to the level of the pump spout only. They are used where the water is to be delivered into a bucket, trough, tank, or other open receptacle at the pump location. Such pumps are usually hand or windmill operated. Figures 6-1 through 6-4 illustrate variations of this type of pump. Note that all are open at the top; therefore they cannot be used for pumping against pressure. They are available for use on shallow-well sources as illustrated in Figs. 6-1 through 6-3, or deep-well sources as shown in Fig. 6-4.

Force Pumps

Force pumps are designed to pump water from a source and to deliver it to a higher elevation or against pressure. They are used primarily to pump water into elevated reservoirs and pressure tanks. All pressure-type water systems use force pumps. Figures 6-8 through the end of this chapter illustrate various types of force pumps. Note that all are enclosed so that the water can be forced to flow against pressure. They are available for use on shallow or deep wells to 1500 feet (457 m).

PRINCIPLES OF OPERATION OF LIFT PUMPS

The bucket and chain pumps are classed here as lift pumps although they may not be so designated in manufacturers' catalogues. Their operations are described in the legends of the illustrations.

TABLE 6-I

CLASSIFICATION OF PUMPS MOST COMMONLY USED FOR DOMESTIC AND FARM WATER SUPPLIES

PUMPS

Lift Pumps		Force Pumps	
Shallow-Well	Deep-Well	Shallow-Well	Deep-Well
Bucket	Single-acting, plunger type	Single-acting, plunger type	Single-acting, plunger type
Chain		Differential, plunger type	Differential, plunger type
Single-acting, plunger type -pitcher spout -round spout -set length		Double-acting, piston type -single cylinder -duplex	Double-acting, plunger type
		Centrifugal Single stage Multistage	Jet (with centrifugal)
		Turbine Multistage	Submersible (with multistage centrifugal)
		Jet (with centrifugal or turbine)	Turbine (usually multistage)
		Helical, rotary, Screw type Submersible	Hilical, rotary, screw type

The single-acting plunger type of pump is by far the most common type of lift pump. It is variously referred to as "pitcher spout pump," "cistern pump," and "house lift pump." It consists essentially of a cylinder in which a plunger with a valve moves up and down, and a check valve at the bottom of the cylinder as shown in Fig. 6-3.

Contrary to popular opinion, pumps do not "lift" water up from the source by suction. Rather the pump reduces the atmospheric pressure on the water *in* the suction pipe and the atmospheric pressure on the water *outside* of the suction pipe pushes the water up and into the pump. The principle is the same as that of drawing soda water through a straw, as shown in Fig. 6-5, or of filling a syringe, as shown in Fig. 6-6.

Figure 6-7 illustrates the operation, which is as follows:

1. With the pump primed, as shown at A, the plunger is raised. As air cannot pass the plunger owing to the water seal, a part of the atmospheric pressure is lifted off the water in the pipe. The air and water in the pipe follow the plunger upward. The space in the cylinder below the plunger fills with air from the pipe.

2. At the top of the cylinder the plunger stops, and the check valve closes of its own weight, thus trapping air in the cylinder.

3. On the next downstroke the entrapped air is compressed between the plunger and the bottom of the cylinder. When the pressure becomes greater than the atmospheric pressure above the plunger, plus

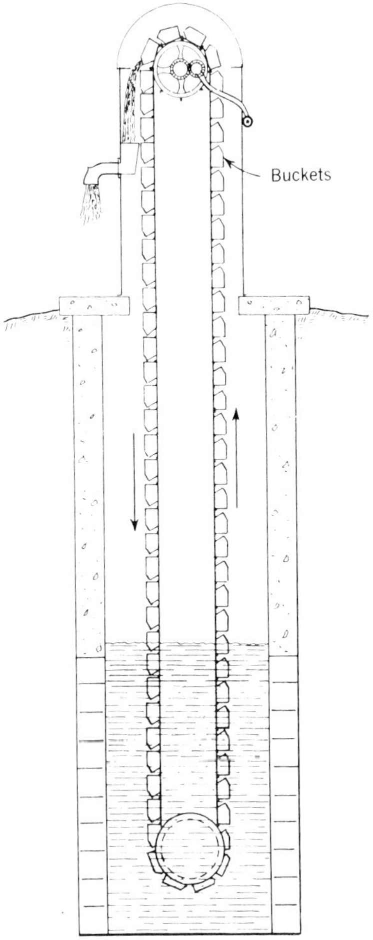

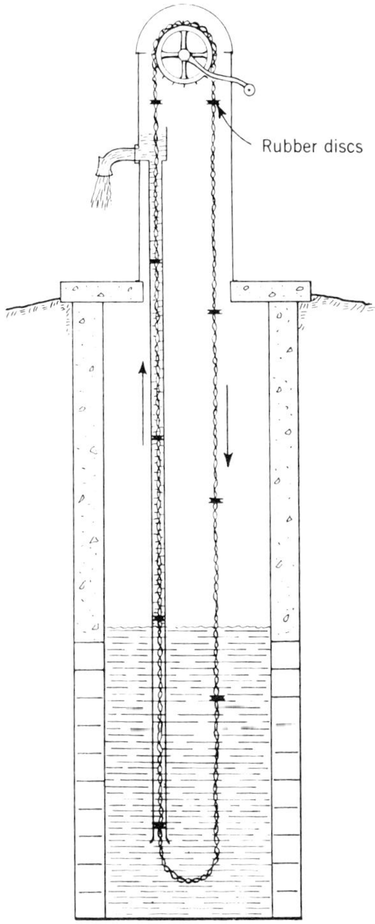

Fig. 6-1. Bucket pump. Small buckets attached to an endless chain are rotated over sprockets as shown so that each bucket dips water from the source at the bottom, carries it to the top, and empties it into the spout as it passes over the top sprocket. Small holes in the bottom of the buckets permit the water to drain back to the source after pumping to prevent freezing. Used mostly on cisterns and shallow dug wells.

Fig. 6-2. Chain pump. Rubber discs attached to endless chain running over a sprocket at the top are pulled upward through a pipe to lift water mechanically up to the spout. Small holes through the rubber discs permit the water to drain to the source after pumping to prevent freezing. Like the bucket pump, it is used mostly on cisterns and shallow dug wells.

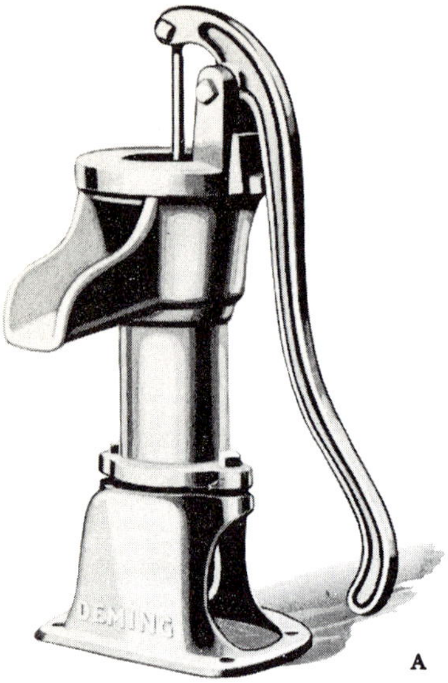

A

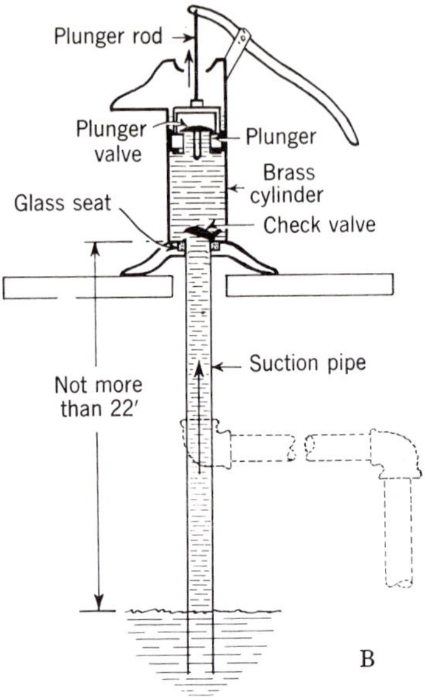

B

Fig. 6-3A courtesy Deming Co.

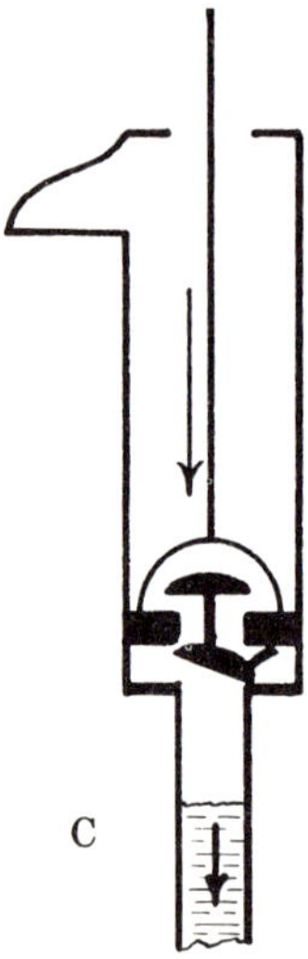

C

Fig. 6-3. A single-acting pitcher spout shallow-well lift pump. Can deliver water only at the spout. Can be drained to prevent freezing by lifting the handle all the way up as indicated at C. Unless in excellent condition the pump must be reprimed with water each time before using. If necessary, the suction pipe can be run latterly for a distance to the water as indicated by the dash lines in B. Maximum suction lift is 25 feet (7.62 m.) including friction head.

the weight of the valve, the air will lift the valve and escape through the priming water as shown at B.

4. On the next upstroke more air will be drawn out of the pipe and the water will rise higher, eventually flowing into the cylinder under the plunger as shown at C.

5. With the cylinder and pipe full of water as at C, the check valve closes, trapping water in the cylinder.

6. On the next downstroke the plunger and valve pass through the water as shown at D.

7. When the plunger reaches the bottom of the cylinder and stops, the plunger valve closes, thus trapping the water above the plunger, as shown at E.

8. On the next upstroke the water above the plunger is lifted out of the pump as shown at F. At the same time more water is drawn into the cylinder through the check valve.

9. On each successive downstroke step E is repeated, and on each successive upstroke step F is repeated. Thus the pump delivers water on each upstroke.

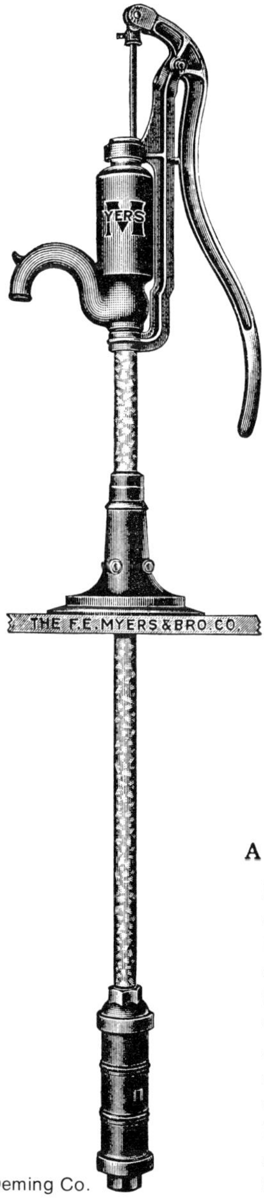

Courtesy Deming Co.

A

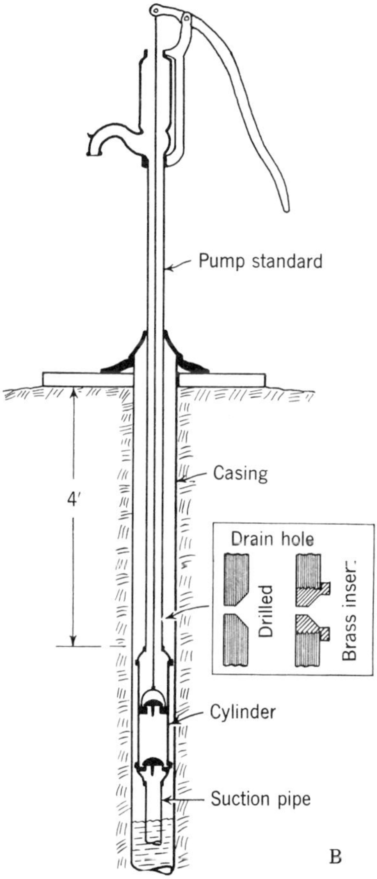

B

Fig. 6-4. A set length lift pump. Cylinder hangs about 4 feet below pumping head to place it below frost. Where the installation must be out of doors in cold climates a small drain hole is made in the pipe as shown in the inset in B so that the water will automatically drain out of the pipe after pumping. The base forms a seal at the top of the casing. This pump can be used on moderately deep wells by placing the cylinder at lower levels. Note that the drain hole is counter sunk. A brass insert is better than a plain drilled hole as it will not fill up with rust.

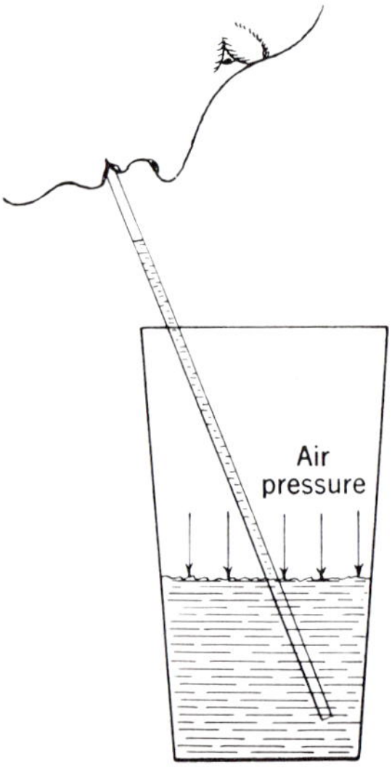

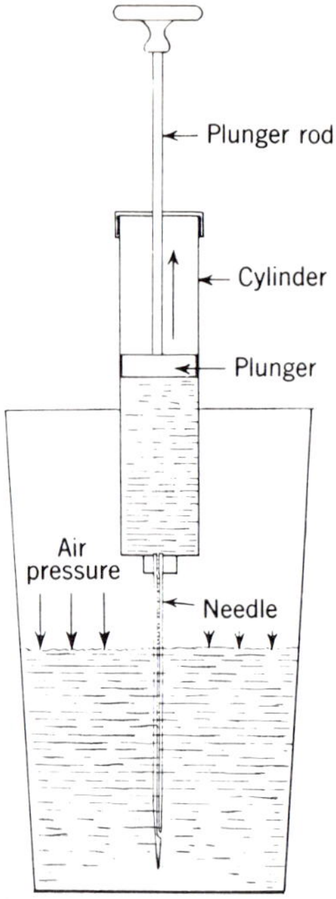

Fig. 6-5. Atmospheric pressure pushes the soda water up through the straw when the air is drawn out of the straw.

Fig. 6-6. Atmospheric pressure on the liquid in the glass forces the liquid up into the syringe when the plunger is raised.

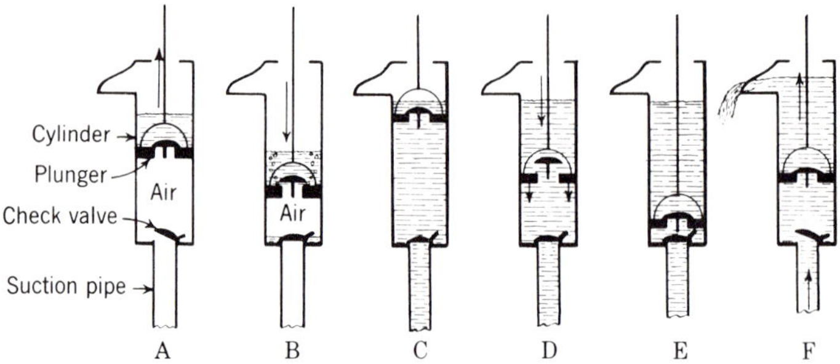

Fig. 6-7. Illustrating the stages in the cycle of operation of a plunger type of shallow-well lift pump

PRINCIPLES OF OPERATION OF FORCE PUMPS

There are many different types of force pumps used for pumping water for homes and farms. Table 6-I indicates the more common ones.

Reciprocating Types

Single-acting shallow-well force pumps.

This pump is illustrated in Fig. 6-8. Its principle of operation is the same as that of the single-acting plunger type of lift pump except that it is enclosed at the top and therefore can be used to force the water to higher elevations, or against pressure. Also, such pumps usually have an air chamber to even out the discharge flow. On the upstroke of the plunger the air in the air chamber is compressed and on the downstroke the air expands to maintain a flow at the discharge while the plunger goes down. The trap tube serves to trap air in the air chamber so it cannot leak out around the plunger rod. The pump is called single acting because the cylinder discharges only on the upstroke.

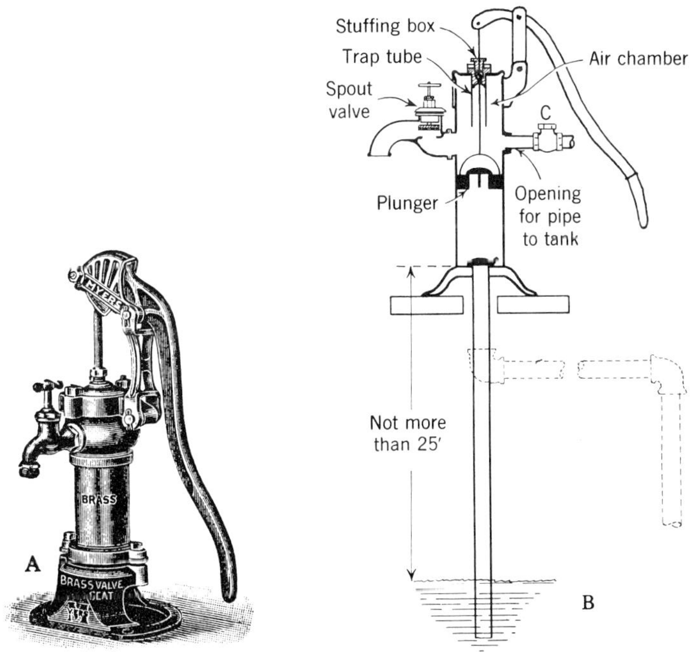

Fig. 6-8. A single-acting shallow-well force pump. This pump can be used to deliver water under pressure at the spout or, by closing the spout valve, may be used to deliver water through check valve C to an elevated storage tank. The check valve prevents back flow of tank water when it is desired to pump fresh water at the spout. The pump can be offset from the source as indicated by the dash lines in the drawing. Note that the top of the pump is sealed by means of a stuffing box.

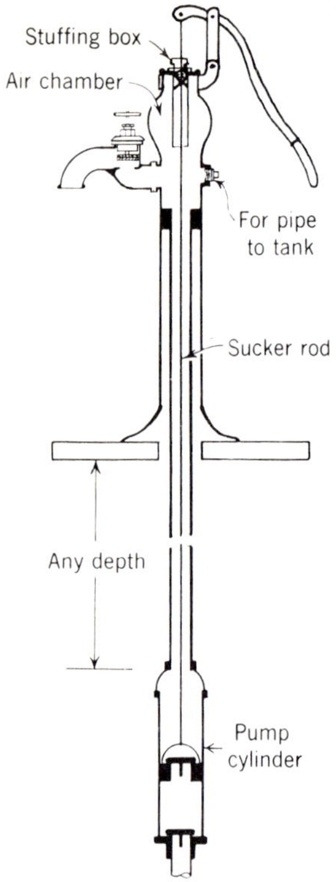

Fig. 6-9. A single-acting deep-well force pump. Note that the cylinder is located down in the well. Available also with double-acting cylinder. See Fig. 6-12.

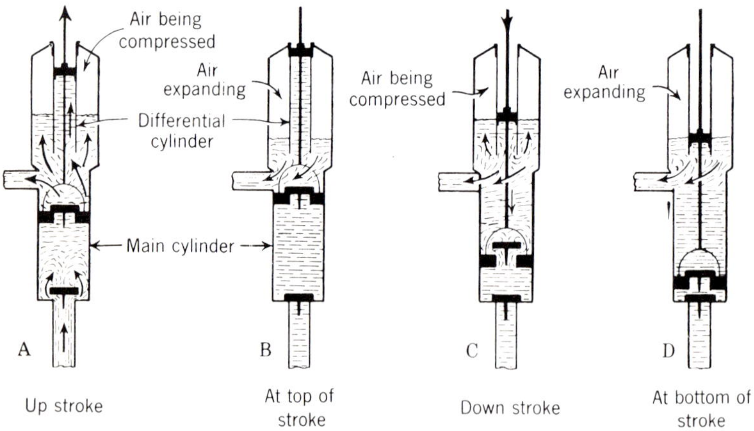

Fig. 6-10. Operation of a differential force pump. Note that the differential cylinder helps discharge the water, takes the place of a stuffing box, and in this case serves as a trap tube for the air in the air chamber.

Single-acting deep-well force pumps.

The operation of this pump is the same as that of Fig. 6-8. The principal difference is in the location of the cylinder. With the cylinder down in the well it can pump from a depth greater than 25 feet. See

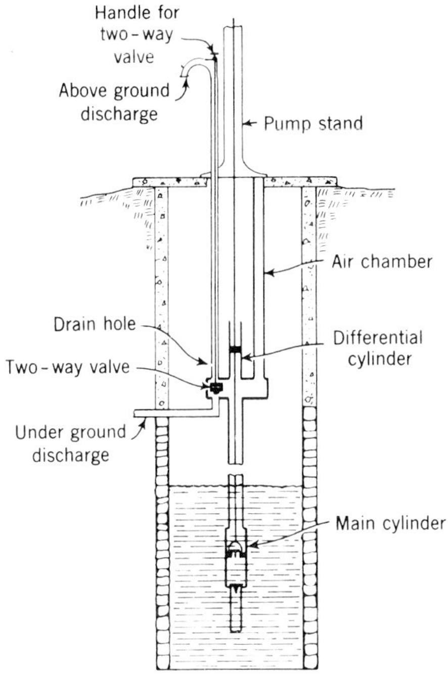

Fig. 6-11. A differential force pump with nonfreezing drop head. Such a pump is frequently used with a windmill. Its large size at the two-way valve limits its use to wells of fairly large diameter at the top. The main cylinder can be lowered in a relatively small drilled well. The two-way valve makes it possible to pump to the spout or to a storage tank. Can be used on deep wells or shallow wells.

Fig. 6-9. Therefore it is a deep-well pump. A nonfreezing drip hole can be drilled in the pipe below the frost line as shown in Fig. 6-4B.

Differential force pumps.

Differential force pumps are similar to the single-acting force pumps previously described except that they have a differential cylinder, or an enlarged plunger rod, which evens out the discharge flow, reduces the necessary power for operating the pump, and in some cases serves as a trap tube. Also the differential cylinder and plunger take the place of a stuffing box. Figures 6-10 through 6-11 illustrate this type of pump. Commonly used with windmills.

Since electric power is almost universally available now the hand operated lift and force pumps are seldom installed these days. However, there are thousands of them still in use.

Double-acting shallow-well piston type of force pumps.

This pump was once used extensively on domestic water supply systems, but has now been largely replaced by jet pumps and submersibles. In large sizes it is used for small community water supplies, for camps, for spray water, and for places where high pumping heads are needed. Due to the positive action of the piston and valves

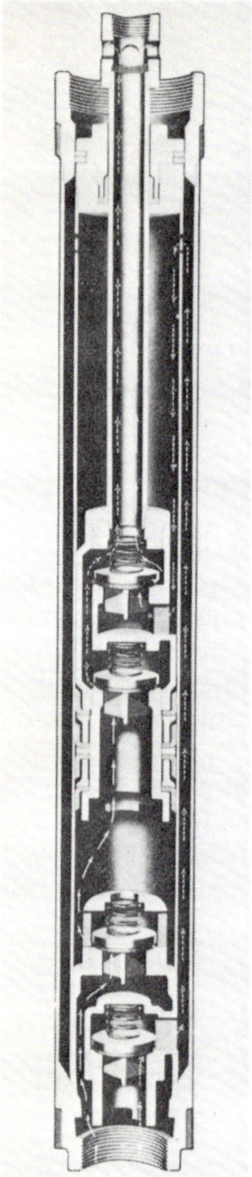

Fig. 6-12. A double-acting deep-well cylinder. Recommended for use in small-diameter wells where more capacity is required than can be obtained with a single-acting cylinder. Size for size it will deliver about 80% more water than the single-acting cylinder.

it delivers a nearly constant volume of water, up to its maximum suction and pressure head. See Fig. 6-13. For its size it can handle more water than the single-acting pump.

Because of the reciprocating action of the pump it tends to be noisy, especially where long pipes are used, or if the air chamber becomes waterlogged.

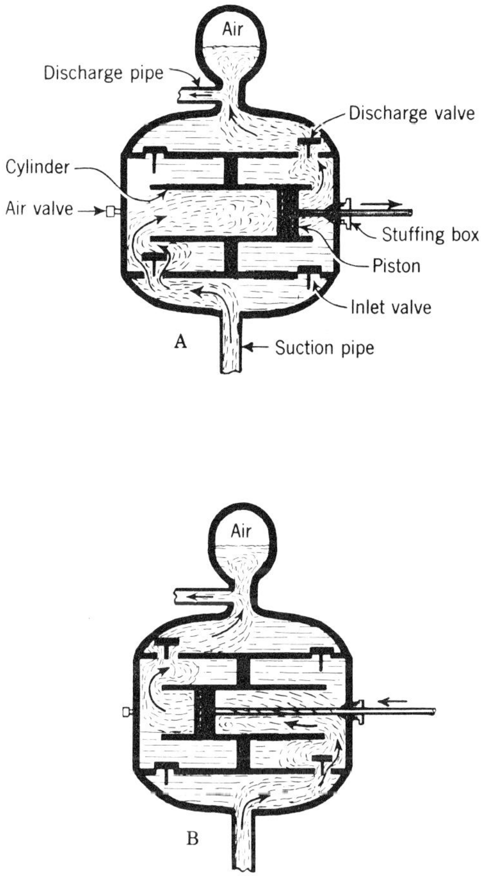

Fig. 6-13. Two stages of operation of a double-acting piston type of shallow-well force pump. At A the intake is on the lower left and the discharge is on the upper right. At B on the next stroke the intake is on the lower right and the discharge is on the upper left. Suction lift is 25 feet. (7.62 m.)

Principle of Operation

As shown in Fig. 6-13 the pump has one cylinder, one piston with two cup leathers, and two sets of valves. The piston moves back and forth within the limits of the cylinder. On one stroke as shown at A, water is drawn in from the source through the intake valve at the left and simultaneously water is discharged from the cylinder through the discharge valve at the right. On the reverse stroke intake and discharge are through the other set of valves as shown at B. Thus water is drawn in and discharged on each stroke of the piston, hence the name "double-acting."

In the two-cylinder (duplex) pump the operation of each cylinder is the same as above but the cylinders intake and discharge 180 degrees apart, thus giving a more uniform flow.

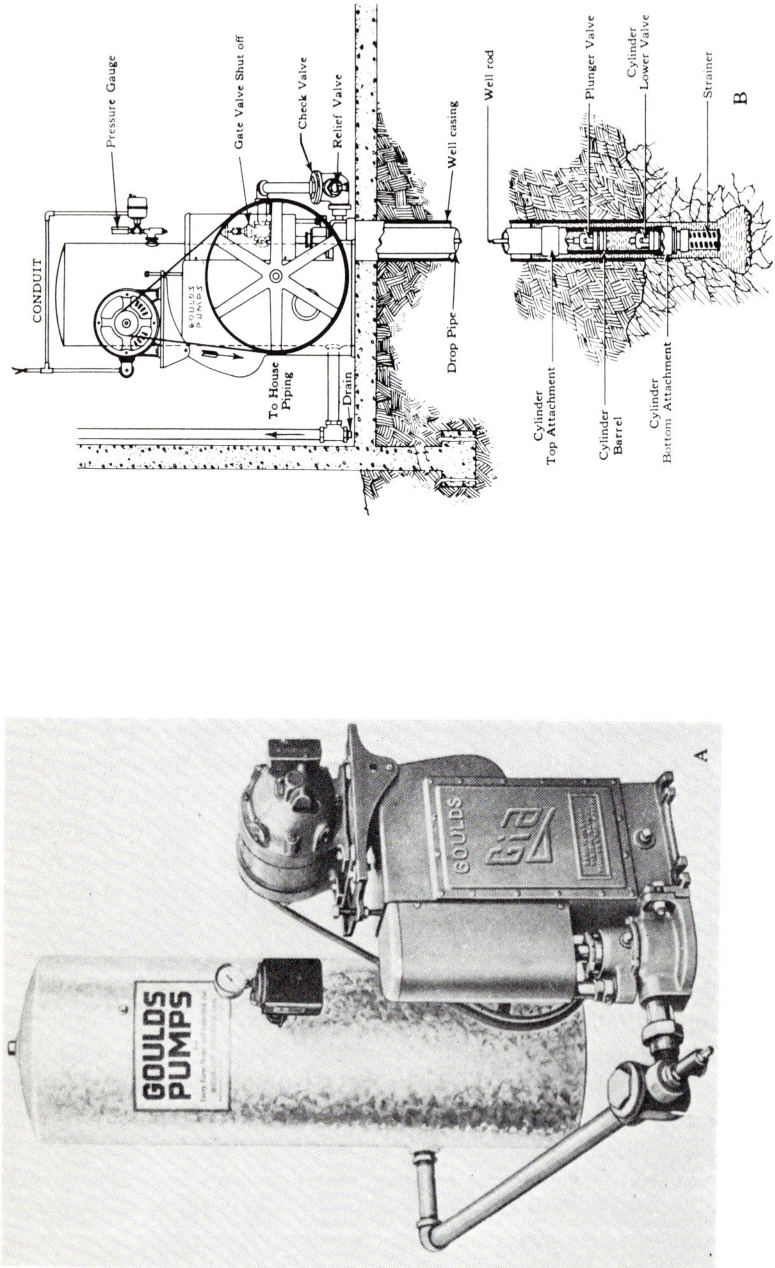

Fig. 6-14 A & B.

Courtesy Goulds Pumps, Inc., Seneca Falls, N.Y. W.J. Romano, Communication Specialist.

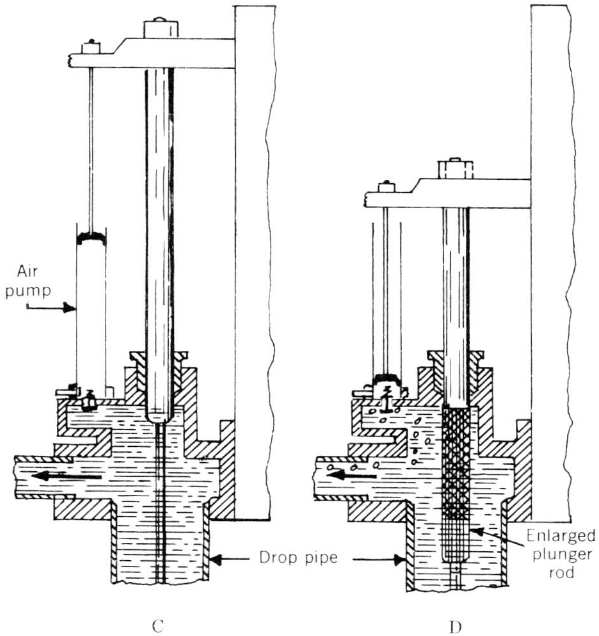

A & B Courtesy Goulds Pumps, Seneca Falls, N.Y. through Mr. W.J. Romano.

Fig. 6-14-C & D.

A power-driven deep-well reciprocating pump with differential characteristics. Instead of a differential cylinder this pump has an enlarged section of the plunger rod at the top which displaces its volume of water on the down stroke. Thus the pump discharges on both strokes, giving it the advantages of the differential cylinder. The plunger rod has a large-diameter stuffing box for longer life. The air pump is needed only when pumping into a pressure tank.

Note that the drop pipe is large enough to permit the withdrawal of the main plunger and lower cylinder valve by means of the plunger rod. This makes it possible to repair there parts without pulling the heavy drop pipe. See at B.

Details of differential feature. At C, up stroke. At D, down stroke. Cross-hatched portion of plunger rod at D indicates approximate volume of water discharged on down stroke.

Centrifugal Types

Centrifugal force pumps.

The centrifugal type of force pump has wide application on farms and in homes. The following are some examples:

1. Water supply, particularly in conjunction with jets and in submersibles.
2. Irrigation.
3. Drainage.
4. Cellar drains (sump pump).
5. Washing machines.
6. Dishwashers.
7. Milk coolers.
8. Water-circulating pumps on hot-water types of heating systems.
9. Air-conditioning equipment.
10. Circulation of coolant in internal-combustion engines.
11. High pressure service for washing vehicles, cleaning floors, fire fighting, etc.
12. Sewage and sludge pumps.

The centrifugal pump is most efficient for handling large volumes of water at low pressures and low suction heads. As it has no valves it can handle a wide variety of liquids and, if designed for the purpose, can handle liquids with considerable sediment. It is relatively inexpensive and is efficient in operation if used for the purpose for which it was designed. In no other pump is it more important that the design exactly suit the needs.

Unlike the plunger and piston pumps the capacity of a centrifugal decreases as the total working head (suction head and discharge head) increases. See Fig. 6-15. For this reason, in choosing a centrifugal pump consideration must be given to the discharge pressure as well as to the suction head.

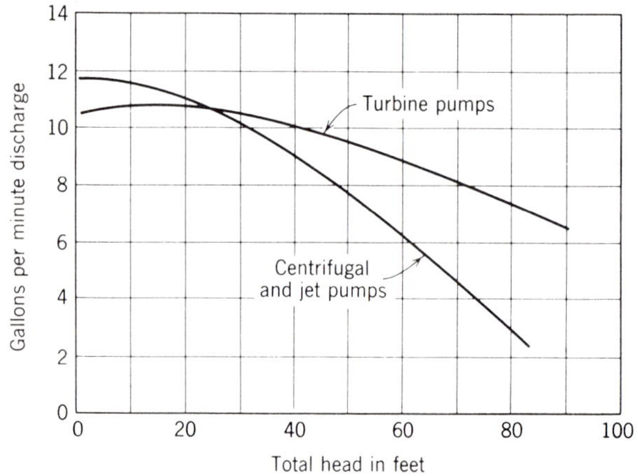

Fig. 6-15. Curves showing general discharge characteristics of centrifugal, jet, and turbine pumps.

Principles of operation. The centrifugal pump consists of an impeller mounted in a housing or volute as indicated in Fig. 6-16. The impeller is driven at fairly high speed (1750 or 3450 rpm) within the housing and is the only moving part of the pump. Where clearance between the impeller and the housing is wide, as indicated in the drawing, the pump can handle liquids with some sediment, but will not pump against high heads. It is the type used extensively for circulating liquids where the pump is submerged or located below the liquid level.

As illustrated in Fig. 6-16, the impeller has vanes which radiate from the hub. In domestic water system pumps the vanes are enclosed between shrouds as indicated in Fig. 6-17. The shrouds make it possible to pump against higher heads.

With the pump full of water (primed) when the impeller is rotated, the water that is between the vanes is thrown outward by centrifugal force. This builds up a pressure around the inner surface of the housing, which pressure-forces the water out the discharge.

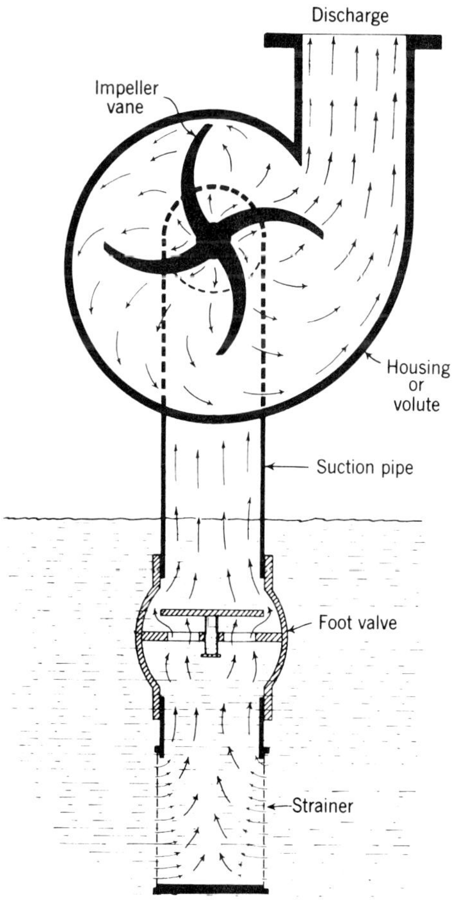

Fig. 6-16. A centrifugal force pump in cross section.

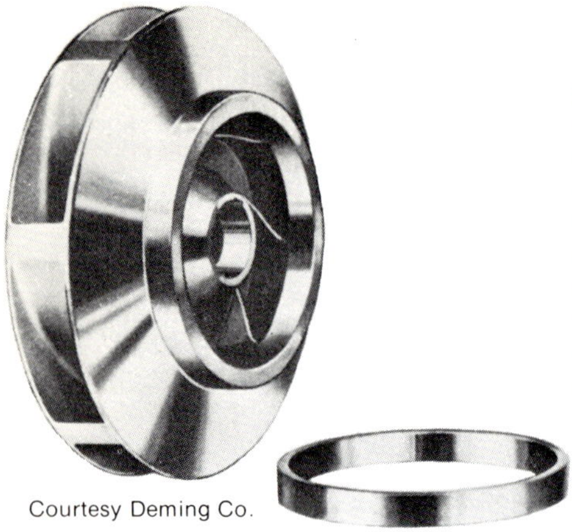

Courtesy Deming Co.

Fig. 6-17. An enclosed impeller with shrouds on each side of the vanes. This type of impeller is used extensively on domestic water systems for pumping clear water, especially in conjunction with jets as indicated in Figs. 6-18 and 6-20. The water enters at the large hole in the center and is discharged at the periphery.

When water is thrown from the center of the impeller, a partial vacuum exists at that point. This permits atmospheric pressure on the water at the source to force water to flow in from the source and fill the space between the vanes. With continual rotation of the impeller this water is in turn thrown outward, is replaced by more water from the source, and so a continuous stream of water is caused to flow through the pump. There are no pulsations or reciprocating parts to set up vibrations; therefore the pump is relatively quiet in operation. This is an advantage where a pump is installed in a home. Figure 6-18 illustrates a centrifugal pump used in conjunction with a jet for pumping from deep sources.

Multistage centrifugals. Centrifugal pumps are frequently used in series is illustrated in Figs. 6-18 and 6-26. Each impeller and housing so arranged in series is called a *stage* and each stage adds to the pressure at the discharge. Thus by increasing the number of stages in a centrifugal pump the discharge pressure can be built up to almost any value. However, regardless of the number of stages and the pressure the discharge *capacity* in gallons per hour will be approximately the same as that for one stage. Multistage centrifugals are used extensively with jets for wells from 100 to 300 feet (30.5 to 91.5 m) in depth and as submersible pumps as illustrated in Fig. 6-26.

Turbine pumps.

Turbine pumps are modified forms of centrifugal pumps. That is, centrifugal force is used to move the water through the pump, but the design of the impeller and housing is such that much higher pressures and suction heads are obtainable than with straight centrifugal pumps of the same size. The capacities are somewhat lower, but are more constant with varying heads.

Deep-well turbines. Figure 6-22 illustrates a deep-well turbine pump. The pump consists of a series of turbines called stages ar-

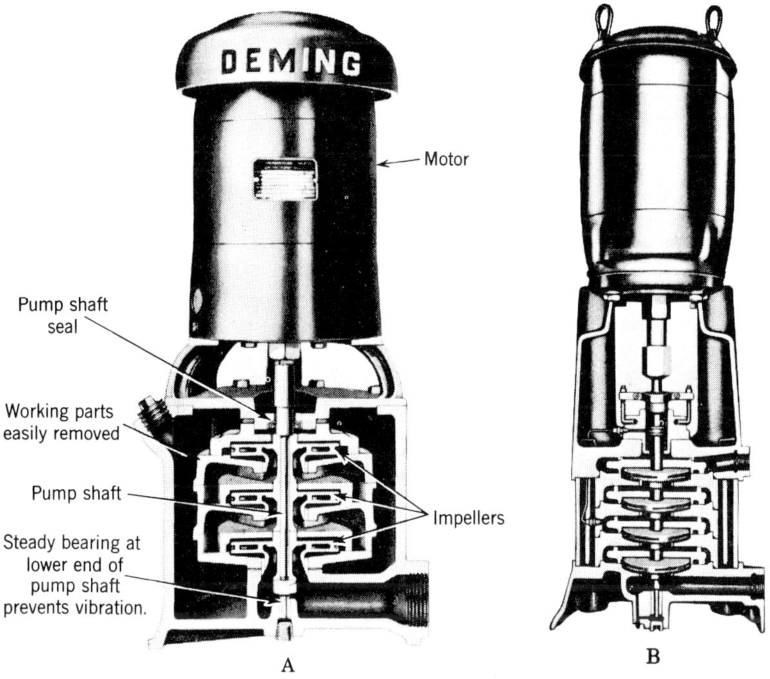

Courtesy Deming Co.

Fig. 6-18. Three- and four-stage centrifugal pumps of a type usually used for deep well jet pumping.

ranged one above the other with a drive shaft extending to the surface. The discharge pressure increases with the number of stages in the pump. The deeper the well the more stages required.

This type of pump is used primarily for pumping large quantities of water from deep wells for irrigation and for municipal and industrial water supplies. It is rarely used for domestic water supply.

Jet Pumps

Construction. So-called jet pumps are a combination of a conventional water pump of some kind, usually a centrifugal pump, and an ejector or educer, which is commonly referred to as the "jet." The jet must be placed within suction distance of the water (usually not over 20 feet (6 m) for shallow-well jets; some are limited to 15 feet (4.5 m)). Deep-well jets are usually placed in the water near the bottom of the well as indicated in Figs. 6-23 and 8-7.

The motor and pump can be placed in any convenient place at the surface. For shallow-well operation the jet is installed within the pump housing as indicated in Fig. 6-19.

Some of the jet pumps now available are so designed that the same pumping unit can be used for either shallow or deep wells simply by installing the jet in the pump housing or in the well as the situation demands.

Jet pumps should be carefully selected from manufacturer's Selection Tables to suit the existing operating conditions. This applies particularly to deep-well jets. The design of the pumps and the educers varies for different depths and operating heads.

The jet pump offers a special advantage for deep-well operation in that the motor and pump can be offset from the well as indicated in Figs. 6-20, 6-23, and 8-7. This greatly simplifies frost protection as the pumping unit can be placed in an existing building instead of in a specially constructed frostproof structure as is often required where the conventional reciprocating deep-well pump illustrated in Fig. 6-14 is used. Moreover, the jet pump is less expensive than the conventional deep-well pump of the same capacity; has no reciprocating parts, so is much quieter; and if plastic pipe is used to the jet in the well, installation and repairs are much easier.

Another advantage of jet pumps is that they can be installed in crooked wells without interfering with their operation and without being unduly noisy. There are no rods or shafting to bind, wear, or make noises.

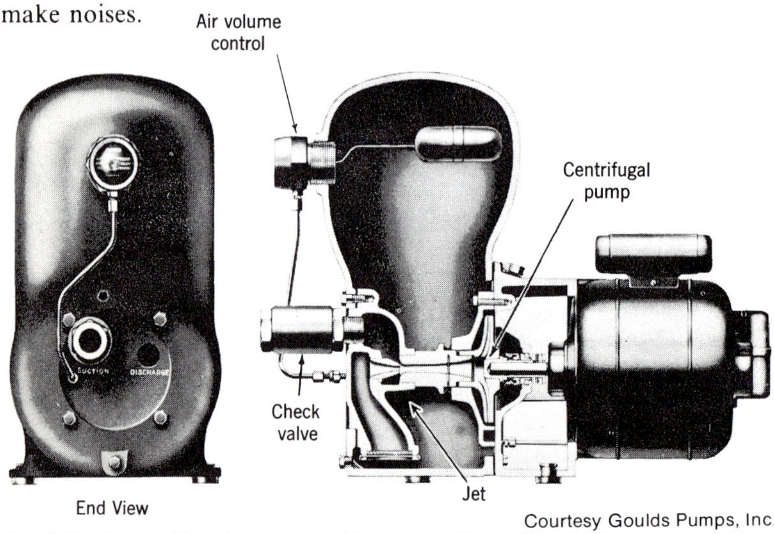

Courtesy Goulds Pumps, Inc.

Fig. 6-19. A centrifugal pump used in conjunction with a jet for pumping from shallow sources. The illustration is that of a so-called "tankless" water system. The enlarged air dome serves as the only storage tank. The system is suitable for boosting pressures, or for use where a limited amount of water is to be employed such as supplying one faucet, a summer cottage, or soft water from a cistern to hot-water faucets only.

The pump is designed with a "balanced flow" feature, which means that the discharge varies according to the amount of water being drawn. Thus the pump does not stop and start frequently when small amounts of water are being drawn even though there is no pressure tank. However, a pressure tank of any size can be used between the pump and faucets. See also Fig. 7-9.

Fig. 6-20. A two-stage centrifugal pump used with a "jet." A one-pipe jet is available for wells of small diameter.

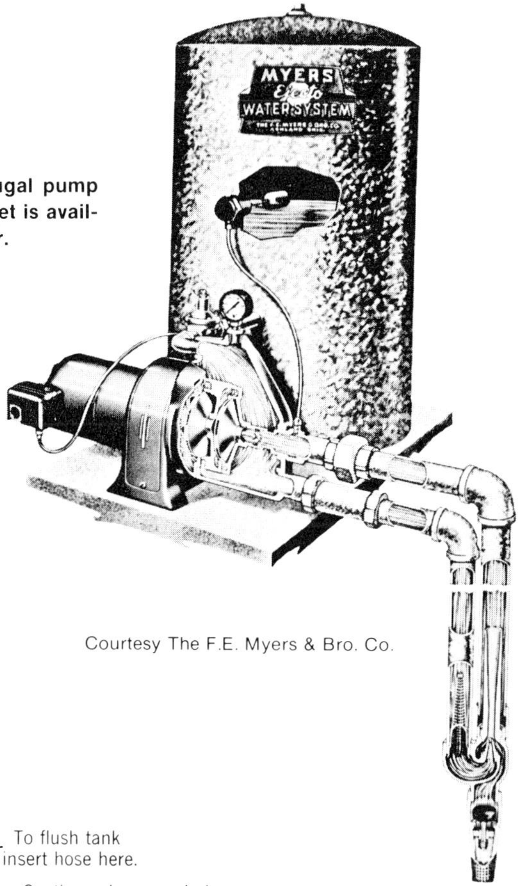

Courtesy The F.E. Myers & Bro. Co.

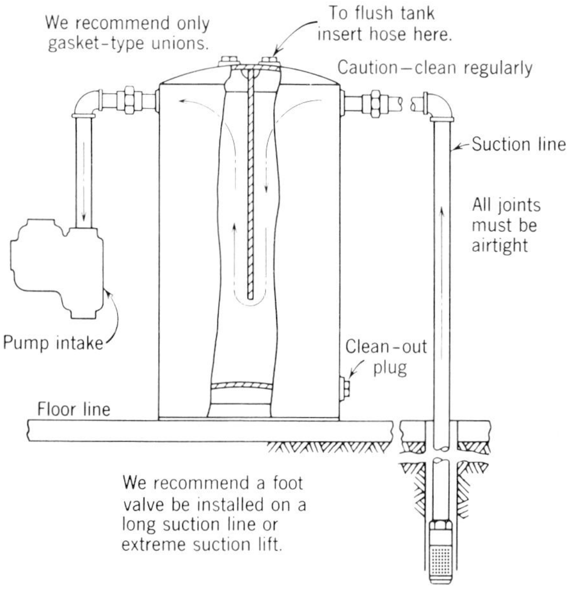

Courtesy Decatur Pump Co.

Fig. 6-21. A sand trap installed in the suction line of a pump.

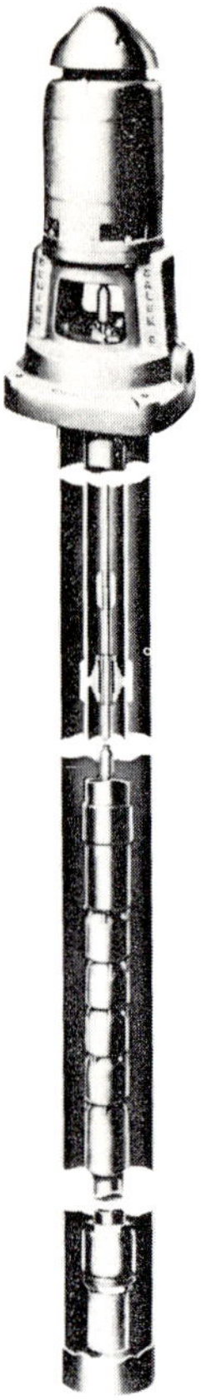

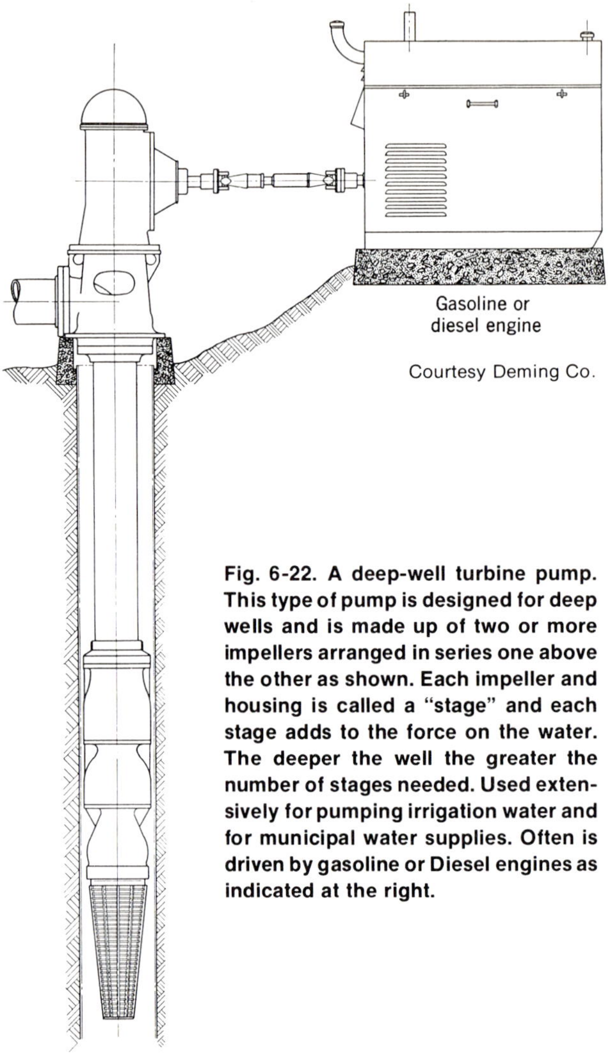

Fig. 6-22. A deep-well turbine pump. This type of pump is designed for deep wells and is made up of two or more impellers arranged in series one above the other as shown. Each impeller and housing is called a "stage" and each stage adds to the force on the water. The deeper the well the greater the number of stages needed. Used extensively for pumping irrigation water and for municipal water supplies. Often is driven by gasoline or Diesel engines as indicated at the right.

Operation of the jet. It is the function of the jet to lift the water from the source to within suction distance (25 feet or less) of the pump at the top. Figure 6-24 illustrates how a jet pump could be rigged up by use of a centrifugal pump and a garden hose. Water under pressure from the discharge side of the pump will flow through the hose and out the hose nozzle (the jet) at high velocity. If the nozzle is placed within a restricted area (the venturi) as shown, the high-velocity discharge will cause water to rise in the pipe to within suction distance of the pump. The pressure regulating valve on the discharge pipe serves to maintain the correct pressure on the jet regardless of the pressure in the tank. This valve can be adjusted for various depths of water; thus the pump, with the aid of the jet, can get water from

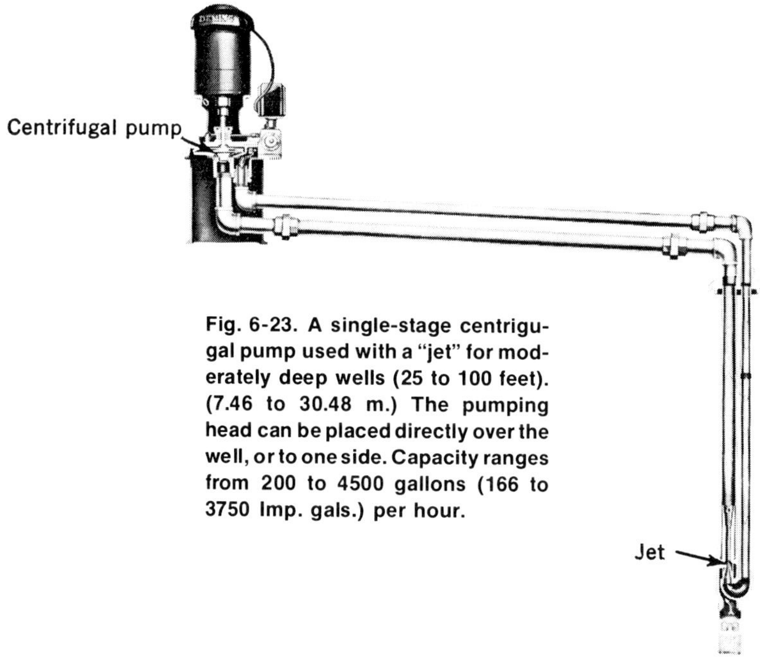

Fig. 6-23. A single-stage centrifugal pump used with a "jet" for moderately deep wells (25 to 100 feet). (7.46 to 30.48 m.) The pumping head can be placed directly over the well, or to one side. Capacity ranges from 200 to 4500 gallons (166 to 3750 Imp. gals.) per hour.

Courtesy Deming Co.

depths beyond the suction limits of the centrifugal pump alone. The deeper the well the higher the velocity must be at the nozzle in order to force the water to within reach of the pump, hence the multiple-stage pumps for wells over 100 feet (30.48 m) to water.

The crude jet shown in Fig. 6-24 would not be practical for a permanent installation. As sold on the market, jets are assembled units as illustrated in Fig. 6-25. There are threaded openings to take the necessary piping.

Referring to Fig. 6-25, the high-velocity stream from the nozzle discharges into a restricted passage called the venturi tube or educer. The high-velocity stream pulls the water upwards around the tip of the nozzle. This in turn creates a suction at that point. The suction draws in more water from the source which in turn is carried upward with the high-velocity stream. Thus, as long as water is pumped through the nozzle more water will be drawn in from the source in a continuous stream. The water from the source passes up through the venturi at high velocity along with the jet stream. As these two volumes of water pass upward into the enlarged portion of the venturi the velocity decreases and the pressure increases. In other words, velocity is converted to pressure. It is this pressure that forces the water up to within suction distance of the pump.

These two mixed volumes of water (that from the nozzle plus that from the source) flow to the intake of the pump and are forced out the discharge side of the pump by the impeller. There is a by-pass

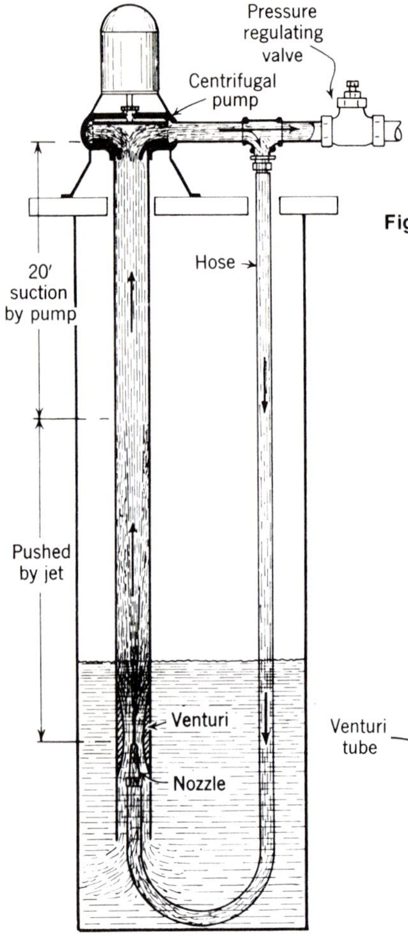

Fig. 6-24. The principle of a jet pump.

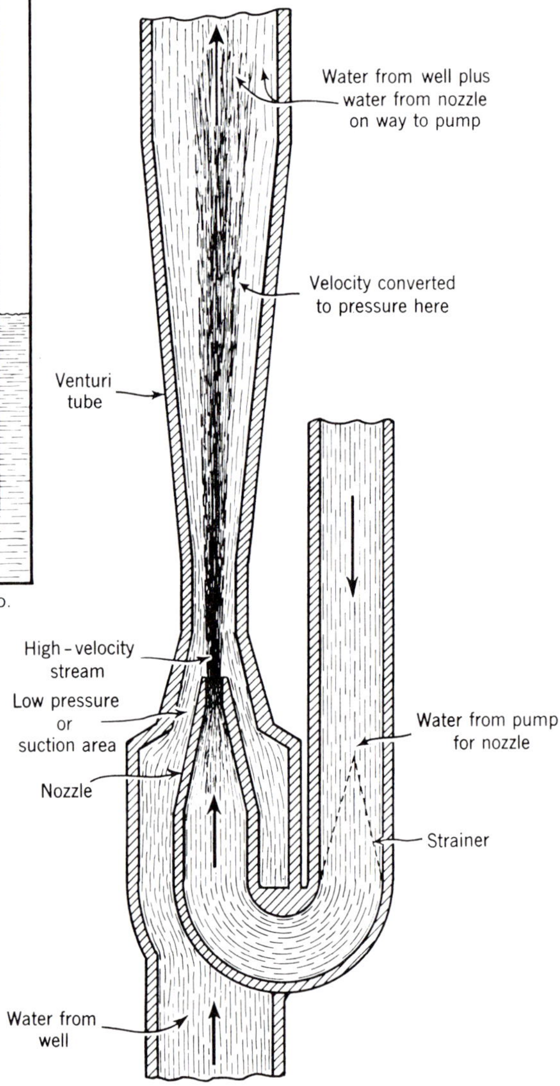

Fig. 6-25. Details of a "jet."

leading back to the nozzle; see Fig. 6-24. At this point the discharge flow divides, that portion required for operation of the jet going back down to the nozzle and that portion which was drawn in from the source going to the storage tank. Thus a portion of water is constantly recirculating through the pump and the jet in order to transfer another protion from the well to the tank. This recirculation of water somewhat reduces the efficiency of the pump.

Submersible Pumps

Submersible pumps for domestic water supply are a comparative recent development and they have considerable promise for future applications. Some of its special advantages are: (1) its exceptional quietness of operation because of being submerged, (2) it needs no priming as it is under water, (3) it is easy to install and easy to remove, (4) costs of frostproofing or other superstructures are largely eliminated, (5) requires only one drop pipe in the well, (6) the motor and pump are water-cooled, and in some models also water lubricated. At least one make on the market has the motor sealed in a bath of oil while the pump itself is water lubricated. In either case no periodic oiling or greasing is required. (7) Is more efficient than jet pumps as it does not recirculate any of the water, (8) can be installed in any position from horizontal to vertical, (9) can be used on any water source: deep wells, shallow wells, ponds, lakes, streams, springs, etc. It is a popular pump for summer cottages along streams and lakes, or for summertime irrigation or lawn sprinkling because the pump can be easily removed from the water in the fall and easily installed in the spring. In case it is necessary to leave the pump installed during freezing weather and the discharge pipe cannot be buried below the frost line, as would be the case along a rocky shore, then the discharge pipe can be drained to the water line by installing a bleeder valve near the tank and a heating cable inside of the pipe at the water level of the source as indicated in Fig. 8-12. Placing the heating cable inside of the pipe gives it protection from floating ice along the shore.

Some of its limitations are: (1) it should not be installed on a source which might be pumped dry. The pump is water-cooled; therefore if the source is pumped dry the motor and pump might be burned out. (2) If installed in a well, the well hole must be at least 4″ in diameter, (3) they are especially susceptible to damage by lightning. For this reason some models have built-in lightning protectors.

As protection from pumping the source dry, special sensors can be installed in the well along with the pump which will shut the pump off if the water level drops too low, and this same device will turn the pump on again when the water level rises.

As indicated in Fig. 6-26 the pump and motor are assembled as a unit with the motor on the lower end. The pump is a multistage centrifugal. The assembly is attached to the lower end of the well pipe and is submerged *in* the water as indicated in Fig. 7-25. Thus the pump forces the water all the way up the pipe and there is no suction problem.

These pumps are available for wells from 4 inches in diameter upward and for pumping from depths to 820 feet (250 m). As in the case of jets, the submersibles should be carefully selected from manufacturer's Selection Tables to suit the existing operating conditions.

Utility Pumps

In addition to the pumps discussed so far, there is on the market a group of utility pumps designed for special purposes. The following are some of the most important of these.

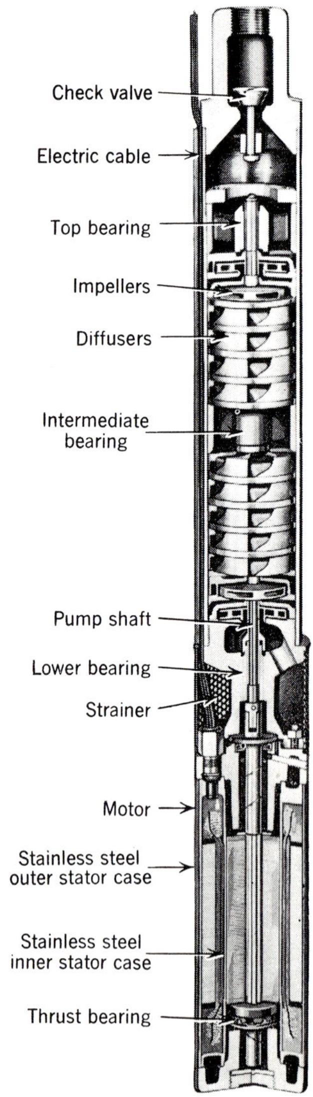

Fig. 6-26. A submersible pump. Consists of a multistage centrifugal type of pump with submersible motor attached to form pumping unit. The unit is suspended at the lower end of the drop pipe under water. A waterproof cable supplies the motor from connections at the surface. The motor of this particular pump is designed to run in water, is lubricated and water cooled. The windings are enclosed in watertight stainless steel casings. The rotor runs in water. On some models the motor is sealed in watertight housing and runs in an oil bath.

Courtesy Deming Co.

High pressure pump.

See Fig. 6-27. This pump is designed to boost the pressure from an ordinary water system. It can be connected to a hose outlet and will add up to 140 pounds (63.64 kg) pressure to the intake pressure, depending on the model used. It will also pump from any shallow well source.

It is a useful pump for such purposes as cleaning floors in animal shelters, cleaning paved driveways, swimming pools, tennis courts, and window screens. For spraying insecticides and disinfectants, for washing cars, trucks, tractors, boats, etc. For extra pressure for fire fighting. The unit is portable and weighs only about 40 lbs. (18.2 kg). Operates on 115 volt, 60 cycle AC current and draws 10 amperes.

Fig. 6-27. Goulds Water Gun Model HB05.

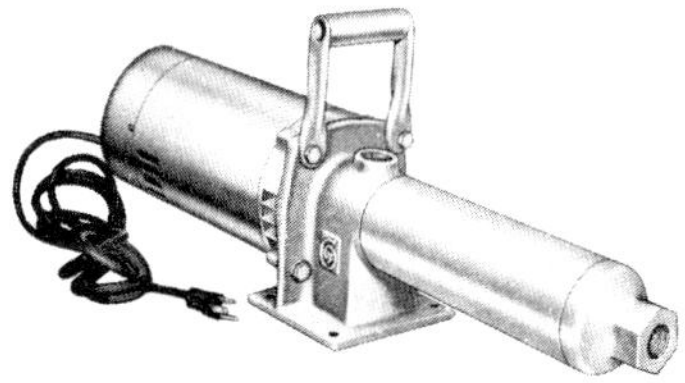

Courtesy Goulds Pumps, Inc.

Cellar drainers and sump pumps.

See Fig. 6-28. The model on the left is for use in shallow sumps. The motor is not waterproof. It is designed for continuous operation, has thermal overload protection. The float operates the switch to turn the pump on when water rises in the sump.

The models on the right are submersible and can be used in shallow or deep water. They are pre-lubricated and automatic in operation.

All these models are corrosion resistant.

Fig. 6-28.

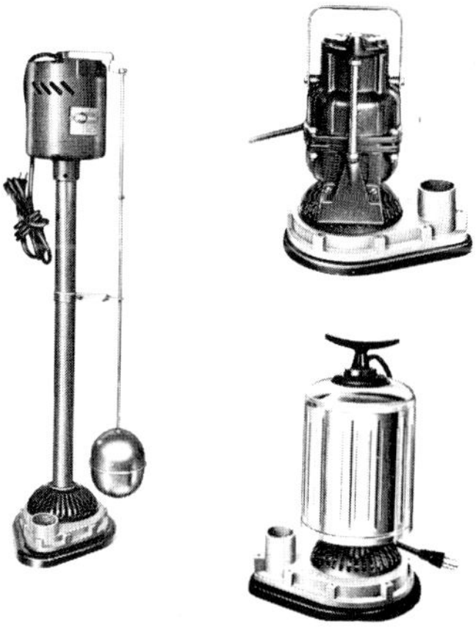

Courtesy Goulds Pumps, Inc.

Sewage and sludge pumps.

See Fig. 6-29. This pump can be used for homes, farms, trailer or mobile homes, camps, motels, schools, sewage plants, hospitals, or any place where there is a need for such things as flood control, sewage and waste removal, land drainage, sump drainage, or most any liquid transfer. The pump will handle solids up to 1 inch (2.5 cm) in diameter. It can be run dry without damage. The motor is sealed in high grade transformer oil and needs no other lubrication. It has over load protection.

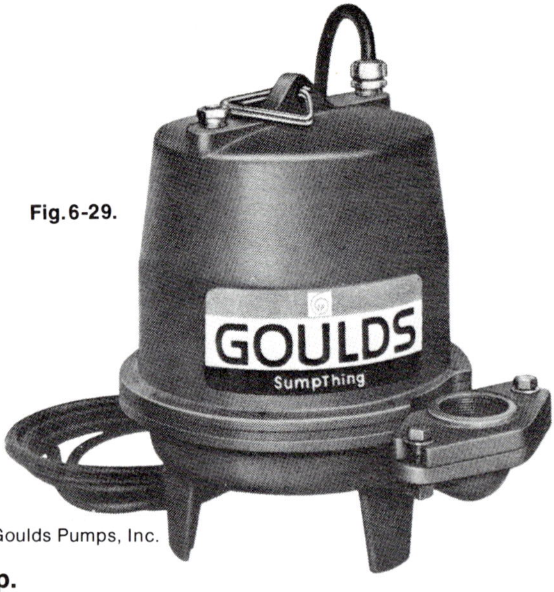

Fig. 6-29.

Courtesy Goulds Pumps, Inc.

Lawn sprinkling pump.

See Fig. 6-30. This pump is designed for operating sprinklers for watering lawns, gardens, etc. It is self priming after the initial use. Has no tank or pressure switch. Is designed for continuous operation. Available in a range of sizes.

Portable gasoline engine powered pump.

See Fig. 6-31. A pump designed for use where electric power is not available. It can be used for such purposes as filling spray rigs from ponds, lakes or streams, for small scale irrigation, for fire fighting, and for emergency water supply during power failure. It is portable, and can be carried by one man. It has a suction lift of 25 ft. (7.62 m) and capacities up to 85 U.S. gals. (71 Imp. gals.) per minute.

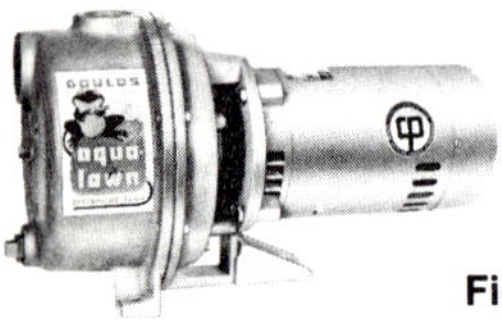

Fig. 6-30.

Courtesy Goulds Pumps, Inc.

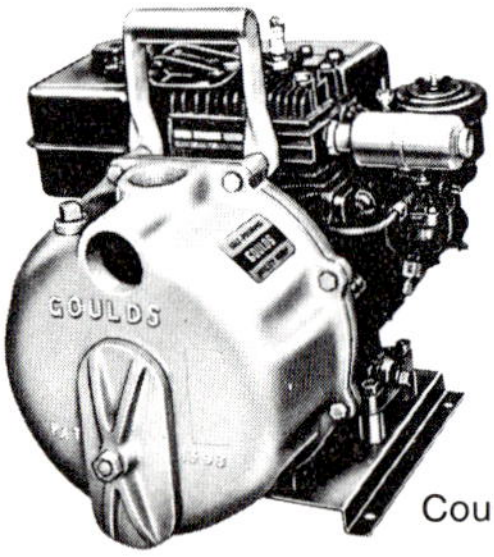

Fig. 6-31.

Courtesy Goulds Pumps, Inc.

Water Systems Types and Principles of Operation 7

DEFINITION OF A WATER SYSTEM

The term "water system" as used here designates the facilities and equipment used for delivering water from a source or sources to a system of supply plumbing. These would include pumps, reservoirs, tanks, connecting pipes, fittings, valves, and controls.

IMPORTANCE OF A WATER SYSTEM

Without a water system, water must be dipped, bailed, pumped, and carried by hand. Figures 7-1 and 7-2 illustrate various ways in which this has been and is being done. Pumping and carrying by hand are strenuous and sometimes unpleasant, especially in cold weather when there is ice and snow to contend with. The result is that a minimum amount of water is used. This is not good for health and sanitation, and on a farm it is not good for profits.

Handling water by hand is also expensive. Figure 7-2 illustrates the amount of work and the costs involved for a household supply. On a farm where water is also used for animals and crops the amount of water needed can be several times as much as for a household alone. For these reasons it is much better and cheaper to use a water system of some kind in conjunction with a system of supply plumbing. Pumps for water systems can be powered by electric motors, gasoline engines, windmills, water wheels, etc.

TYPES OF WATER SYSTEMS

Domestic water systems are of (1) the *natural gravity type,* (2) *pumped gravity type,* (3) *hydropneumatic* or *pressure type,* or (4) a *combination of both* gravity and pumped.

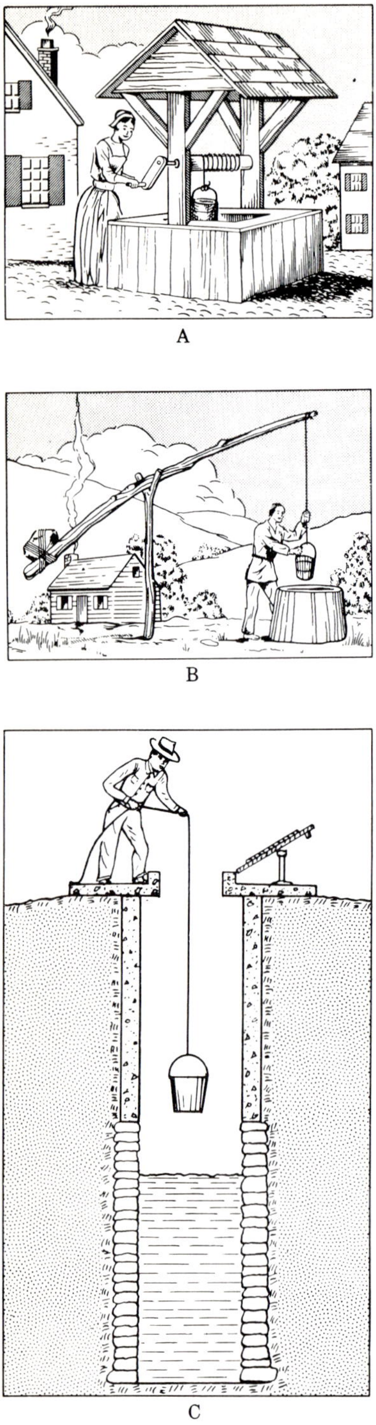

Fig. 7-1. Pioneer methods of drawing water. A — Windlass well; B — pioneer well; C — bucket and rope.

Figs. 7-1A and B courtesy Wm. C. Popper & Bo.

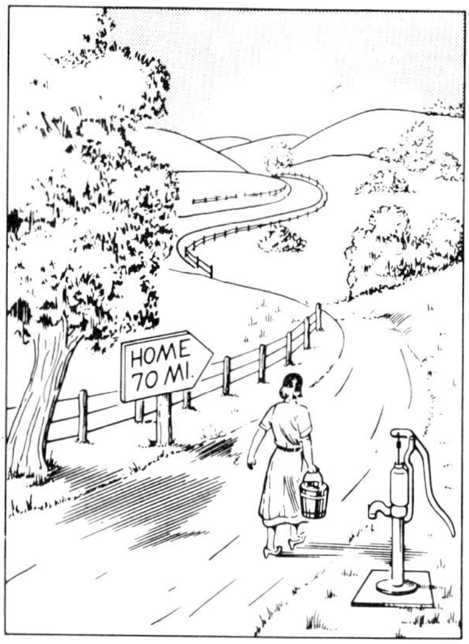

It is estimated that a farm housewife, without a water system, walks 70 miles (112.7 km.) a year between the hand pump and the house, carrying approximately 70 tons (63.6 metric tons) of water.

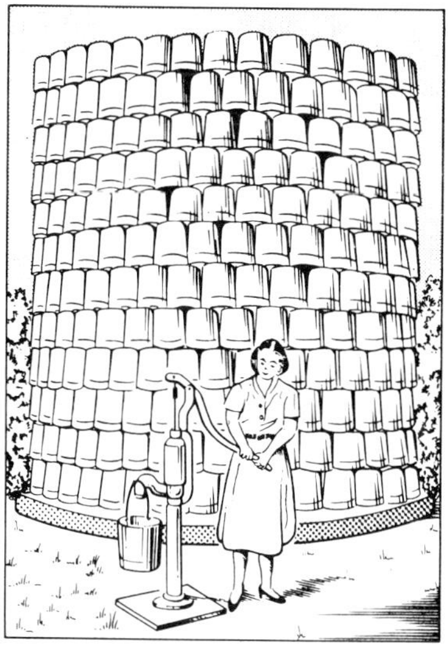

This mountainous pile of 465 buckets was actually built in Hudson, Mich., to show the amount of water an average farm family has to pump and carry each month.

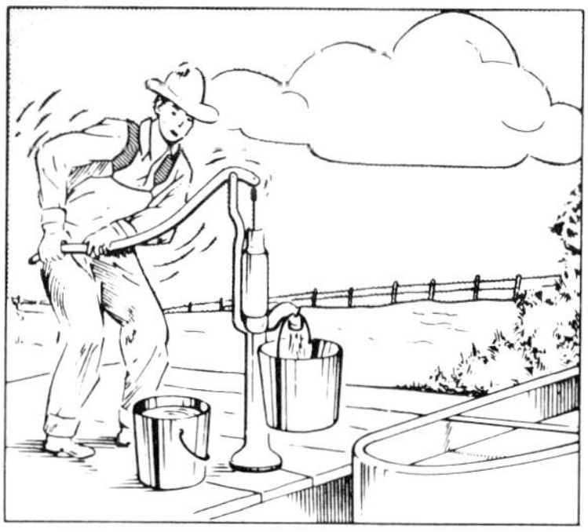

Pump and carry system costly. It takes nearly 40 minutes a day to pump and carry water by hand for the average home. A year's supply requires about 240 hours. This equals 24 full working days of 10 hours each. At wages of $2.00 per hour, the cost would be $480.00.

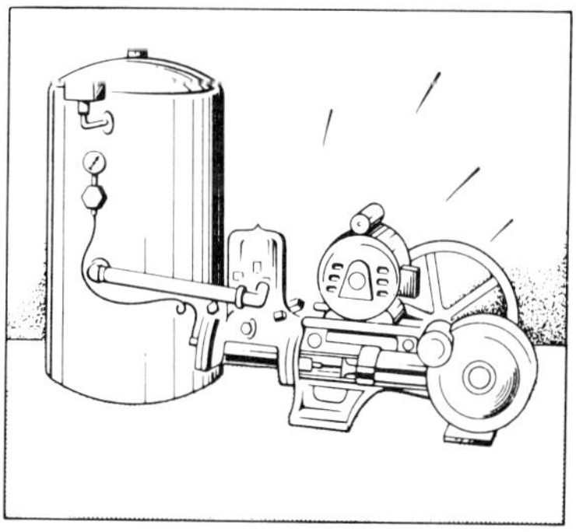

Water system much cheaper. At average electrical rates, the power to run a home water system costs only a few cents a day!

Courtesy Wm. C. Popper & Co.

Fig. 7-2. Handling water by hand is strenuous.

Natural Gravity Type

A natural gravity water system is one having a source and storage reservoir located higher than the faucets from which water can flow to the faucets by the force of gravity. A spring on a hill is an example. See Fig. 7-3.

The natural gravity system should be considered only when the source of water is high enough above the buildings to give adequate flow, when the yield of water at the source is adequate for the needs, and then only when the cost of development is not excessive over the cost of a well and a pressure system. An elevation of 20 feet will provide a satisfactory flow for moderate demands if the pipe is short and large enough. However, for long distances higher elevations are desirable so that smaller and less expensive pipe can be used. A source to be developed should provide an adequate year-round supply of good quality water. Special attention should be given to catchment basins, size of pipe to use, frost protection and protection from contamination or pollution.

One distinct advantage of this system is that there is no energy cost for operation. Also, such systems are very simple mechanically and therefore have a low maintenance cost.

Pumped gravity system.

This type of water system is commonly used where the pump is driven by a windmill or a gas engine, or where large volumes of water must be stored. The pumped gravity system is very satisfactory where windmill power is used because a large storage capacity can be had at a relatively low cost. A large storage capacity is desirable to provide

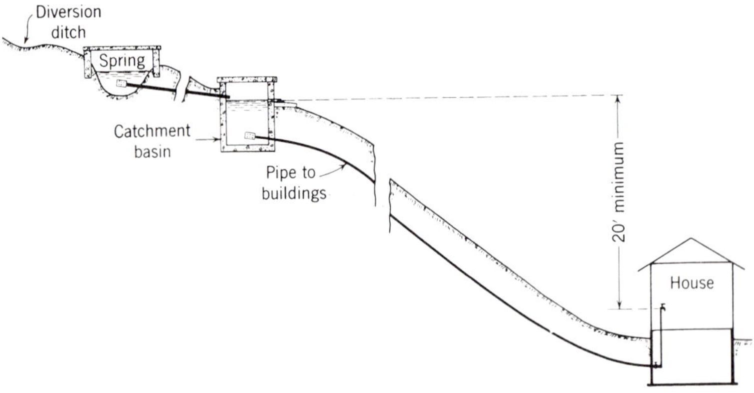

Fig. 7-3. A natural gravity water system. A spring located at a higher elevation than the buildings can supply water by gravity. Unless the spring has a strong flow a catchment basin should be built below the spring as shown. For a satisfactory flow there should be at least 20 feet (6 m.) of elevation on the highest faucet. If the distance to the spring is great, more than 20 feet of elevation would be desirable.

water for days when there is no wind. With gasoline engine power a large storage tank means less frequent starting of the engine.

City water systems are often of the pumped gravity type because of the large volumes of water used. See Figs. 7-5 and 7-6.

Hydropneumatic or "Pressure" Type

The hydropneumatic or pressure type of water system is the most adaptable to a wide variety of water situations. For this reason it is used more than any other type of system.

Advantages of Pressure Systems

1. They are compact and require little room.
2. They can be installed in almost any convenient location.
3. They can supply pressures up to 70 pounds. (32 kgm.) Higher pressure systems are available at extra cost.

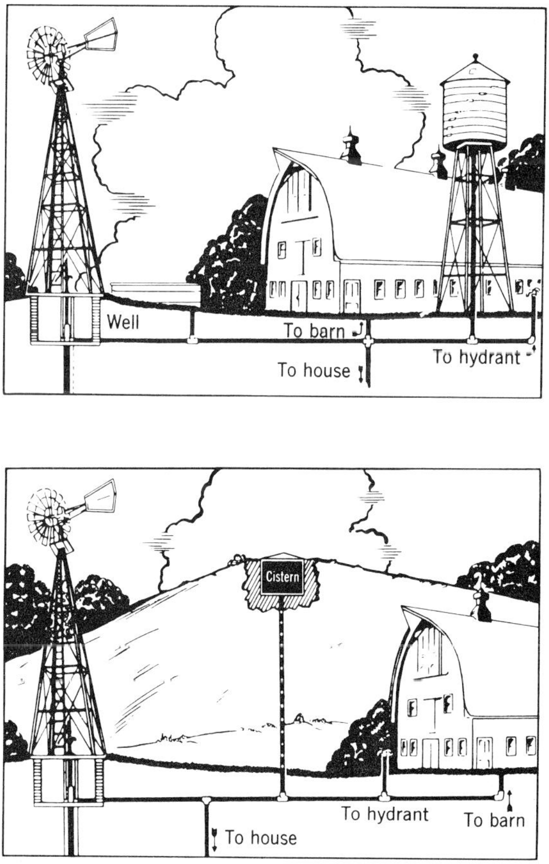

Courtesy National Association of Domestic and Farm Pump Manufacturers

Fig. 7-4. Two pumped gravity water systems using windmills as power units.

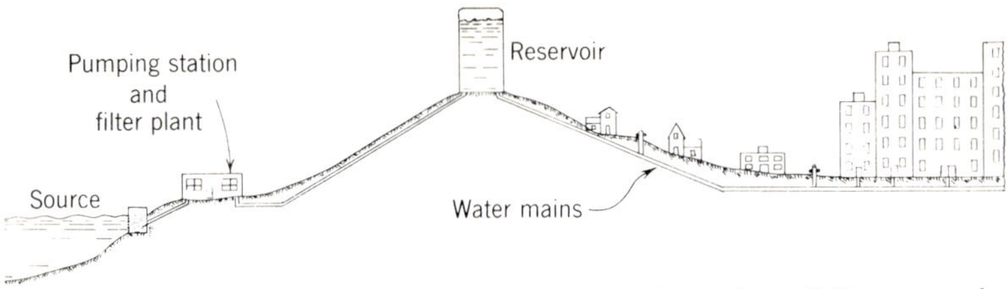

Fig. 7-5. A pumped gravity type of city water supply system. If the source is higher than the city so that the water will flow directly from it to the city, then pumping of raw water can be omitted. In some cases the source of water is clear enough to be used without filtering but the water from such a source should always be chlorinated.

4. Because of the possible higher pressures they are very satisfactory for such uses as sprinkling, car washing, and to some extent fire fighting.

5. The higher pressures available make it possible to use smaller pipes to the faucets than are required with low pressures.

6. As the water is not exposed to the atmosphere they are more sanitary than the open gravity systems.

7. When correctly installed the electrically driven systems make very little noise and require a minimum of attention.

8. Being electrically driven they are completely automatic. They provide a water service comparable with that from city mains.

9. Operating cost is very low.

10. The initial cost is moderate.

There are a great variety of makes and designs of pressure water systems on the market. The systems illustrated in the rest of this chapter are examples. Selection and installation for various water situations is discussed in Chapter 8.

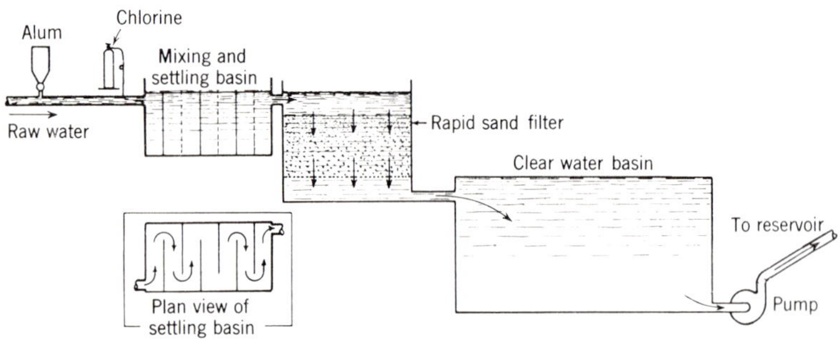

Fig. 7-6. Schematic drawing of a rapid sand filter plant such as is used by many cities for treatment of their water supply. Alum (aluminum sulphate) is used to produce a flock for removing sediment. The flock and sediment settle out to a large extent as the water slowly moves through the settling basin. Chlorine is used to kill bacteria. The sand filter removes the remaining flock and sediment after which the water is held in the clear water basin long enough for the chlorine to take effect. The water is then pumped to the reservoir.

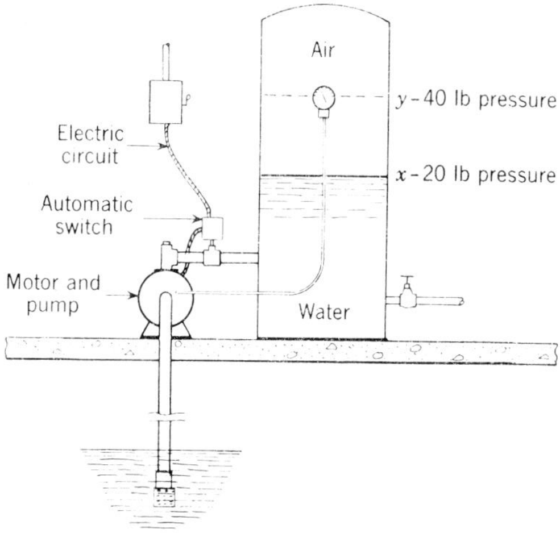

Fig. 7-7. A pressure type of water system illustrating the cycle of operation. Pump starts at 20 pounds' (9 kg.) pressure and stops at 40 pounds' (18 kg.) pressure. Other pressure ranges can be obtained by adjustment of the controls.

All pressure systems use a force pump of some kind. They are available for deep or shallow sources.

Principle of operation.

Regardless of the wide differences in designs of these systems the principle of the cycle of operation is the same for all. Referring to Fig. 7-7 it will be seen that the pressure tank is normally filled with water in the lower part and air in the upper part. The water is pumped into the tank near the bottom, compressing the air above it. The usual pressure range is 20 psi minimum to 40 psi maximum. That is, when the pressure drops to 20 pounds the pump starts and when the pressure reaches 40 pounds the pump stops. On most systems the pressure range can be varied by adjustments on the pressure switch.

Starting with the pressure in the tank at 20 pounds, the cycle of operation is as follows:

1. At 20 pounds' pressure the water level in the tank will be low as indicated at line *X* in Fig. 7-7. At this point it is desirable to pump more water; therefore the pressure-operated switch closes and starts the pump.

2. The pump draws water from the source and forces it into the tank. The rising water level compresses the air above it.

3. When the water level in the tank has reached a higher level, as at line *Y*, the pressure will be high enough to trip the automatic switch and stop the pump.

4. The compressed air above the water in the tank constantly presses down on the water like a giant spring. This pressure will cause the water to flow out of the tank through the pipes whenever a faucet is opened.

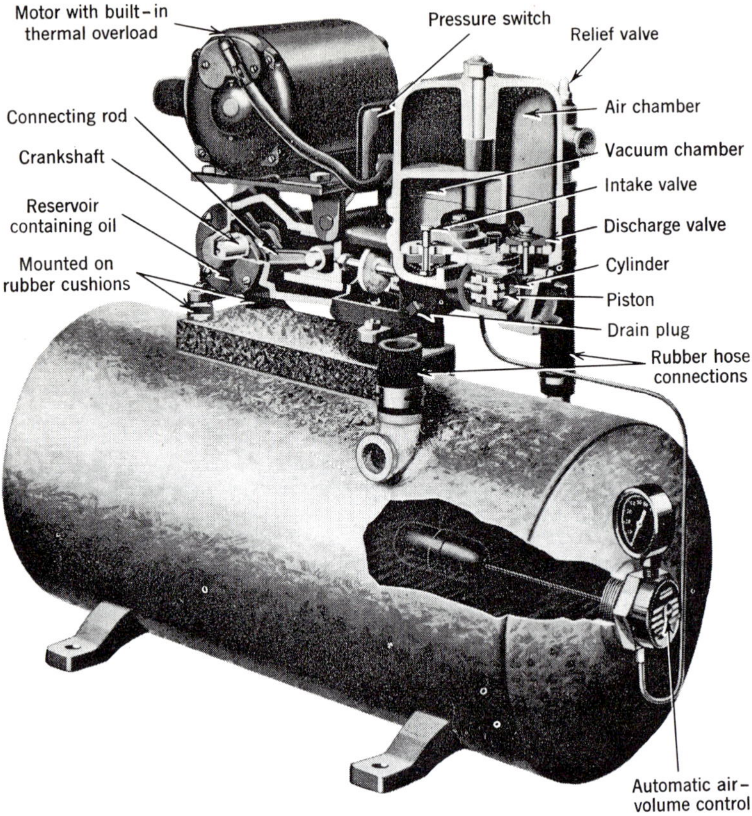

Courtesy Deming Co.

Fig. 7-8. A shallow-well pressure system with a double-acting piston pump. Maximum practical suction lift is 25 feet (7.62 m.) at sea level including friction losses in the pipe. Suitable for installation on shallow wells, springs, or cisterns. This particular system has a capacity of 250 U.S. gallons (208 Imp. gals.) per hour. Note the rubber mounts and hose connections for silencing.

5. As water leaves the tank the air is allowed to expand. As the air expands its pressure drops. When the water level has dropped to line *X* the pressure will again be at 20 psi and the switch will close to start the pump.

In this manner these systems automatically maintain a satisfactory pressure so that water can be drawn at the faucets at any time.

Volume of water from tank per cycle of operation.

The amount of water which can be drawn from a tank between 40 and 20 pounds of pressure depends upon the size of the tank and the initial air-water ratio within the tank. The most common size tank is 42 U.S. gallons. (35 Imp. gals.) Figure 7-10 illustrates the volume of water which can be drawn from such a tank with four different air-water ratios. Note that the less air the less the volume of water which can be drawn off between 40 and 20 pounds of pressure. If there were no air in the tank the pressure would go up to 40 pounds and down to 20 pounds just the same, but as water is practically noncompressible only a very small volume of water (about 1 ounce (28.35 g)) could be drawn off before the pump started. This condition of no air in the tank is called a "waterlogged" condition. It is indicated by the pump starting every time a faucet is opened. Under this condition the system would work just as well without the tank. The frequent starting and stopping of the pump takes more electric energy and may soon cause motor failure.

From the foregoing it is obvious that *the function of the air in the tank is to make it possible to draw off an appreciable amount of water between the stopping and starting of the pump.* However, there is a practical limit to the amount of air a tank without a diaphram should have. If the air voluem is too great the water level will drop below the outlet pipe before the pressure drops to 20 pounds. This results in air escaping into the pipes and out the faucets, as indicated in Fig. 7-11. With tanks of the types shown in Figs. 7-9 and 7-18 this cannot happen.

Table 7-I indicates the approximate volume of water which can be drawn off between high and low pressures with various sized tanks. The volume of discharge can be varied (1) by adjustment on the automatic switch to increase the cut-in and cut-out pressures, and on some systems the range of pressure can be changed, as from 20-40 lbs. to 20-50 lbs. (2) by precharging the tank with air above atmospheric pressure. This can be done by pumping extra air into the tank before

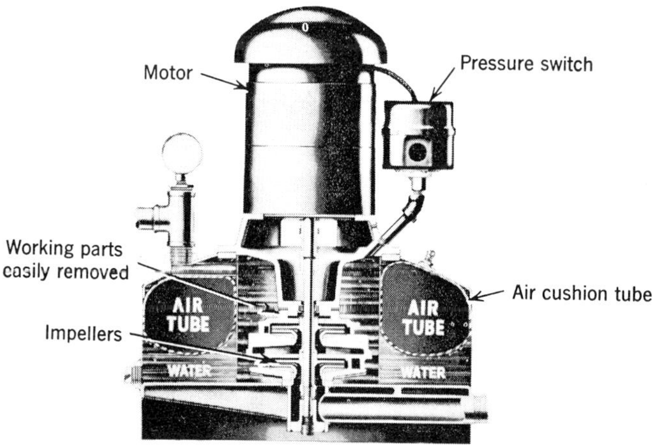

Courtesy Deming Co.

Fig. 7-9. A shallow-well pressure system with a two-stage centrifugal pump. The air is confined in a rubber tube located on the inside of the tank. As the water cannot absorb the air in the tube no air volume control is needed. This system id designed to be used for boosting pressure, or for places where water demands are moderate as for a cottage or just a kitchen sink.

TABLE 7-I

APPROXIMATE U.S. GALLONS OF WATER AVAILABLE BETWEEN HIGH AND LOW PRESSURE RANGE OF HYDROPNEUMATIC TANKS*

Operating Range, lb. Cutin Cutout	% of Tank Filled With Water at Cutin Pressure	Cutout Pressure	Tank Size, U.S. Gallons Capacity** 12	30	42	80	120	220	315	530	1000
20 to 40	25	53	3.3	8.2	11	22	33	60	87	146	275
	33	58	2.9	7.3	10	19	29	53	77	130	245
	50	68	2.2	5.5	8	15	22	40	57	97	183
30 to 40	25	39	1.6	4.1	6	11	16	30	43	73	137
	33	45	1.5	3.7	5	10	15	27	38	65	122
	50	59	1.1	2.7	4	7	11	20	29	48	91
30 to 50	25	48	2.8	7.0	10	19	28	51	73	123	232
	33	54	2.5	6.2	9	16	25	45	65	109	206
	50	65	1.8	4.6	6	12	18	34	48	82	154
40 to 50	25	37	1.4	3.5	5	9	14	26	37	62	116
	33	43	1.2	3.1	4	8	12	23	32	55	103
	50	58	0.9	2.3	3	6	9	17	24	41	77
40 to 60	25	45	2.4	6.0	8	16	24	44	63	106	200
	33	51	2.2	5.4	7	14	22	40	57	95	180
	50	63	1.6	4.0	6	11	16	29	42	71	134
50 to 60	25	35	1.2	3.0	4	8	12	22	31	53	100
	33	42	1.1	2.7	4	7	11	20	28	48	90
	50	57	0.8	2.0	3	5	8	15	21	35	67

Example: First line, Cutin pressure 20 pounds, tank 25% full of water. Cutout pressure, 40 pounds, tank 53% full of water. Under column headed "42-gallon tank" it shows that 11 gallons may be drawn off during the time the pressure drops from 40 to 20 pounds.

*Courtesy Deming Co.

**For Imperial gallons divide U.S. gallons by 1.2.

water is pumped in or later at a time when the pressure is low. Air can be pumped into the tank by means of a hand or power pump connected to a Schrader valve on the air-volume control or to such a valve installed on the tank or the piping for that special purpose.

Note: Some types of pumps, particularly the centrifugals and jets with centrifugal pumps, may not be able to deliver the required amount of water at higher pressures.

Air-volume controls.

When water and air are confined together under pressure there is a tendency for the water to absorb the air. Consequently, as water is drawn from the tank it carries with it some of the air. If this air is not replaced the tank becomes waterlogged, as indicated at *A* in Fig. 7-10.

There are a number of designs for air-volume controls available. Figures 7-12 through 7-16 illustrate some of the more common ones.

Figure 7-12 illustrates a *float type* of control for shallow-well systems. If the suction lift on a piston pump is high this type of control will at times affect the capacity of the pump because one side of the pump may pump only air. When used on jet pumps as indicated in Fig. 7-13 the capacity of the pump is affected very little.

In the *water displacement type* of control air is drawn in by water displacement, as shown in Fig. 7-15.

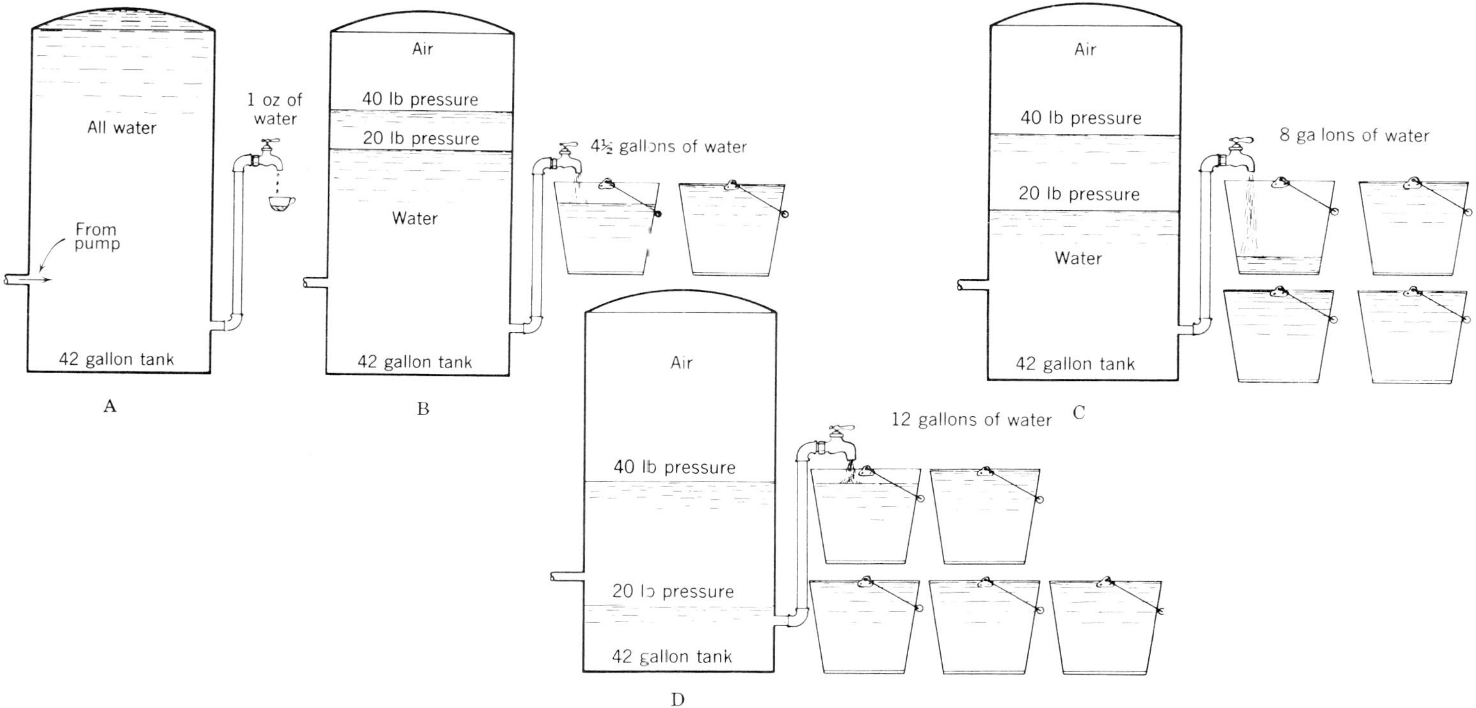

Fig. 7-10. The amount of water which can be drawn from a pressure tank between the stopping and starting of the pump varies with the air volume in the tank.

A — No air. Pressure drops from 40 pounds to 20 pounds when very small amount of water is drawn. Tank is of no use. Pump will start every time a faucet is opened.

B — One-quarter of tank filled with air at 40 pounds' pressure. 4½ U.S. gallons (3.75 Imp. gals.) can be drawn before pump starts.

C — One-third of tank filled with air at 40 pounds' pressure. 8 U.S. gallons (6.67 Imp. gals.) can be drawn off before pump starts.

D — One-half of tank filled with air at 40 pounds. 12 U.S. gallons (10 Imp. gals.) can be drawn off before pump starts.

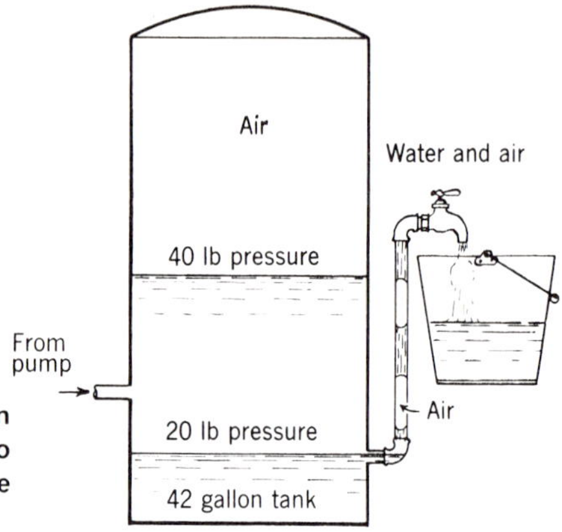

Fig. 7-11. If there is too much air in the tank some of it will escape into the discharge pipes and cause spurting at the faucets.

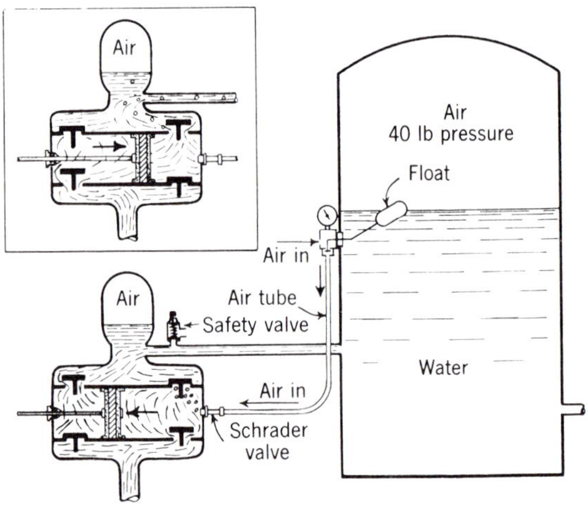

Fig. 7-12. Air-volume control on a pressure system with a shallow-well double-acting piston pump.

Just before the pump shuts off, when the water level in the tank is approaching its highest level, the float rises to open a valve in the upper end of the air tube. This permits one side of the pump to suck air as well as water. On the reverse stroke the air and water are discharged into the tank as shown in the inset. Some of the air goes to the air chamber on the pump to keep that charged with air. A Schrader valve on the pump prevents air and water from flowing back through the air tube.

To prevent this, automatic air-volume control devices function to maintain automatically the correct volume of air in the tank at all times regardless of how much is drawn off with the water. Air absorption can be reduced by means of a floating barrier in the tank which almost completely separates the air from the water. See Fig. 7-17. If the inside of the tank becomes rough with rust blisters the float will not move up and down freely with the water level.

Air absorption can be completely eliminated by means of air tubes in the tank as shown in Fig. 7-9 or by means of a diaphram as shown in Fig. 7-18.

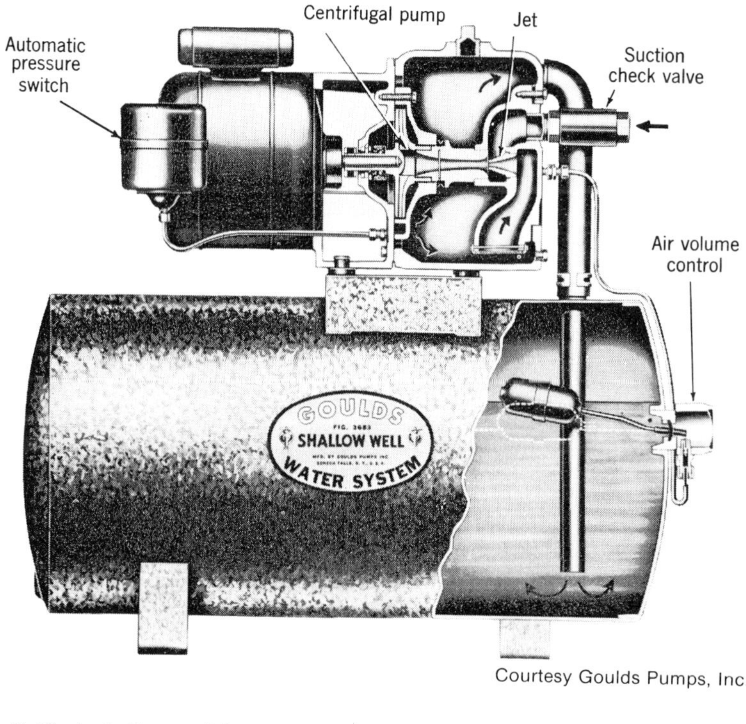

Courtesy Goulds Pumps, Inc.

Fig. 7-13. A shallow-well jet system. Maximum suction lift is 25 feet (7.6 m.) at seal level including friction losses. Capacity ranges from 150 U.S. gallons (125 Imp gals.) per hour to 520 U.S. gallons (433 Imp gals.) per hour with a 10-foot suction lift and a discharge pressure of 15 pounds.

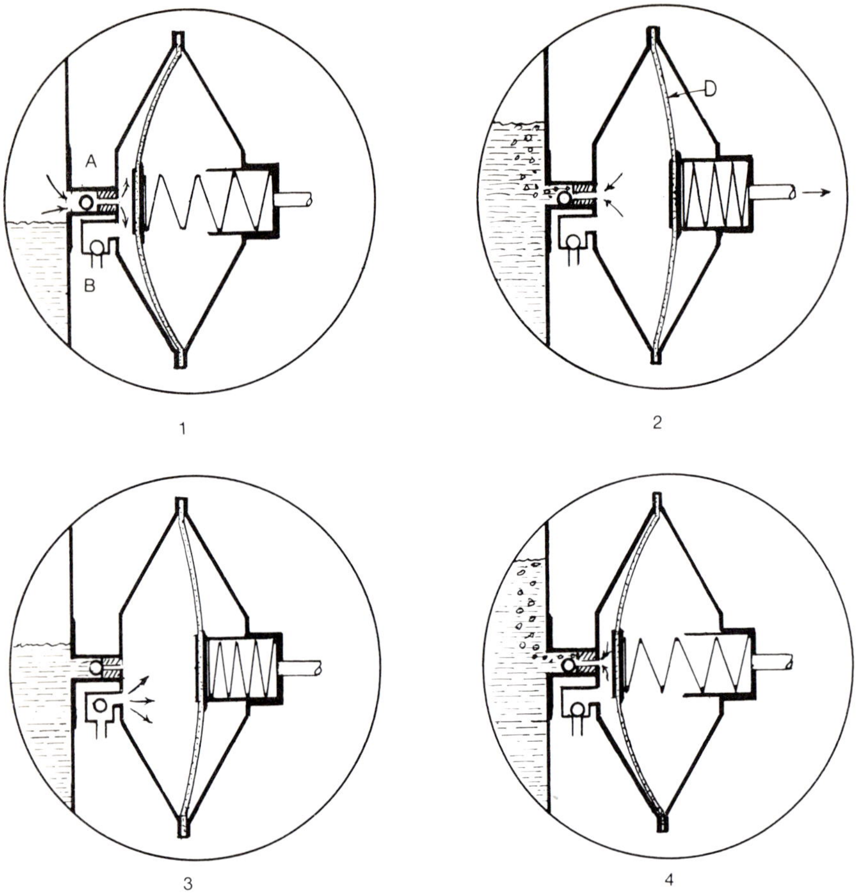

Fig. 7-14. A diaphram type of air volume control.

At (1) tank has enough air. The water level in the tank is below valve A and valve A is open. When the pump starts suction from the pump pulls the diaphram D to the right against the pressure of the spring. Air is drawn *from the tank* through valve A. When the pump stops the spring pushes the air back into the tank as shown at (2). No air added.

At (3) the tank needs air. Water level is high. Valve A is closed. When pump starts the suction of the pump pulls the diaphram to the right. Valve B is drawn open and *outside air* is drawn into the control, as shown. When the pump stops the spring pushes the diaphram to the left forcing the outside air into the tank as shown at (4). Thus air is added to the tank each time the pump runs until the tank has enough air.

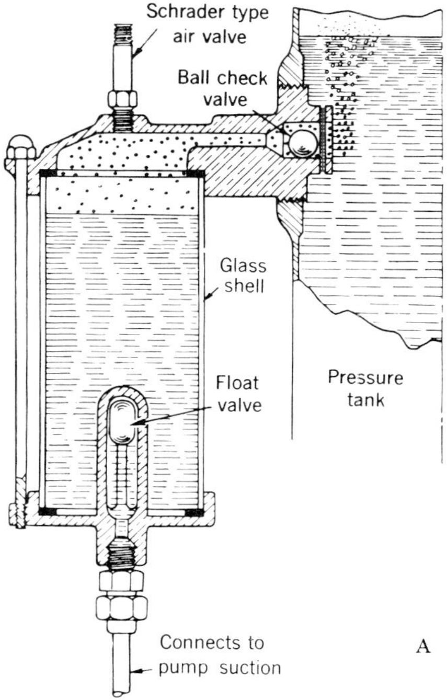

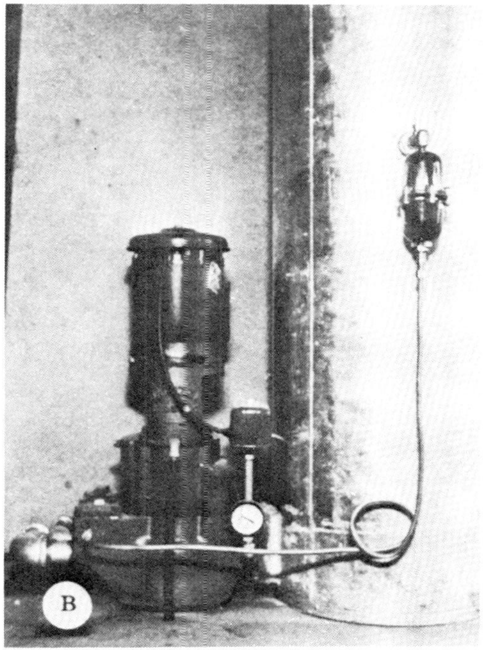

Courtesy National Association of Domestic and Farm Pump Manufacturers

Fig. 7-15. Water-displacement type of air-volume control. When the pump starts water is drawn out of the glass or plastic shell, creating a partial vacuum at the top. If the tank water level is above the ball check valve, this valve closes to prevent water from entering the control from the tank. Air is then drawn in through the Schrader air valve.

When the pump stops, the pressure equalizes in the glass shell and in the tank. The air drawn in passes through the ball check and bubbles to the top of the water in the tank. As the air escapes water rises and refills the glass shell.

If the tank water level is low enough (plenty of air in the tank) the ball check valve remains open and as the water is drawn down in the glass shell air enters from the tank instead of through the Schrader valve. At the end of the pumping period this air re-enters the tank without increasing the air volume.

This type of control mounted on a multistage deep-well jet system is shown in B.

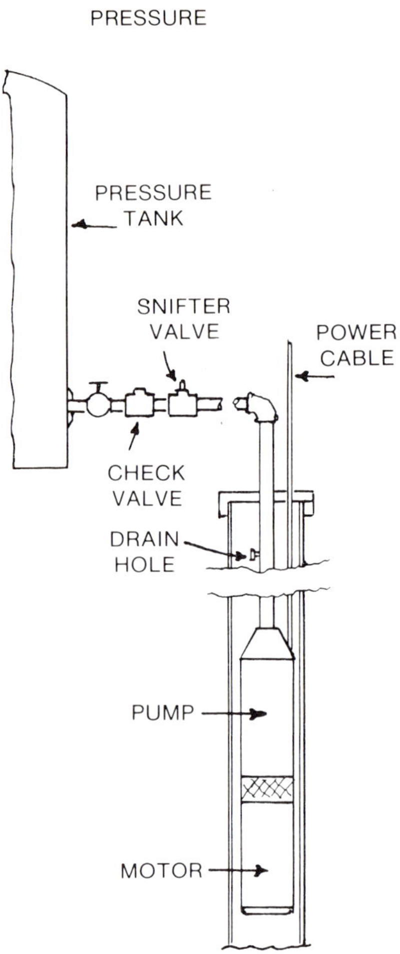

Fig. 7-16. *Air-volume control for submersibles.* **Her the pump is submerged in the water and cannot pump air. Air-volume control can be obtained by means of a combination of a snifter valve installed on the pump side of the check valve as shown. A drain hole in the pump discharge pipe a little farther toward the pump, and a float operated air blow-off valve the same as used on the deep well reciprocating pump system shown in Fig. 7-19. With this arrangement, when the pump stops the water in the pipe will leak out down to the level of the drain hole. At the same time air will enter the pipe through the snifter valve. When the pump starts again the air thus drawn into the pipe will be forced into the tank ahead of the water. As the same amount of air is put into the tank each time the pump starts the tendency is to add too much air to the tank. The float controlled air blow-off valve functions to release the excess air.**

The controls of Figs. 7-12 and 7-15 will not function properly unless the pump has some suction. Where water flows to the pump by gravity or underground pressure so that the pump does not "suck" to get water it is necessary to place a valve or other restricting device in the suction line to make the pump suck. See Fig. 7-20.

The Schrader valves used on air-volume controls are similar to those used in automobile tires *except they have a much lighter spring.* See Fig. 7-21. Tire valves will not function properly because of the stronger spring and should never be substituted for the water system type.

Air-volume controls for plunger pump deep-well systems. Deep-well jet systems can use the shallow-well types of air-volume controls, as just described. With the plunger type of pump where the pumping unit (cylinder) is submerged in the water down in the well, the water pump cannot be used to pump air. Therefore a separate air pump is

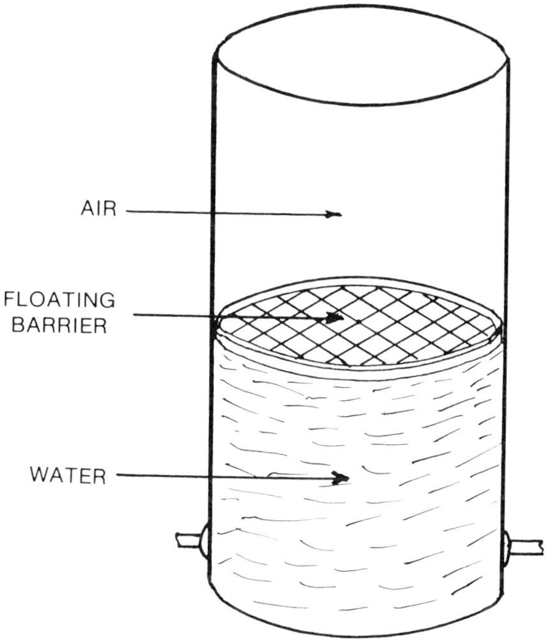

Fig. 7-17. A pressure tank with a floating barrier between the air and the water which greatly reduces air absorption. The barrier floats up and down with the changes in water level.

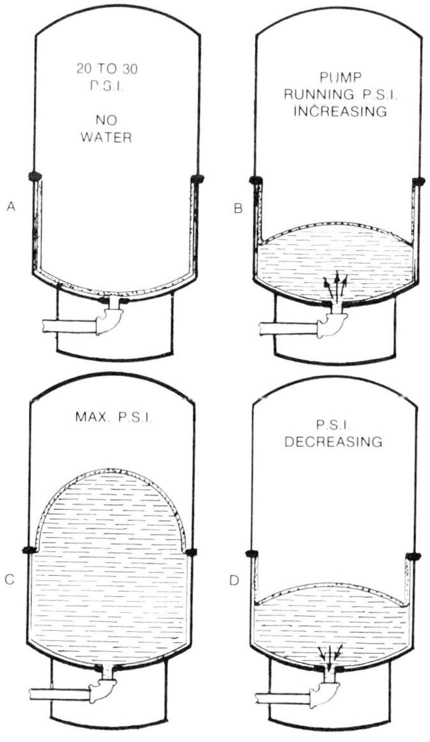

Fig. 7-18. A pressure tank with a flexible diaphram which completely separates the air from the water. No water logging. No air volume control needed. The lower part of the tank which is in contact with the water has a corrosion resistant lining.

At A, no water in the tank. Tank precharged with 20 to 30 pounds of air pressure.

At B, the pump is delivering water into the tank under the flexible diaphram and is increasing the pressure.

At C, the pressure has been increased to the maximum and the automatic switch has stopped the pump.

At D, water is being drawn off at the outlets. The pressure decreases until the pump starts.

usually mounted on the system above ground level. See Fig. 6-14 *C* and *D*. As the air pump operates whenever the pump is running, the tendency is to pump too much air into the tank. The control illustrated in Fig. 7-19 is designed to blow off excess air. There is no connection to the pump.

Size of system to install

The size of system to install depends largely upon the demands for water as determined from Table 3-I. Also the combined capacity of the pump and storage tank should be enough to meet the peak demands.

Combination of Gravity and Hydropneumatic Types

Combinations of gravity and hydropneumatic pressure systems are not common. However, under certain conditions they are of considerable value. Figures 3-3 and 3-4 illustrate a combination where the pressure system is used to boost the pressure from a spring. Figure 7-28 shows a system which can be used on a weak well to supply a large volume of water for peak demands. The gravity storage tank could be placed on a tower or underground on a hill as shown in Fig. 7-4. In cold elimates the storage tank should be protected from freezing.

Safety devices.

All electrically driven hydropneumatic pressure systems should be equipped with an automatic switch which is actuated by pressure changes in the tank. See Fig. 7-27. This device is the primary safety device. However, such switches are subject to failures. If the pump is of the plunger or piston type and the switch fails to stop the pump, dangerous pressures can be built up in the tank. An exploding pressure tank can wreck a building and of course may cause loss of life. For these reasons a system with a plunger or piston pump should *always* be equipped with a pressure relief valve, in addition to the pressure switch. Figures 7-24 and 7-26 show pressure relief valves installed on the discharge side of the pump. These valves should be checked at least twice a year to see that they are in working order.

Most systems using a centrifugal or turbine pump cannot build up excessive pressures because of slippage within the pump. For this reason pressure relief valves are usually omitted on such systems.

On most high-quality systems an overload protective device is also provided for the electric motor. This device may be an integral part of the automatic switch, as shown in Fig. 7-27, or it may be installed in or on the motor as shown in Fig. 7-29. Its purpose is to open the electric circuit and stop the motor if for any reason the motor becomes overloaded or too hot. Some forms of this device automatically reset and start the motor again when it has cooled off; others must be reset Figure 7-30 illustrates a method of protecting motors by means of delayed-action fuses.

In areas where severe lightning storms occur it is good practice to install lightning protectors, especially if a submersible pump is used.

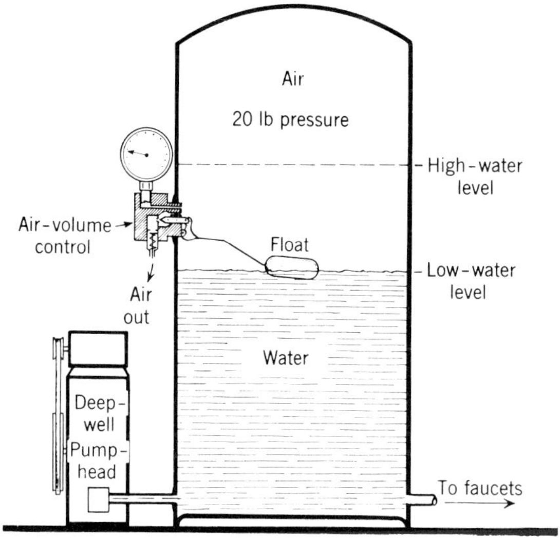

Fig. 7-19. Automatic air-volume control for single- and double-acting deep-well plunger, and submersible pumps. An air pump attached to the pumping head pumps air into the tank throughout the pumping period. This tends to put too much air in the tank. When the water level in the tank reaches its lowest point and just before the pump starts, the float pulls the needle valve in the air-volume control open and allows the excess air to escape.

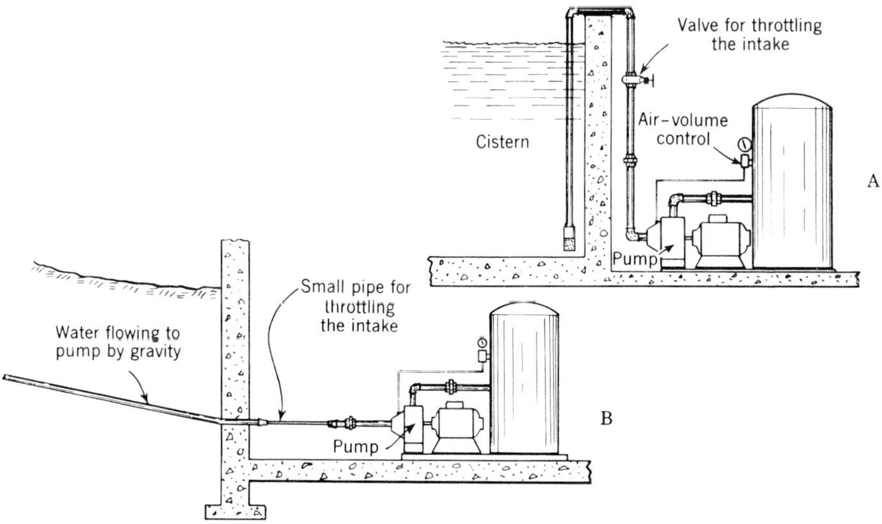

Fig. 7-20. Two methods of throttling the intake so that the pump will suck air. A — A valve in the suction line which can be partially closed. B — A small-diameter pipe in the line. The friction losses in this small pipe increase the suction head on the pump.

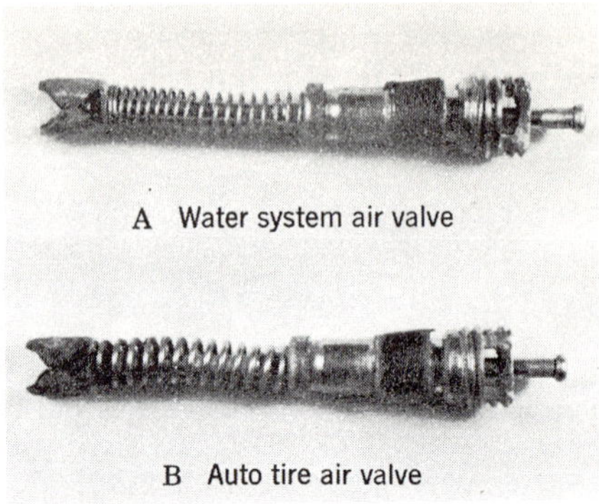

Fig. 7-21. Schrader valves. A — Shows the light-spring type used on water system air-volume controls, B — The heavy-spring type used in automotive tires. The latter should not be used on water systems.

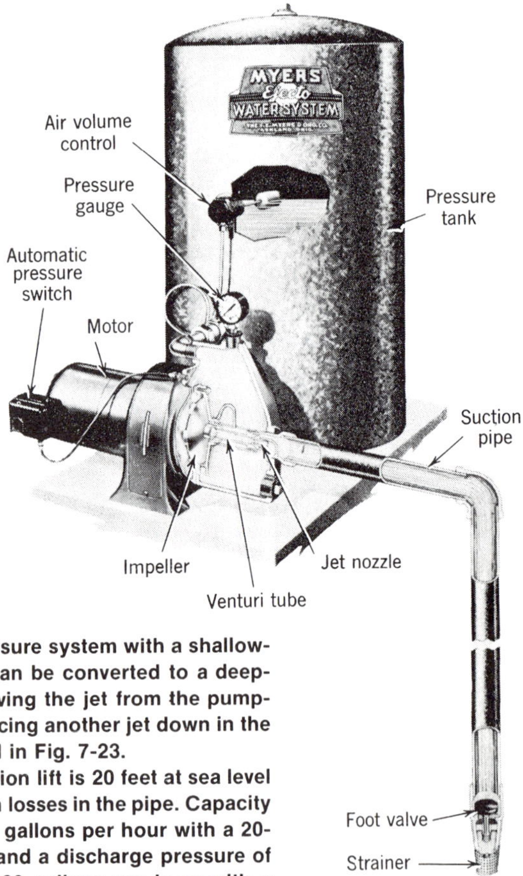

Courtesy The F.E. Myers & Bro. Co.

Fig. 7-22. A pressure system with a shallow-well jet pump. Can be converted to a deep-well jet by removing the jet from the pumping head and placing another jet down in the well as indicated in Fig. 7-23.

Maximum suction lift is 20 feet at sea level including friction losses in the pipe. Capacity ranges from 180 gallons per hour with a 20-foot suction lift and a discharge pressure of 50 pounds to 1620 gallons per hour with a 10-foot suction lift and 20 pounds of discharge pressure.

1-foot = 0.3048 meters.

1-U.S. gallon = 0.833 Imperial gallons.

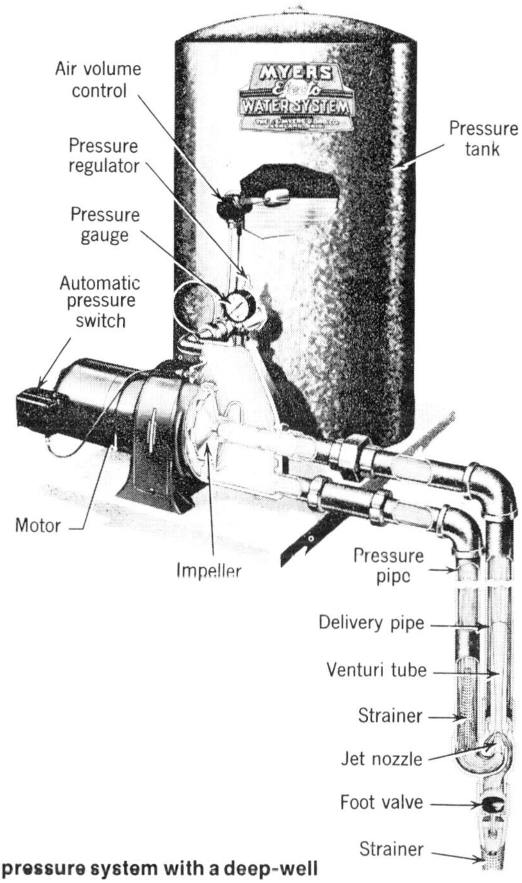

Fig. 7-23. A pressure system with a deep-well jet pump. Suitable for depths to 100 feet (30.5 m.) The pumping head and tank are the same as shown in Fig. 7-22 and can be offset from the well as indicated.

For depths below 100 feet (30.5 m.) a multistage pump should be used.

Courtesy The F.E. Myers & Bro. Co.

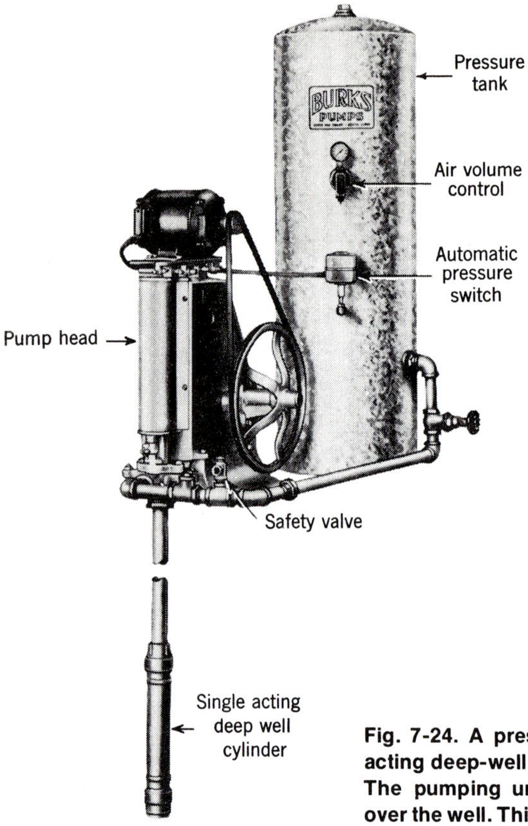

Fig. 7-24. A pressure system with a single-acting deep-well plunger type of force pump. The pumping unit must be placed directly over the well. This type of system can be used on wells of almost any depth and has a wide range of capacities depending upon the size of cylinder, length of stroke, and number of strokes per minute. The horsepower rating and size of the pumping head increase with depth of well and rate of pumping. This type of system is now being largely displaced by deep-well jets, turbines, and submersible pumps.

Courtesy Decatur Pump Co., Decatur, Ill.

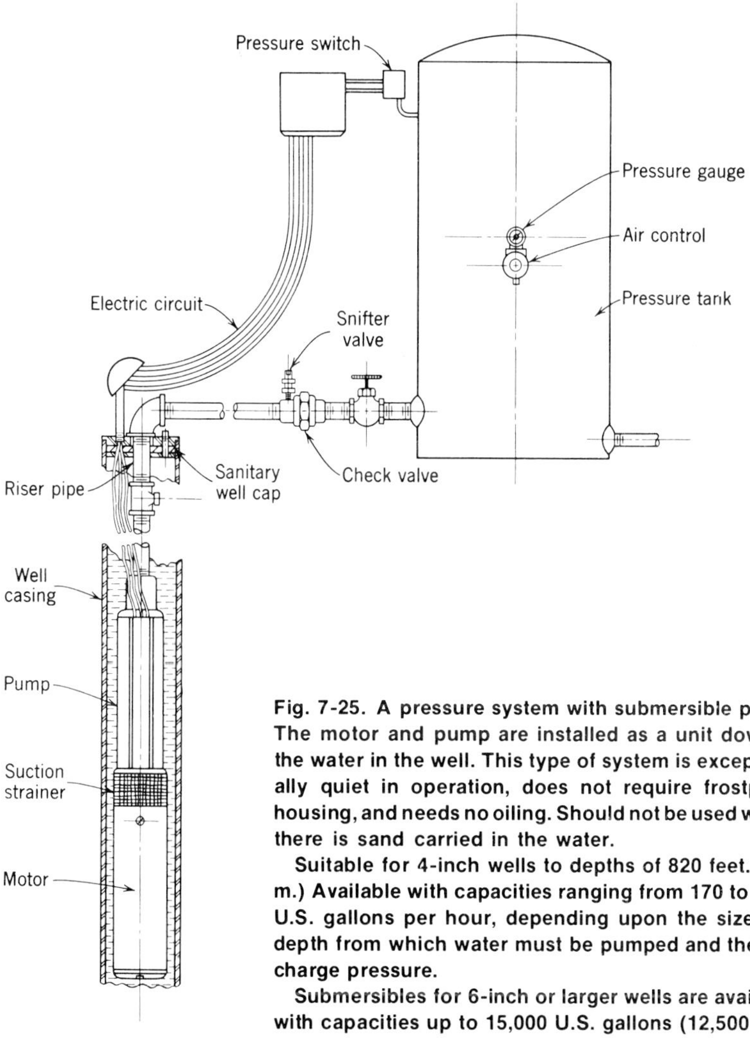

Fig. 7-25. A pressure system with submersible pump. The motor and pump are installed as a unit down in the water in the well. This type of system is exceptionally quiet in operation, does not require frostproof housing, and needs no oiling. Should not be used where there is sand carried in the water.

Suitable for 4-inch wells to depths of 820 feet. (250 m.) Available with capacities ranging from 170 to 3000 U.S. gallons per hour, depending upon the size and depth from which water must be pumped and the discharge pressure.

Submersibles for 6-inch or larger wells are available with capacities up to 15,000 U.S. gallons (12,500 Imp. gals.) per hour, can develop pressures to 400 p.s.i.

Courtesy Deming Co.

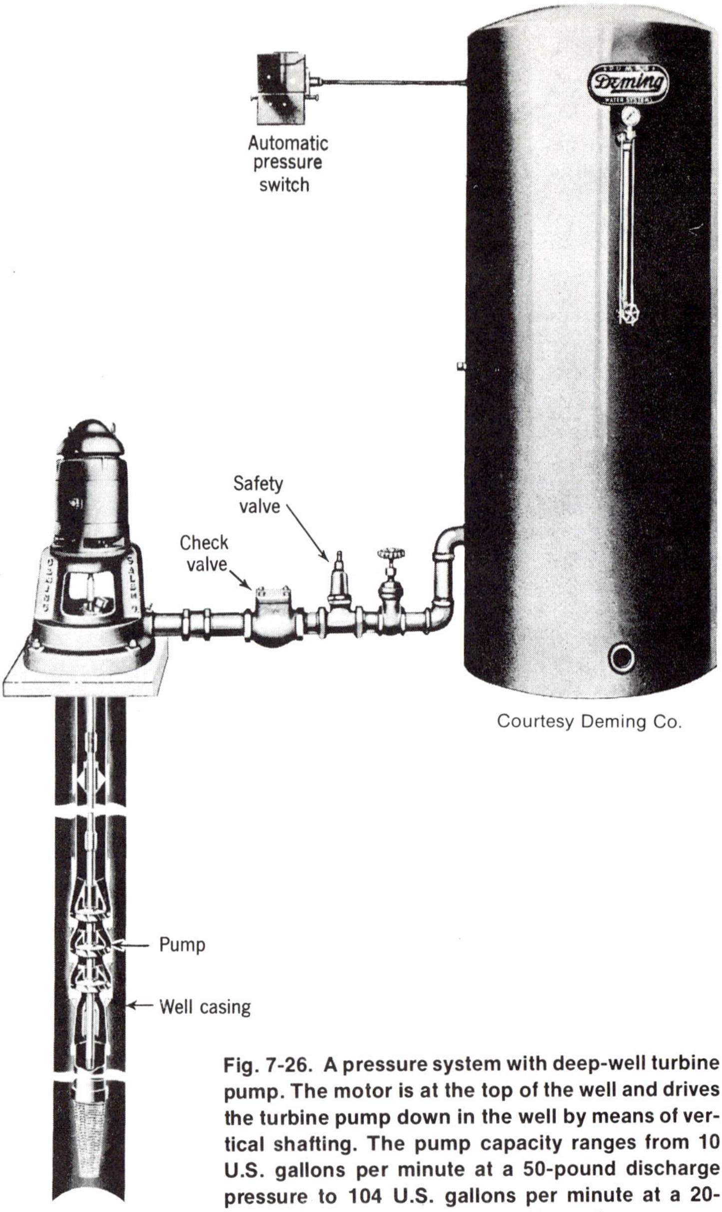

Courtesy Deming Co.

Fig. 7-26. A pressure system with deep-well turbine pump. The motor is at the top of the well and drives the turbine pump down in the well by means of vertical shafting. The pump capacity ranges from 10 U.S. gallons per minute at a 50-pound discharge pressure to 104 U.S. gallons per minute at a 20-pound discharge pressure. Motor horsepower ranges from 1½ to 5. Used mostly where large volumes of water must be pumped. This system can use the same type of air-volume control as the submersibles.

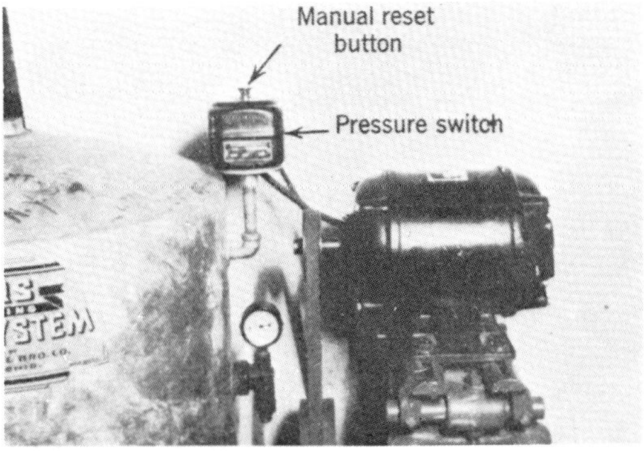

Fig. 7-27. Motor overload protective device built into the pressure switch. The button pops up and opens the circuit in case of an overload. The button must be pushed down to reset.

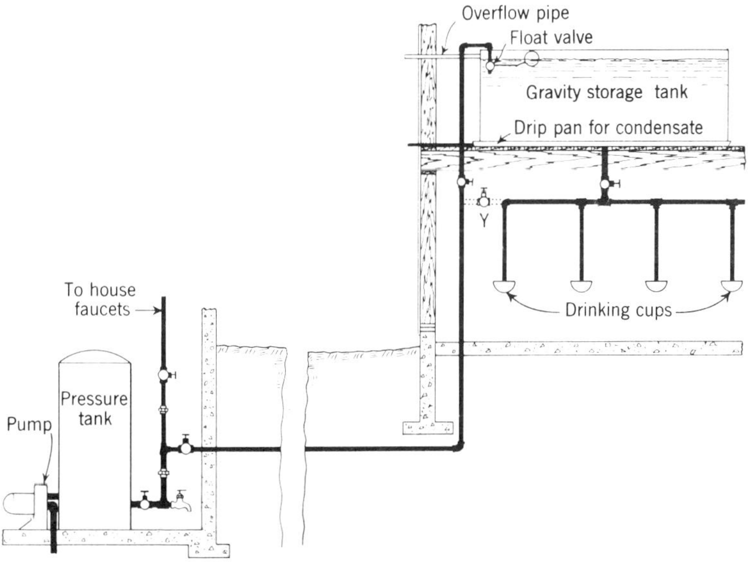

Fig. 7-28. A combination gravity and hydropneumatic pressure system for supplying a dairy herd or for other short-period heavy demands for water. It is especially suitable where the well has a weak but steady flow. A small-capacity pump can be used to fill the gravity tank between peak demand periods. This system can also be used to eliminate water hammer noises in the house plumbing when such noises are caused by drinking cup action in the barn. Cross connection at Y is optional. It is recommended that the gravity storage tank have a capacity of at least 1000 U.S. gallons.

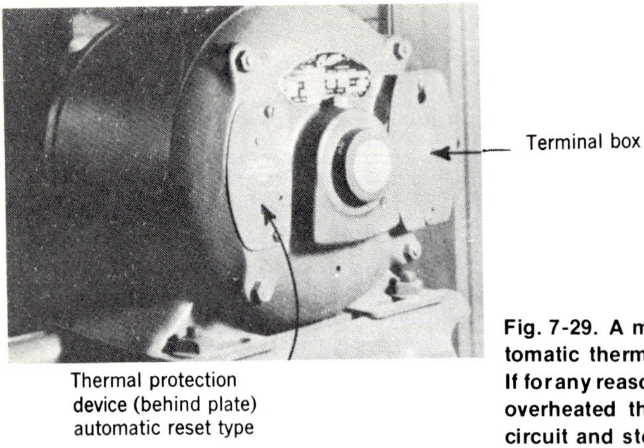

Fig. 7-29. A motor with built-in automatic thermal protection device. If for any reason the motor becomes overheated this device opens the circuit and stops the motor. When the motor has cooled the device closes the circuit and starts the motor again.

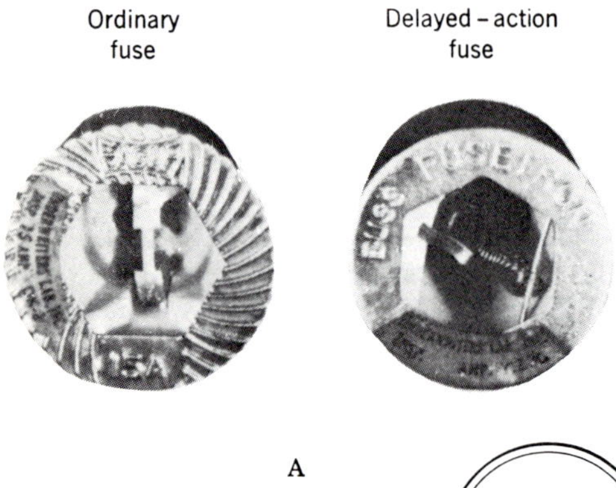

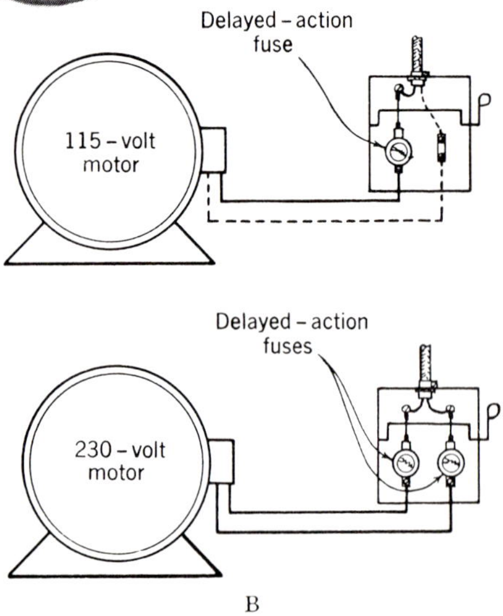

Fig. 7-30. Delayed-action fuses give overload protection for motors. A — A delayed-action fuse compared with a regular circuit fuse. B — Wiring diagram for use of these fuses. No other load should be connected between the fuses and the motor.

Typical Water System Installations 8

The following examples of water system installations are intended as a guide for the selection of systems and the procedures for installation under various conditions of source and demand. Pipe sizes are calculated according to the instructions in Job 6. Elevations can be measured according to instructions in Job 8.

INSTALLATIONS OF NATURAL GRAVITY SYSTEMS

In hilly or mountainous areas where there is ample rainfall there are often good opportunities for developing natural gravity systems from springs, streams, lakes, and ponds. If correctly developed, with ample storage and large enough pipe, they can be very satisfactory. See Figs. 3-2 through 3-6, 7-3 and 8-1. Fig. 8-2 illustrates one which was a failure because of poor design.

Installation of System Shown in Fig. 8-1

Here a pond or lake serves as a source of water and as a reservoir. See Chapter 3, pages 49-52, for development of ponds. This same type of System can be used to bring water from a spring. No pump is needed. See also Fig. 7-3.

For this installation the following conditions are assumed:

1. Gravity head available = 47 feet at low water level.
2. Equivalent length of pipe = 800 feet (includes allowances for elbows, valves, and other fittings).
3. Maximum rate of flow to be 12 U.S. gallons per minute.*
4. Water to be used for livestock only.

---

*Imp. gals. = U.S. gallons ÷ 1.2
1 ft. = 0.3048 m.
1 in. = 2.54 cm.

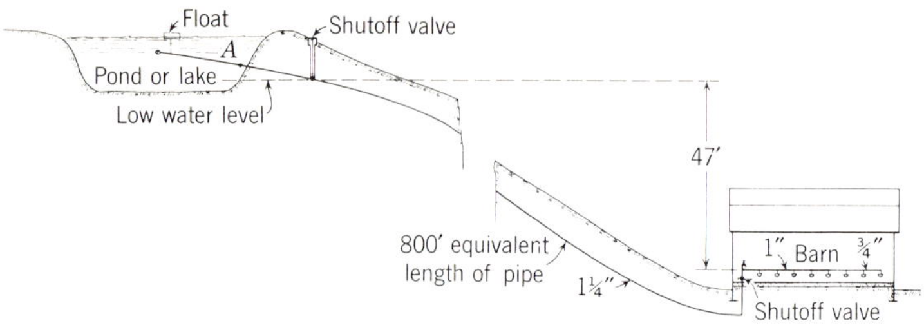

Fig. 8-1. Natural gravity flow from a pond or lake. The elevation of the source should be at least 20 feet (6 m.) above the highest faucet. A float on the intake end of the pipe will keep the pipe near the surface for better quality water. Pipe A can be hinged as shown, or flexible plastic pipe can be used.

From Table J-6-II on page 279, we find that if we use 1-inch pipe for a rate of flow of 12 U.S. gallons per minute the head required to overcome friction would be 126.0 feet (8 × 15.76 feet). Only 47 feet of head is available; therefore 1-inch pipe is too small. The rate of flow would be only about 4 gallons per minute. However, if 1¼-inch pipe is used the loss of head due to friction would be only 33.0 feet (8 × 4.13). This would leave 47 — 33 or 14 feet of head for the pipe and drinking cups in the barn; therefore 1¼-inch pipe should be used to the barn. In the barn 1-inch pipe and ¾-inch pipe could be used to supply the drinking cups.

A good strainer should be provided at the pond end of the pipe.

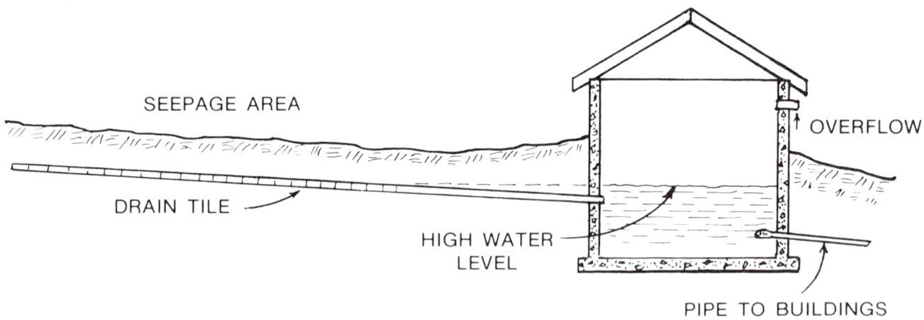

Fig. 8-2. An example of an expensive natural gravity flow water system that was a failure because of faulty design. There was plenty of water in the seepage area, a good system of underground collecting tile was installed, a large concrete reservoir was built, and 1200 feet (365 m.) of the best (and most expensive) copper pipe was laid underground to the farm buildings. When the collecting tile was led into the reservoir the water level would not rise above the half way mark because the upper half of the reservoir was higher than the seepage area. If the reservoir had been built 5 feet (1.5 m.) deeper in the ground the farmer would have had a first class water system for his home and farm.

Shutoff valves should be provided as indicated.

Steel, copper, or plastic piping can be used. See Chapter 10 for description of piping. Standard weight steel pipe would be strong enough, but if copper or plastic tubing is used it should be of the heavy-duty grade because of possible high pressures due to surges in the long pipe.

If the installation is in a cold climate the pipeline should be placed underground below the frost zone. See Table 3-II, page 28. In warm climates the pipe can be laid on the surface, but placing it under the sod protects it from the hot sun and from surface damage. If laid under cultivated fields it should be well below plowing depth.

Trenching for the pipe can usually be done cheaper by machinery than by hand. The trench bottom should have a fairly uniform grade and should be firm to support the pipe. The pipe should be laid in the trench and tested for leaks with normal pressure before backfilling. In backfilling, first cover the pipe with at least 1 foot of soil or sand which is free of sizable stones. This is especially important if plastic or copper tubing is used.

INSTALLATIONS OF PUMPED GRAVITY SYSTEMS

Conditions Favorable for Pumped Gravity Systems

Where large volumes of water must be stored as in the case of windmill or gas-engine operated pumps, an elevated gravity tank provides economical storage space.

The reservoir must be high enough to give adequate flow at the faucets. It is desirable to have it as near to the faucets as practical to avoid the use of long lengths of large pipe.

In cold climates the reservoir must be protected from freezing and in warm climates it should, if possible, be protected from the hot sun. In all cases it should be protected from pollution and contamination.

The common locations for reservoirs are (1) on a nearby hill, (2) in the attic of a house, (3) in a barn, and (4) on a tower.

A tank set in the ground on a nearby hill, if available, as shown in Fig. 7-4, is a preferable location because there it is protected from frost in the winter, from the heat of the sun in the summer, and from winds at all times, and leaks are not damaging to buildings. There is, however, a danger of pollution and contamination unless the tank is well built and protected from surface waters.

Underground tanks are usually made of cast-in-place concrete. Tanks for buildings are generally of galvanized steel and should have drip pans with drains to catch water from the "sweating" of the tanks. Tanks for outside towers may be of wood stave or, preferably, steel construction. A light-colored paint such as aluminim gives considerable protection from the heat of the sun.

The reservoir should be large enough to hold at least ½ day's supply of water. Usually it is made large enough for at least 1 day's supply.

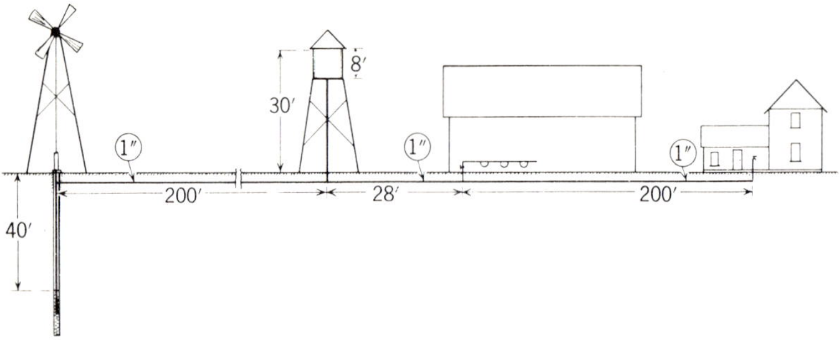

Fig. 8-3. A pumped gravity system with a deep-well, windmill-powered pump and a reservoir on a tower near the buildings.

The type and size of pump to use depends upon such factors as (1) volume of water to be pumped, (2) nature of source of water such as depth of well, flow of well, and distance from storage tank, (3) pressure to be pumped against, (4) kind of power available, etc. Types of pumps are described in Chapter 6.

The piping can be of steel, copper, or plastic. In any case it is important to use the correct sizes.

Installation of System Shown in Fig. 8-3

Assumed conditions:

1. Daily demand for water, 850 U.S. gallons. (708 Imp. gals.)
2. Flow of well, 6 U.S. gallons (5 Imp. gals.) per minute at 40-foot (12 m.) level.
3. Rate of flow from reservoir to barn, 16 U.S. gallons (13.3 Imp. gals.) per minute.
4. Rate of flow to house, 8 U.S. gallons (6.66 Imp. gals.) per minute.
5. Highest faucet is 20 feet (6 m.) below bottom of tank.
6. Located in a warm climate.
7. Pump windmill-operated.

Windmill power should be considered only where the prevailing winds are strong enough and dependable enough to pump the required amount of water almost every day, or where no other form of power is available or practical. With windmill power the reservoir should, if possible, be large enough to supply the water needs over any ordinary period of calm. This might be for several days. If longer periods of calm are common it is questionable if the windmill should be considered at all unless it can be supplemented with some other source of power such as a stand-by gas engine. For this installation we will provide storage facilities for 3 days' supply or about 3000 U.S. gallons. (2500 Imp. gals.)

The pump will have to be a deep-well pump suitable for windmill operation. The pump shown in Fig. 6-11, is of this type. The pump must be of a size which can be driven by the available wind and will not pump the well dry. As we have specified for this problem that the well will deliver 6 U.S. gallons (5 Imp. gals.) per minute at the 40-foot (12 m.) level, we could pump up to 6 U.S. gallons (5 Imp. gals.) per minute or 360 gallons (300 Imp. gals.) per hour.

Windmills are available in various designs. Some are self-regulating in speed and especially constructed to withstand gale winds. For satisfactory operation the millwheel should be 15 to 20 feet (4.526 m.) above the level of buildings, trees, knolls, or other wind obstructions which are within 400 or 500 feet (122 to 152 m.) of the tower. The horsepower requirements will depend upon the rate of pumping and the total head. As the pump and windmill should be chosen together, it is suggested that in any particular case a manufacturer or a dealer for such equipment be consulted on the exact models and horsepower to use.

The selection and installation of the pipe and the sanitary measures would be on the same basis as for the gravity system of Fig. 8-1. The correct sizes of pipe to use as calculated from the friction table on page 279 are indicated on the drawing.

INSTALLATIONS OF PRESSURE SYSTEMS

The types and principles of operation of pressure water systems are explained in Chapter 7.

Conditions Favorable for Pressure Systems

If natural gravity is not available at reasonable cost and if only moderate amounts of water need to be stored, the pressure system is the logical choice, particularly so where electric power is available for the operation of an automatic pump.

The principal problems of installation of pressure systems are, (1) type of pump to use, (2) capacity of pump, (3) size of pressure tank, (4) location of the system, (5) type and size of pipes to use, (6) installation procedures such as installing the piping and wiring for the motor, and (7) housing and sanitary measures.

Type of pump to use.

The types of pump available for pressure systems are described in Chapter 6. As indicated on pages 92-103, the centrifugal, submersible, turbine, and jet pumps deliver larger volumes of water at low pressures; therefore, if the rate of flow at the source is limited as in the case of a weak shallow well or a spring, these pumps are likely to pump the source dry and cause loss of priming. Furthermore, when the discharge of the pump is greater than the flow into the well even though the well is not pumped dry, the level of the water in the well will drop, thus decreasing the capacity of the pump and increasing the cost of operation. The farther the water must be lifted the more it costs to pump it.

As plunger and piston pumps have a fixed rate of discharge, they can be tailored to the flow of the well. For example, if the rate of flow of the well is 2 gallons per minute a plunger or a piston pump having a discharge capacity of 2 gallons per minute or less can be used without danger of lowering the water level or pumping the well dry. Other types of pumps, such as centrifugals, and submersibles can be used if sensors are installed in the well to stop the pump when the water level drops too low and to start it again when the water level rises.

Capacity of the pump.

If there is plenty of water at the source the pump should be large enough to supply the daily demands as calculated from Table 3-I in 2 hours of pumping. This size with a 42-U.S. gallon tank, will insure adequate water to meet ordinary peak demands. A large-capacity pump is an advantage for fire fighting, small-scale irrigation, filling spray rigs, etc.

As previously indicated, if the supply of water at the source is limited it may be necessary, in order to avoid pumping the source dry, to use a small-capacity pump and a large storage tank. The discharge capacity of the tank plus the capacity of the pump should equal the peak demand. See page 122-135 for tank discharge capacities.

Jet pumps can be used on weak wells without pumping them dry by using a 35-foot (10 m.) drop pipe below the jet. See Fig. 8-4. As suction head increases, the capacity of jet pumps drops off toward zero; therefore, at some point below the jet and within the limits of the 35-foo (10 m.) drop pipe the capacity of the jet will just equal the flow into the well. Although this arrangement will work it may mean pumping a large portion of the water at low efficiency and therefore at greater expense. A submersible pump with water level sensors in the well might be a better choice.

Size of pressure tank.

Pressure storage tanks are available in a wide range of sizes. The most common sizes together with their respective normal discharge capacities are indicated in Table 7-I. If there is plenty of water at the source, if there are no unusually high peak demands, and if the pump is automatic, a 42-U.S. gallon tank is a satisfactory size. Smaller tanks are satisfactory with low peak demands, a large-capacity pump, and a plentiful supply of water. For exceptionally high peak demands or where the water supply is so limited that a very small pump must be used, large tanks in the order of 1000 U.S. gallons (833 Imp. gals.) or more may be needed.

Location of the system.

In general it is best to install the pump and tank close together. This simplifies the plumbing, the wiring, and the controls. Many systems are factory-assembled with pump, tank, and controls in one pack-

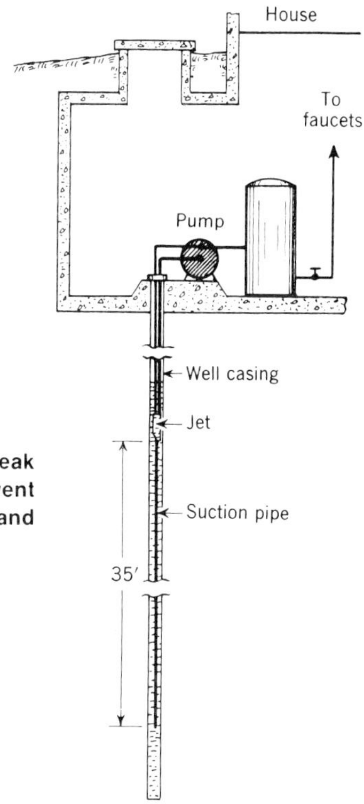

Fig. 8-4. A jet pump installation on a weak well. The long suction pipe will prevent the pump from pumping the well dry and losing its priming.

aged unit as indicated in Figs. 7-8, 7-9, and 7-13.

In areas where freezing temperatures are encountered the pump and tank must be protected from frost. In warm climates they should be protected from sun and rain.

If the system can be housed in an existing building such as a house or a barn, the cost of special housing is eliminated. Where suction lift or distance from the source makes the use of existing housing impractical special housing should be provided. See Fig. 8-8. Here again, using a submersible pump may eliminate the expense of frostproof housing.

Type and size of pipe to use.

As in the case of gravity systems, steel, copper, and plastic piping are used for pressure systems. The type to use should be determined by the existing local circumstances. See Chapter 10 for a description of piping. Drop pipes for conventional deep-well plunger pumps should be made of steel. The size of pipes or tubing to use can be calculated from the friction table on page 279 and will be illustrated later.

The size of suction pipe for shallow-well pumps should not be selected according to the size of the tapped opening on the pump except for short lengths. Use the friction table on page 279 to calculate the correct size. In case it is necessary to throttle the intake for air-volume control, refer to Fig. 7-20.

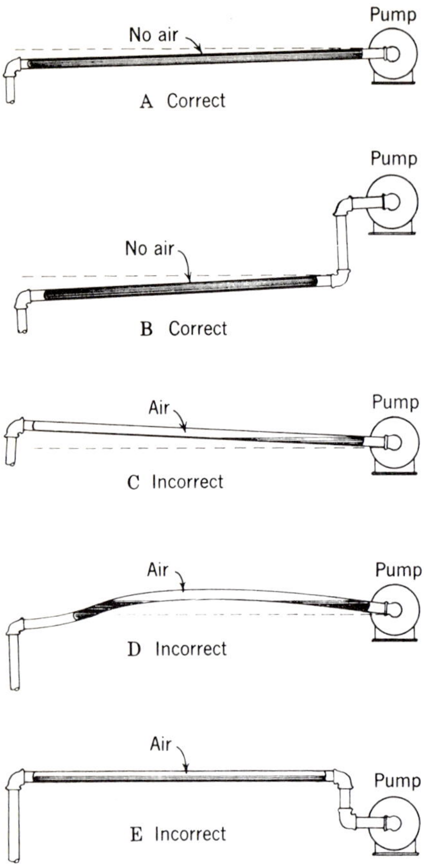

Fig. 8-5. The suction pipe for a pump should be graded continuously downward from the pump to the water as shown at A & B.

The suction pipe should be graded continuously downward from the pump to the water. See Fig. 8-5. High points in the suction line collect air and may cause loss of priming. If a long suction pipe is used on a reciprocating plunger pump a vacuum chamber should be installed on the suction pipe near the pump. The vacuum chamber will reduce pounding noises and will relieve strains on the pump. All joints in a suction line should be airtight. Threaded joints should be carefully "doped" and unions should be absolutely tight. See Job 2. The entire suction line should be as straight as possible. Copper or plastic tubing is ideal for long suction lines because it is available in long lengths without fittings, and can be bent on long sweeping curves to reduce friction losses.

In most cases a foot valve and strainer should be installed on the lower end of suction pipes.

To facilitate repairs on deep-well plunger pumps it is common practice to have the drop pipe larger than the cylinder so the plunger and valves can be removed by means of the plunger rod without pulling the drop pipe. See Figs. 6-14 at *B*.

For well depths beyond 100 feet (30 m.) a wooden plunger rod should be used instead of steel. The wooden rod is more rigid, is not so noisy if it hits the drop pipe, and is lighter than water, therefore tends to float. For wells of considerable depths this difference in weight may make an appreciable difference in the horsepower requirements.

For the same discharge capacities the deep-well pumps require more horsepower than the shallow-well pumps because the water must be lifted through greater distances.

Deep-well jet pumps are usually installed with two pipes into the well as indicated in Figs. 7-23, and 8-7. For small-diameter wells two concentric pipes can be used. The well casing is often used as one of the pipes.

The discharge pipe from the pump to the tank should never be less than ¾ inch. For large-capacity pumps or for long lengths of pipe the size should be calculated from a friction table. See Job 6.

Wiring the motor.

If electric power is used to drive the pump it is very important that the wires be large enough to supply the rated voltage and amperage to the motor. The size of wires to use depends upon (1) the horsepower of the motor, (2) the length of the circuit, and (3) the voltage on the circuit. The wiring should be installed by a compitent electrician and in accordance with the National Fire Insurance Underwriters Code and should include overload and low-voltage protective devices. In areas where electrical storms are common lightning protection should also be provided.

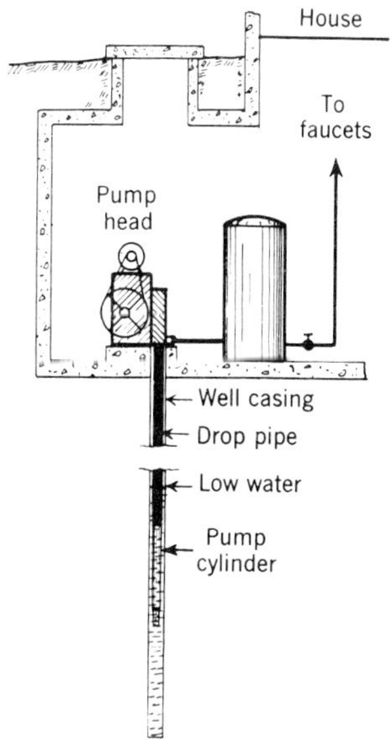

Fig. 8-6. A plunger-type deep-well pump installed on a well close to the building. The well pit opening into the basement makes access easy and provides good ventiliation for the motor and the pumping head. An opening should be provided directly over the well so the drop pipe and pump can be removed for repairs.

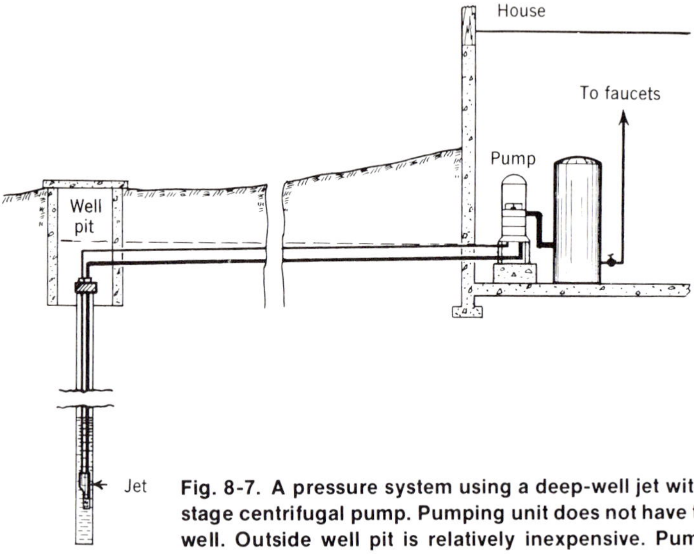

Fig. 8-7. A pressure system using a deep-well jet with a multi-stage centrifugal pump. Pumping unit does not have to be over well. Outside well pit is relatively inexpensive. Pump proper and jet should be selected from manufacturer's Selection Tables. Pressure relief valve not necessary. Well pit should have a drain to surface if possible. See Fig. 8-8 for alternate arrangements of well pit.

Sanitary measures and housing.

Every precaution should be taken to protect the water from contamination or pollution at all points, from the source to the faucets. See Chapter 3. Such matters as well seals, floor drains, ease of cleaning, ventilation, and housing should have special attention. Health officers are usually glad to advise on such matters.

The water system installations shown in this chapter and elsewhere in this book illustrate at least reasonably good sanitary measures. Figure 8-8 illustrates a series of comparative illustrations for pump housing which merit study.

Installation of System Shown in Fig. 8-9

Assumed conditions:

1. Demand for water as calculated from Table 3-I is 600 gallons (500 Imp. gals.) per day.
2. The flow of the well is 2 U.S. gallons (1.7 Imp. gals.) per minute at a water level 10 feet below pump.
3. The storage capacity of the well is 200 gallons. (167 Imp. gals.)
4. Water is potable and not highly corrosive to steel.
5. Horizontal distance from well to pump is 30 feet.
6. Suction lift of pump is 22 feet. (6.7 m.)
7. Freezing temperatures are common in the winter.
8. Electric power is available for operation of the pump.

Selection of the type of pump.

Under these conditions any shallow-well pump or submersible should work if the correct size of pipe is used. One of the packaged units of the types illustrated in Figs. 7-8, 7-9, and 7-13 would be satisfactory. The pump should have a capacity of about 300 gallons per hour.

Size of pressure tank.

As there is plenty of water at the well and as only a house is to be supplied, a 30- or 42-U.S. gallon tank would be satisfactory.

Location.

The logical location for a shallow well pump and tank is in the basement of the house as indicated. This gives frost protection, provides ventilation, and makes wiring easy, and the system is easily accessable for servicing. If a submersible is used the pump would be in the water in the well.

Type of piping.

Steel, copper or plastic piping can be used.

Size of suction pipe.

With a 300-U.S. gallon (250 Imp. gals.) per-hour pump the rate of flow would be 5 U.S. gallons (4 Imp. gals.) per minute. The length of pipe would be 30 feet (9.1 m.) horizontal run plus 10 feet to water plus 5 feet under water plus elbow and strainer, or the equivalent of about 50 feet. (15.2 m.) As the pump has a suction lift of 22 feet (6.7 m.) there would be 12 feet (3.7 m.) of suction lift to overcome friction head. Referring to the friction table on page 279 we see that with 5 gallons per minute a ¾-inch pipe would be adequate. However, if 1-inch pipe is used the pump will have less work to do and if a jet, centrifugal, or submersible pump is used the rate of pumping would be higher. For these reasons 1-inch pipe should be used.

Accessories.

The system should be equipped with an automatic pressure switch, an air-volume control, either a foot valve in the well or a check valve at the pump, and if a piston pump is used a safety valve should be used on the discharge side of the pump. The motor should have overload and low-voltage protection.

Installation procedure.

If the well is in poor repair it should be waterproofed down 6 or 8 feet (2 or 4 m.) from the top to eliminate surface water, should have a tight cover, and the ground surface should be graded up to the cover as indicated in Fig. 8-9. After repairing the well the water should be tested and chlorinated if necessary.

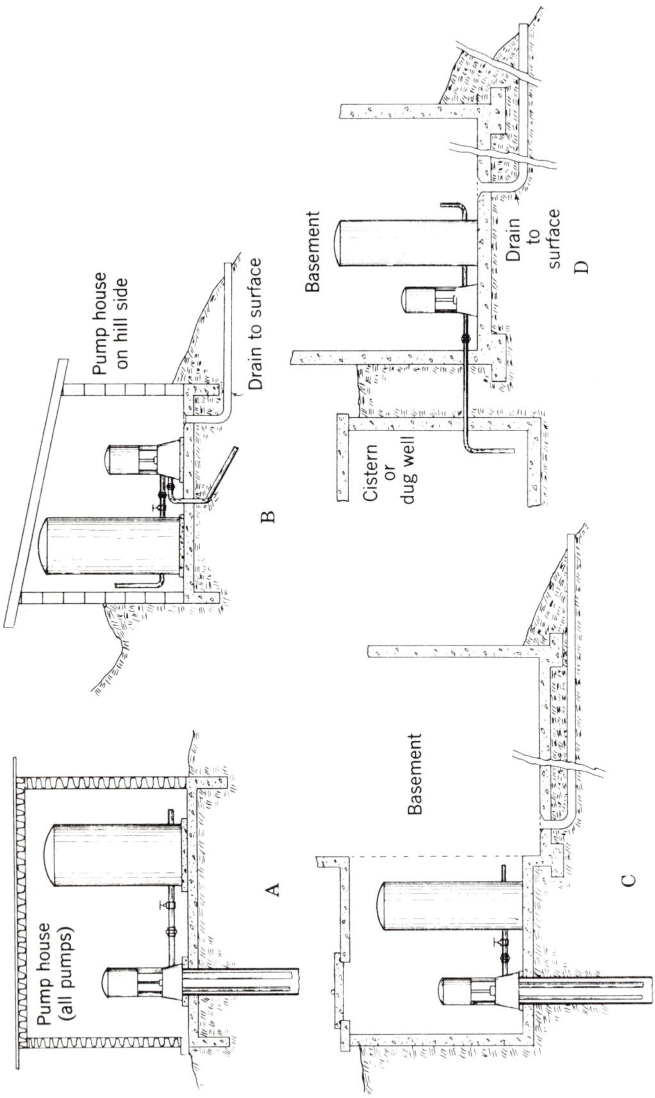

Courtesy Prof. G.E. Henderson, Athens, Ga.

Fig. 8-8. See page 144 for legend.

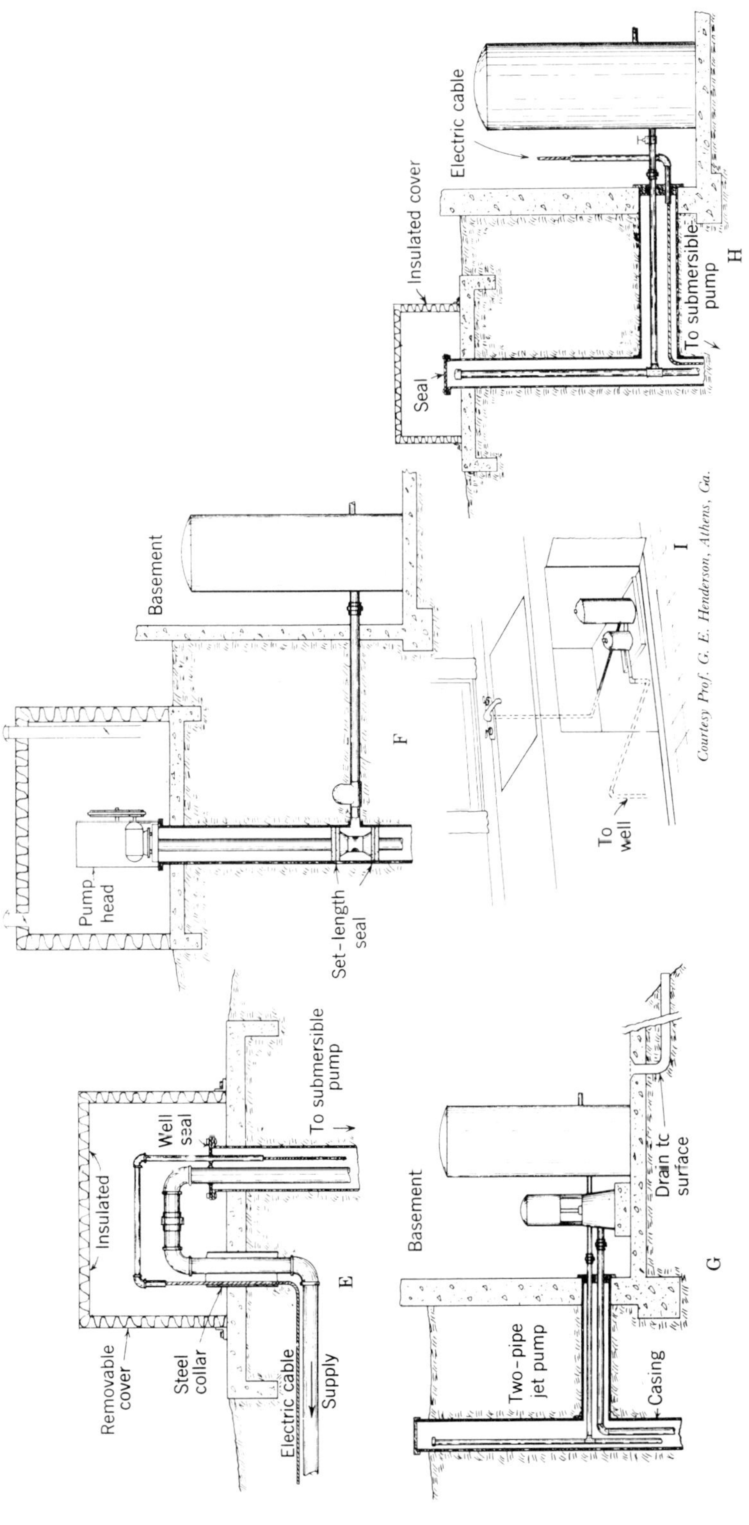

Fig. 8-8. See page 144 for legend.

Courtesy Prof. G.E. Henderson, Athens, Ga.

Fig. 8-8. Types of pump protection enclosures and their relative merits.

RECOMMENDED

A — Surface pump house.

Protection from temperature extremes: Excellent if well insulated or automatically heated.

Drainage: Excellent.

Ventilation: Can be excellent through open doors and windows or through rafter vents.

Ease of cleaning and ease of servicing: Excellent.

Adaptable for pumping from: All sources of water.

B — Recessed pump house.

Has some qualities as pumphouse A. Used mostly for pumping from springs, ponds, and lakes.

C — Basement extension.

Protection from temperature extremes: Excellent, especially if basement is heated.

Drainage: Excellent if basement is well drained.

Ventilation and ease of cleaning: Excellent.

Ease of servicing: Excellent if opening on top of extension is over well and large enough to pass equipment through it easily.

Adaptable for pumping from: All sources, but especially from deep wells close to building.

D — Basement installation.

Protection from temperature extremes: Excellent.

Drainage: Excellent if basement is well drained.

Ventilation, ease of cleaning, and ease of servicing: Excellent.

Adaptable for pumping from: All sources with shallow well or jet pumps.

E — Surface-connected submersible.

Protection from temperature extremes: Excellent if well insulated or automatically heated.

Drainage: Excellent, but not much of a problem with this type of pump.

Ventilation: Not a problem.

Ease of cleaning and ease of servicing: Excellent.

Adaptable for pumping from: Wells of 4-inch diameter or larger, but especially wells over 100 feet deep.

F — Pitless frostproof set length.

Protection from temperatures extremes: Excellent as water does not rise above set length seal. Pump head is exposed to temperature extremes unless cover is insulated.

Drainiage: Excellent, but not much of a problem.

Ventilation: Not much of a problem except for cooling in hot weather. If vent pipes are used dampers in vents can be set as needed.

Ease of cleaning: Excellent.

Ease of servicing: Excellent except in case of deep snow.

Adaptable for pumping from: Steel cased wells with deep-well plunger pumps.

G — Basement installation with extended well casing.

Protection from temperature extremes, drainage, ventilation, ease of cleaning, and ease of servicing: Excellent.

Adaptable for pumping from: All types of drilled wells with shallow-well and jet pumps.

H — Subsurface-connected submerisble.

Protection from temperature extremes and drainage: Excellent.

Ventilation: No problem.

Ease of cleaning, and ease of servicing: Excellent.

Adaptable for pumping from: Wells 4 inches in diameter or larger, but especially from wells over 100 feet deep.

I — Undersink installation.

Protection from temperature extremes: Excellent if room is always heated in cold weather.

Drainage: Should have a drip pan under pump and tank to carry stuffing box drip and condensation to outside.

Ventilation: Usually satisfactory.

Ease of cleaning: Satisfactory.

Ease of servicing: Satisfactory if connected with unions for ease of removal.

Noise: May be objectionable unless pump is exceptionally quiet.

Adaptable for pumping from: Any source with shallow-well or jet pumps.

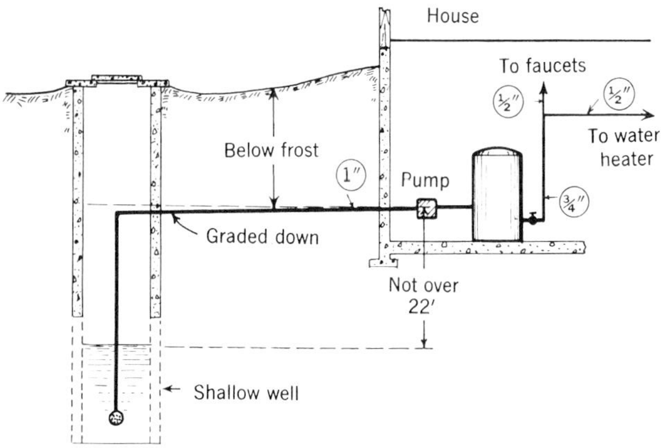

Fig. 8-9. A pressure system for a shallow well or cistern near a building. Well can be dug, drilled, bored, or driven. This same system can be used to pump from a spring catchment basin.

If the soil is free of stones it may be possible to drive a steel suction pipe from the house to the well; otherwise a trench must be dug. In either case the suction pipe must be placed below the frost level and should be graded continuously downward to the water. The pipe should be cast in the concrete or the hole in the well wall where the pipe enters should be sealed with cement mortar or asphalt. Enclosing the pipe in a line of tile sealed at both ends makes replacement easier.

The pump and tank should rest on a solid base such as a concrete floor or slab. The wiring should be large enough and should be installed according to the Underwriters Code. The discharge pipe from the tank should be ¾ inch to the point where the tap is made for supplying the water heater.

Installation of System Shown in Fig. 8-10

Assumed conditions:

1. Demand for water as calculated from Table 3-I is 1000 U.S. gallons (833 Imp. gals.) per day.
2. Source of water is a shallow well with low water level 35 feet (10.7 m.) below basement floor. Pump is 10 feet (3 m.) above water in well.
3. Well is located 90 feet (27.4 m.) from the house.
4. Rate of flow of well is 4 U.S. gallons (3.3 Imp. gals.) per minute.
5. Water is potable.
6. Desired rate of flow at the faucets is 12 gallons per minute.
7. No exceptionally high peak demands.
8. Faucets are 30 feet (9 m.) above low water level in the pressure tank.
9. Freezing conditions in winter.
10. Electric power available.

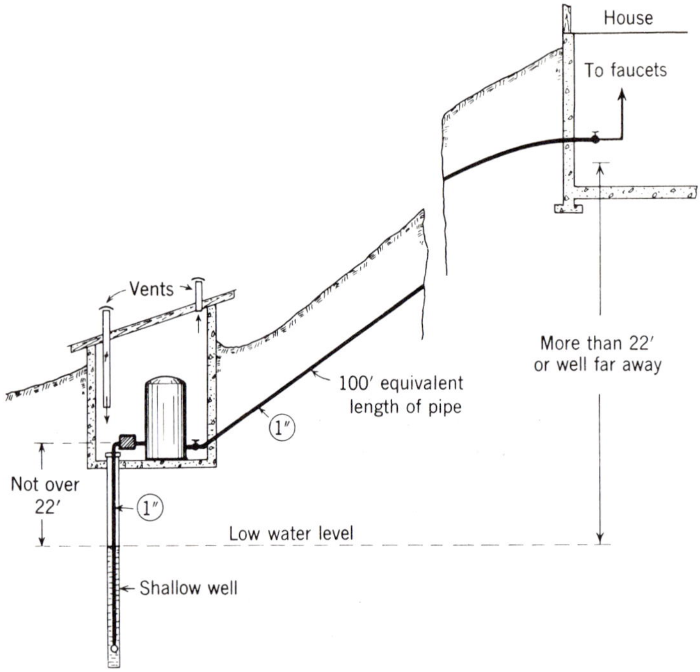

Fig. 8-10. A pressure system for a shallow well or a spring which is either too far away from or too far below the buildings to install the pump in the building. A jet or submersible pump installation as illustrated in Figs. 8-7 and 8-11 could be used on such a source instead of this shallow-well pump.

Good ventilation in the pump house can be had by means of 3- or 4-inch pipe installed through the roof as indicated, or through the sides of the pump house. The air inlet pipe should extend toward the floor and the air outlet extend through the roof or side wall near the highest point. A damper in the inlet pipe makes it possible to control ventilation in extremely cold weather to prevent freezing.

Type and size of pump to use.

Most any of the shallow-well packaged units or a submersible could be used here. The capacity of the pump should be about 500 gallons per hour for a daily demand of 1000 U.S. gallons. (833 Imp. gals.)

Storage tank.

A 42-gallon tank would be satisfactory.

Location of pump and tank.

As the building is beyond the suction range of a shallow-well pump we will place the packaged unit in a pump house built over the well. The pump house should be frostproofed (or heated) and ventilated as shown. Wiring will have to be extended from the building to the pump house.

An alternate arrangement would be a jet pump with the pump and tank in the building or a submersible pump with tank in the building. This would save on the cost of the frostproof structure at the well.

Kind and size of piping.

The suction pipe can be of steel, copper, or plastic. The size of pipe from tank to building should be calculated from the friction table as follows: The distance is 90 feet. Allowing 10 feet for friction in valves and fittings we have an equivalent length of pipe of 100 feet. The rate of flow is to be 12 gallons per minute. The vertical distance from tank to faucets is 30 feet.

With a pressure range of 40 to 20 pounds the minimum pressure of 20 pounds would equal a head of 46 feet; 46 feet minus 30 feet of gravity head leaves 16 feet of head available to force water to the building. Referring to the friction table J-6-II-A we find that 1-inch pipe would require 15.76 feet of head and therefore would be the correct size.

Referring to the metric table J-6-II-B, we find that 1-inch pipe having a rate of flow 10 Imperial gallons per minute would require 4.80 meters of head. As we have 4.88 meters of head available the 1-inch pipe would be the correct size.

Wiring for motor.

The size of the wires should be determined and the installation made according to the Underwriters Code.

If overhead wires are used to the pump house they should be supported high enough above the ground to clear farm machinery, trucks, etc, which might pass under them. If underground cable is used it can be buried in a trench.

There should be a manual cutout switch and fuses in the pump house. The motor should have overload protection.

Installation of System Shown in Fig. 8-11

Assumed conditions:

1. Well 210 feet (64.00 m.) deep and located 40 feet from the tank.
2. Flow of well is 3 gallons (2.5 Imp. gals.) per minute when water level is at 180 feet (54.86 m.) below the surface.
3. Water rises and stands 100 feet (30.48 m.) deep in well when not being pumped.
4. Well hole is 6 inches (15.24 cm.) in diameter.
5. Well is free of sand.
6. Demand for water is 1200 U.S. gallons (1000 Imp. gals.) per day.
7. Peak demand is 200 gallons per hour.
8. Freezing conditions in winter.
9. Electric power available.

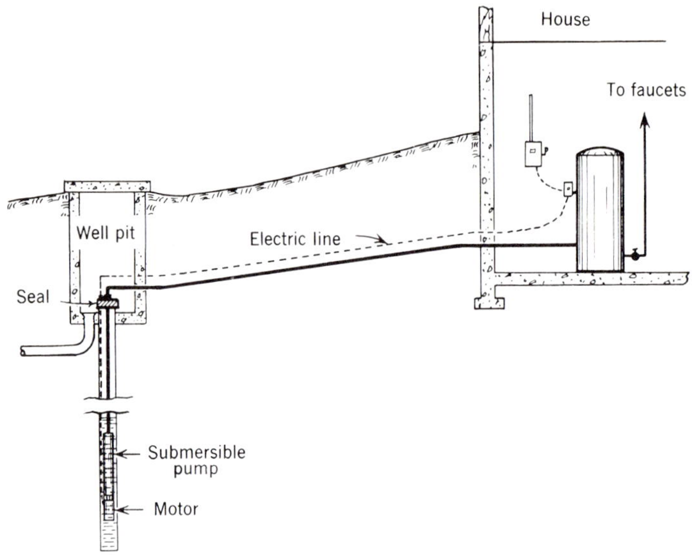

Fig. 8-11. A pressure system using a submersible pump. Pump and motor are in water in the well; therefore operation noises are reduced to a minimum. Good for deep wells to 400 feet. Pump should be selected from manufacturer's Selection tables.

Type and size of pump.

A submersible pump is indicated, but a deep-well jet or a reciprocating deep-well plunger pump could be used. To pump a day's supply in 2 hours of pumping would require a 600-gallon-per-hour pump.

Installation of the System Shown in Fig. 8-12.

There are numerous homes and cottages around lake shores and along the banks of streams where the lake or stream water is used for domestic purposes and for irrigation. Fig. 8-12 illustrates a practical method of pumping the water with a submersible pump. If the pump is to be used only in warm weather the heating cable would not be necessary. The pump can be removed and the pipes drained when there is danger of freezing.

The home is about 100 feet from the water and is roughly 30 feet above the lake level. Near the water the bed rock is exposed so that the pipe could not be buried, therefore some means had to be devised to keep the pipe from freezing. The engineer who installed the system solved this problem by, (1) removing the foot valve from the pump and installing a standard check valve in the pipeline in the house basement and a snifter valve on the pump side of the check valve. See inset at *A*. This arrangement allows the pipe to drain from the check valve to the water line at the lake. The check valve holds the tank pressure. When the pipe has drained the snifter valve closes. Also this

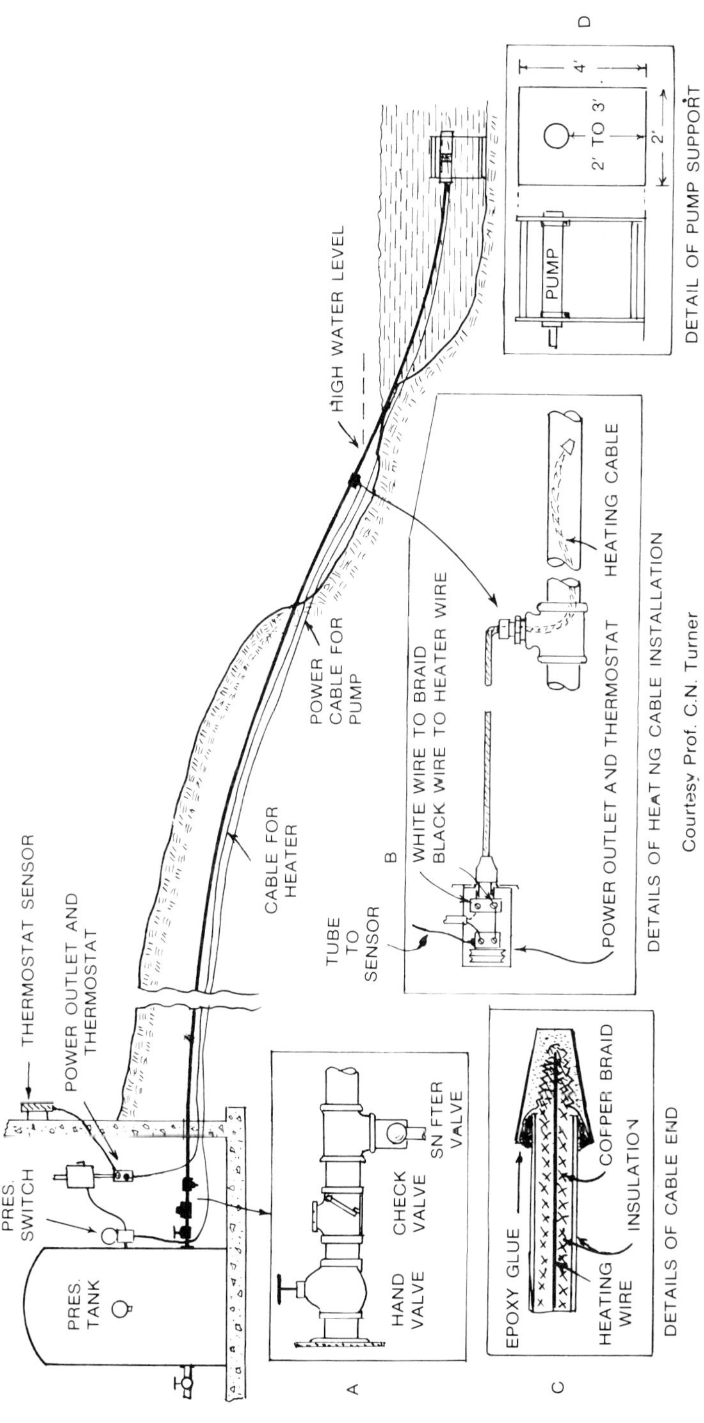

Courtesy Prof. C.N. Turner

Fig. 8-12. An illustration of a water system using a submersible pump for a year-around home on the shore of a lake in New York State. It has been in service, at this writing, for 16 years and has given very satisfactory service.

arrangement supplies adequate air to the pressure tank because the pump forces the air in the pipe into the tank each time it starts. A blow-off type of air volume control releases excess air. (2) As the pipe will not drain below the water level in the lake the water in the pipe at the shore line would freeze in severe cold weather. The heating cable solved that problem. The heating cable was installed in the pipe thru an Appelton fitting in a tee located just above the high water line and is supplied with current thru a waterproof cable laid along the pipe line to the pump. A thermostat sensor installed where it is exposed to outside air temperatures actuates a thermostat in the basement to turn the current on for the heater cable when freezing temperatures prevail. The cable is a commercially available cable with an electrically insulated heating wire in the center, a copper braided armor protects the insulation and a waterproof outer covering keeps the water out. A standard waterproof cable supplies current to the heater cable at the tee. The heater cable extends only from the tee toward the pump to a point well below freezing range.

The copper braided armor serves as the return wire from the outer end of the heating wire. This was accomplished by twisting the copper braid around the bared end of the heating wire and securing the connection by means of a threaded wire nut sealed with epoxy glue. (See inset C).

The submersible pump is supported on a marine plywood rack to keep it off of the bottom of the lake. See inset D. The pump is fastened to the rack by means of clamps. The pump should be located far enough from shore to avoid roily water, deep enough to avoid surface ice and at least 2 ft. below low water level.

To protect the power cable to the pump from abrasion by shelf ice at the water line the cable was run through a length of old steel pipe strapped to the water pipe at the water line.

If the soil were deep enough along the shore the water pipe could be buried below frost line all of the way and the heating cable would be unnecessary.

Installation of System Shown in Fig. 8-13

This figure shows an arrangement for pumping from a well and a cistern.

Assumed conditions:

1. Low water level in well is 15 feet (4.57 m.) below pump.
2. Flow of well is 2 U.S. gallons (1.66 Imp. gals.) per minute.
3. Normal stored volume in well is 300 U.S. gallons. (250 Imp gals.)
4. Demand for cold water is 600 U.S. gallons (500 Imp. gals.) per day.
5. Peak demand for any hour is 100 U.S. gallons. (83 Imp. gals.)
6. Freezing conditions in winter.
7. Cistern in basement with storage capacity of 2800 U.S. gallons (2333+ Imp. gals.) to be used for hot-water supply only.

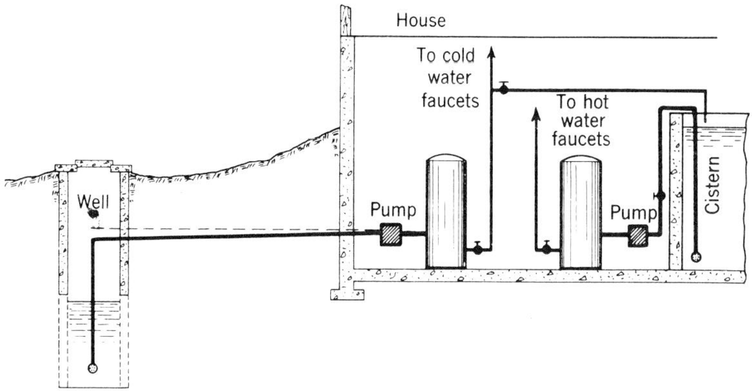

Fig. 8-13. A combination of pressure systems for pumping from two sources such as a well and a cistern. The well water is supplied to the cold-water faucets and the cistern water to the hot-water faucets. Submersible pumps could be used in either installation.

8. Demand for hot water is 80 U.S. gallons (66.66 Imp. gals.) per day.

Type and size of pump.

Any of the shallow-well or submersible pumps could be used on either source. The well pump should have a capacity of about 300 U.S. gallons (250 Imp gals.) per hour. The cistern pump can be of the smallest size available.

The pressure tank for the well water should be a 42-gallon size. A small tank or one of the tankless systems could be used on the cistern. The suction pipe to the well should be 1-inch. If a small-capacity pump is used on the cistern, a ¾-inch or even ½-inch pipe could be used. The small suction pipe on the cistern would increase the suction head on the pump and thus make the air-volume control work better. Otherwise a throttling valve should be installed in the suction line as shown.

A pipe and valve from the well system to the cistern makes it possible to fill the cistern from the well if the cistern supply gets low. This means pumping the hot-water supply twice, but that is better than interconnecting the two systems, as the latter means mixing of the waters so that the cistern water could contaminate the well water.

INSTALLATION OF SYSTEMS FOR FLOWING ARTESIAN WELL

Installation of System Shown in Fig. 8-14.

Assumed conditions:

1. Well flows 4 U.S. gallons (3.3 Imp. gals.) per minute at 10 pounds' pressure at top of casing.

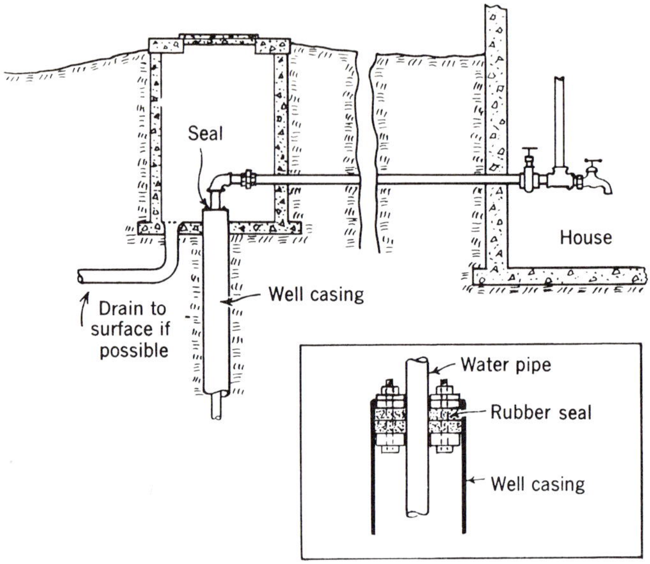

Fig. 8-14. A capped flowing artesian well. A seal for the top of the casing is shown in the inset.

2. Well is 60 feet (18.29 m.) from house.
3. Highest faucet is 10 feet (3.05 m.) above the top of casing.
4. There are 25 feet (7 m.) of pipe inside of building to the faucets.

Size of pipe to use.

The 10 pounds' pressure at the top of casing is equal to 23 feet (7 m.) of head. (10 pounds × 2.3 feet per pound.) This 23 feet (7 m.) minus the 10 feet (3.05 m.) to the faucet leaves 13 feet (3.96 m.) of head to be lost in friction in the pipe and fittings. Total length of pipe is 85 feet; (25.9 m.) allowing for friction losses in the fittings and valves the equivalent length of pipe would be approximately 100 feet. (30.48 m.)

Referring to the friction table J-II-A on page 279 we find that with a flow of 4 gallons per minute through ¾-inch pipe the loss of head due to friction would be 7.0 feet. As we have 13 feet (3.96 m.) of head available the ¾-inch pipe would be adequate.

The well should be capped with a watertight seal as shown in the inset. The piping from the well to the house can be steel, copper, or plastic.

Referring to the metric table J-II-B we find that the flow of 3.3 Imperial gallons per minute thru ¾-inch pipe the loss of head due to friction would be 2.3 meters. As we have 3.96 meters of head available the ¾-inch pipe would be adequate.

Maintenance of Water Systems 9

The fact that a water system is satisfactory when first installed is no guarantee that it will remain that way indefinitely. The owner must keep it in repair and maintain good sanitary conditions in order to assure a satisfactory supply at all times.

MAINTENANCE OF GRAVITY SYSTEMS

Assuming that the source of water has been correctly developed, the principal maintenance problem of gravity systems is to prevent leaks and to maintain an adequate flow through the pipes. Leaks of any kind should be carefully avoided especially where water is in limited supply. Frost or ice may crack a storage tank or reservoir, sometimes underground, and allow water to seep away unnoticed. Likewise, underground pipes may in time leak at joints or from holes rusted through the pipe. Such leaks can sometimes be detected by looking for wet spots along the pipeline. However, a small leak may not produce such evidence. In case of an acute shortage of water, small leaks become important and should be repaired even if it means considerable digging to find them. The best assurance against leaks and other troubles is to use the finest materials available and to install them correctly in the first place.

Leaky valves, faucets, toilets, automatic waterers, etc., can waste a very considerable amount of water in 24 hours. See Fig. J-4-1, page 264. Such devices should be kept in good repair at all times. Jobs 4 and 5 give instructions on such repairs.

Some ground waters cause excessive corrosion and/or scale deposits on the inside of pipes, thus reducing the rate of flow. Also, iron bacteria sometimes grow in steel pipe to such an extent that the flow is practically shut off. The best remedy for these conditions is to replace the old pipe with new, preferably with plastic or copper tubing.

MAINTENANCE OF PRESSURE SYSTEMS

Pressure systems with pumps, automatic controls, safety devices, etc., are more complicated than gravity systems, therefore troubles

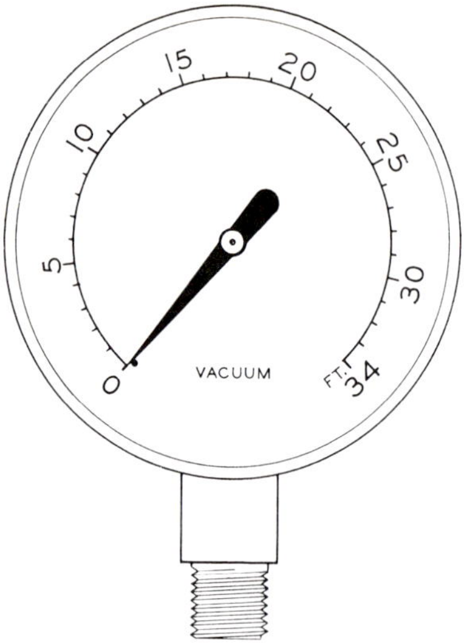

Fig. 9-1. A vacuum gauge calibrated in feet of suction lift.

with them are sometimes more difficult to diagnose. Table 9-I presents the more common troubles together with suggestions for remedies.

Use of vacuum gauge for locating suction pipe troubles.

A vacuum gauge is useful in checking priming and suction pipe troubles on shallow-well pumps. The gauge should be marked in terms of feet or meters of suction head as indicated in Fig. 9-1. It should be installed on the suction side of the pump, either on the pump itself or in pipe *T* near the pump as shown in Fig. 9-2.

Use of vacuum gauge in priming.

With the pump primed and running, the needle on the gauge dial should advance slowly until the pump is delivering water. As long as the needle advances do not stop the pump.

If the needle stops advancing and no water is delivered stop the pump and observe the needle. If it drops back to zero there is probably an appreciable air leak somewhere in the suction pipe or in the pump. If the pump delivers water erratically and the gauge needle fluctuates there is probably a *small* air leak or the water level at the source has dropped below the end of the suction pipe.

If the needle fails to advance at all, (1) the pump may not be properly primed, (2) the suction line may have a *large* air leak, (3) the stuffing box may be too loose, or (4) the well may be dry.

If the gauge advances to 25 feet (7.6 m) or greater and no water is delivered, (1) the water level may be too low for the pump, (2) the suction line may be plugged, or (3) the foot valve may be stuck.

Use of Vacuum Gauge for Locating Pump Troubles

If air leaks are suspected because of a decreased rate of flow from the pump, run the pump until it is delivering water; then stop it and observe the gauge. If the needle remains at a fixed reading above zero there are no leaks. If the needle drops slowly a leak is indicated.

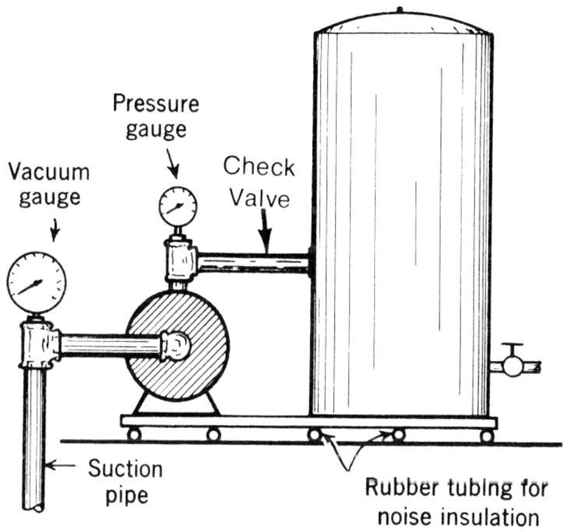

Fig. 9-2. A vacuum gauge installed, either permanently or temporarily, on a pump suction pipe for the purpose of diagnosing pump troubles. Shown also are rubber tubes inserted under the system for dampening pump noises. This is particularly effective if the pump rests on a wooden floor.

If the gauge remains at a fixed reading with the pump stopped it will indicate the approximate number of feet or meters of elevation of the pump above the water level. For shallow-well pumps this should not be over 25 feet (7.6 m); for some pumps, not over 15 feet (4.6 m). If the pump is of the jet, centrifugal, or turbine type a high suction head may account for reduced delivery rate.

The difference between a gauge reading when the pump is running with a normal discharge and when it has stopped indicates approximately the number of feet or meters of suction head lost due to friction in the suction line. If the difference in readings is greater than 5 feet (1.52 m) the friction losses may be enough to reduce the delivery of the pump. The remedy is a larger suction pipe. An old suction pipe may have so filled with scale and rust that the friction losses have greatly increased and thus reduced the output of the pump.

TABLE 9-I

PRESSURE-TYPE WATER SYSTEM TROUBLES AND THEIR REMEDIES*

Trouble	Likely Cause of Trouble	Remedy
1. Pump motor fails to start	Blown fuse or circuit breaker open	Renew fuse or reset circuit breaker. Do not overfuse the circuit
	or	
	Pressure switch not working	Diaphragm may need replacing. Breaker points in switch may be burned or dirty. The tube connecting the switch to pump or tank may be plugged with scale or ice
	or	
	A break in the wiring	Repair the circuit wires
	or	
	Power off	Check by turning on lights. Call power company and report trouble
	or	
	Motor may be burned out, or its starting switch out of order	Inspect and repair motor. This should be done by an experienced motor service man
	or	
	On jet, centrifugal, turbine, or rotary pumps the stuffing box may be binding	This can be checked by turning the shaft by hand. Loosen the packing nut and free the shaft. The nut should be loose enough to allow a slow seepage of water past the packing. The water will serve as a lubricant
	or	
	Scale may be lodged in the impeller housing	Take the pump apart and clean out scale. If the impeller has been damaged it should renewed
	or	
	Pump may have ice in it	Thaw out pump with warm water. Do not use a flame as it may damage pump. Check pump for damage by ice
2. Motor overload switch trips frequently	Motor overloaded due to binding in the pump	Turn pump by hand to see if it is binding. Trouble may be in the stuffing box, in the cylinder or around the impeller
	or	
	Low-voltage condition	Check the voltage at the meter and at the pump while pump is running. If voltage is significantly lower at the pump (10% or more) the trouble is likely to be due to inadequate wiring to the pump. If the voltage is low at the meter the voltage may be down on the powerline. This should be reported to the power company
	or	
	With submersibles, jets and centrifugals the tank pressure may be set too high for the pump so it does not shut off	Lower the tank pressure by adjustment on on the pressure switch
	or	
	Motor connect to wrong voltage, i.e., 115 v instead of 230 v	Check the wiring connections and change if necessary
	or	
	Motor operating in a hot place without good ventilation	Ventilate and insulate the pump house
3. Pump runs but delivers no water	No water at the source. Well dry	Clean and repair well, or develop a new source or sources of water. See Chapter 3
	or	
	Level of water has dropped below suction distance of pump	Can be checked with vacuum gauge or with weighted string. Allow well to fill up or lower pump
	or	
	Well may contain excess amounts of gas or air	Start and stop pump several times

*Working on live wiring near plumbing is especially dangerous. Turn off the current before touching the wires.

TABLE 9-I (continued)

Trouble	Likely Cause of Trouble	Remedy
	Pump has lost ist priming	Can be checked with vacuum gauge. Prime the pump. Most pumps have a priming opening on the discharge side. Follow manufacturer's instructions for priming. If the pump repeatedly loses its priming it may be periodically pumping the well dry, there may be a leak in the suction line, the suction line may have a high point where air accumulates, or the foot valve check valve may be leaking
	or	
	One or more pump valves held open by trash or scale (on reciprocating pumps)	Remove valves and inspect for trouble. With deep-well plunger pumps this may mean pulling the pump cylinder or plunger and valves out of the well
	or	
	With a jet pump the jet may be plugged with trash or scale	Remove jet and clean
	or	
	With a jet or centrifugal pump the impeller housing may be filled with scale or sand	Take pump apart and clean. Install a sand trap on suction line
	or	
	The suction pipe may be plugged with scale or iron bacteria growth or sediment	Can be checked with vacuum gauge. Remove suction pipe and clean or renew
	or	
	The pump cylinder may be cracked (reciprocating pumps)	Renew the cylinder
	or	
	The pump leathers may be worn out (reciprocating pumps)	Renew the leathers
	or	
	The valves or valve seat may be worn or corroded	Renew valves and repair or renew seats
	or	
	With a deep-well plunger pump the plunger rod may be broken	This trouble would be indicated by the pump running freer and probably quieter. Turn the pump over by hand and note if there is resistance on the upstroke. Broken rods must be renewed and this usually means pulling the drop pipe and cylinder out of the well
	or	
	Shutoff valve may be closed	Open vavle
	or	
	On a new installation, motor may be turning in wrong direction	Check this with instruction manual
	or	
	With jets the pressure regulation may not be set high enough to operate the jet at the existing water level	Check the pressure and adjust the regulator according to instruction manual
	or	
	With submerged turbine pumps the pump may be too deep, the propeller shaft may be broken, or the water level may have dropped below the lowest impeller	Check the pump installation and operation against its specifications. Check level of water in the well
4. Pump runs but delivers only a small amount of water (pump runs for unusually long periods of time)	Pump valves leaking	Repair valves
	or	
	Well not yielding enough water	Decrease demands or establish new sources of water
	or	
	Cracked cylinder (plunger or piston pump)	Renew cylinder

TABLE 9-I (Continued)

Trouble	Likely Cause of Trouble	Remedy
	or	
	Plunger leathers badly worn (plunger and piston pumps)	Renew leathers
	or	
	With submersibles, jet or shallow-well centrifugals the water level may have dropped, thus decreasing the capacity of the pump	Lower jet, or pump, or both if possible. Otherwise reduce demands or obtain better source
	or	
	Impeller may be worn	Renew impeller
	or	
	Strainer and/or impeller plugged with scale	Remove and clean
	or	
	Well may contain excessive amounts of gas	Start and stop pump several times
	or	
	Air is in the suction line	Can check this with vacuum gauge. Reduce tank pressure and pump out air if possible. Otherwise repriming may be necessary. If this trouble reoccurs frequently check the suction pipe for leaks and be sure that it is graded continuously downward from the pump. See Fig. 8-5
	or	
	On belt-driven pump, a loose belt will allow the pump to slow down as the pressure builds up	Tighten or renew the belt. See Fig. 9-3 for instructions
	or	
	There is low voltage at the motor. Low voltage will cause the pump to run slower or even to stop (the most common cause of low-voltage conditions is inadequate wiring)	Enlarge the wiring to the pump, or remove other loads on the same circuit or switch from 115 v to 230 v, or get power company to improve voltage on property
	or	
	Screen or foot valve may be obstructed	Remove and clean
	or	
	Suction pipes are too small	Can be checked with vacuum gauge. Install larger pipes
	or	
	Tank pressure is set too high	Lower pressure range
	or	
	With jet pumps scale may be lodged in jet nozzle	Remove and clean jet
	or	
	Foot valve may be out of order	Repair foot valve
	or	
	Pressure regulator for jet may be set too low for existing water level	Set regulator for higher pressure

TABLE 9-I (Continued)

Trouble	Likely Cause of Trouble	Remedy
5. Pump starts and stops to often	Not enough air in pressure tank. Tank waterlogged	For shallow-well pumps, repair or renew air-volume control device. This should include inspection of the Schrader valve on the pump where the air tube is connected. This valve sometimes sticks. If it is defective and must be replaced, be sure to replace it with a *water system valve* and not a tire valve. See page 120 for instructions on this
	or	For deep-well plunger pumps, the air pump may be out of order. Repair air pump
	There is a leaky foot or check valve which allows the water to run back to the well	Repair valve
	or	
	There is a bad leak in the plumbing which runs water to waste. This is especially noticeable with small pressure tanks	Repair the leak. If the leak is underground, considerable digging may be required to locate it
	or	
	Tank may be too small for the demands	Install larger tank
6. Jet pump fails to pump up to full pressure and shut off	Pressure regulator for jet set too low	Set regulator for higher pressure
	or	
	Scale lodged in jet nozzle	Clean jet
	or	
	Water level in well has dropped too low	Decrease demands, obtain a better source, or lower the jet
	or	
	Tank pressure is set too high for pump	Reduce tank pressure by adjusting pressure switch
7. Air spurts from faucet	Too much air in tank	Repair air-volume control device, or check for air leaks on suction side of pump, or be sure well is not being pumped dry periodically
8. Bad leak at stuffing box	Packing worn out or loose	Renew or tighten packing. Leave packing nut loose enough to allow a slow drip of water. The water serves as a lubricant
	or	
	There is a badly scored plunger rod or pump shaft	Renew plunger rod or pump shaft
9. Water leak at air pump on deep-well plunger pump	Check valve in bottom of air pumps stuck open	Repair air check valve
10. Pump is noisy	Pump is waterlogged, or there is a lack of air in expansion chamber of pump if plunger type	Repair air-volume control for shallow-well pump, or air pump on deep-well pump
	or	
	There is a long suction pipe with no vacuum chamber at pump	Install vacuum chamber on suction pipe near the pump

TABLE 9-I (Continued)

Trouble	Likely Cause of Trouble	Remedy
	or	
	Bearings or other working parts of the pump are loose	Tighten or renew parts
	or	
	Motor or pump is loose on mountings	Tighten mountings
	or	
	With deep-well plunger pumps having a steel plunger rod the rod may be slapping against the drop pipe	Use a wooden rod or install guides for rod or straighten drop pipe if crooked
	or	
	With jet, centrifugal, and turbine pumps there may be air in the pump due to leak in suction pipe, or air-volume control out of order, or low water level in the well	Can check with vacuum gauge. Repair air leak or avoid pumping well too low. A 35-foot (10.66 m.) suction pipe below the jet or the pump as indicated in Fig. 8-4 may be the solution
	Some centrifugals and turbines normally make a whirring noise when running. This cannot be avoided	This type of pump noise, and to a certain extent all pump noises, can be reduced by inserting a length of high-pressure rubber hose or plastic tubing in the pipe line between the pump and tank or on the discharge side of the tank as indicated in Fig. 9-4. This reduces the telegraphing of the noise through the plumbing system. The rubber hose will be most effective if installed with a loop or a 90-degree bend in it as shown in Fig. 9-4 at B, C, and D. If the pump rests on a wooden floor rubber pads or lengths of old garden hose placed under the pump will insulate pump noises from the floor. Use a submersible pump

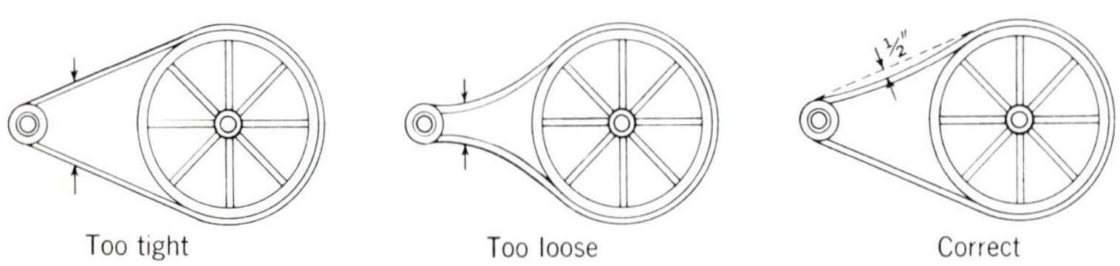

Fig. 9-3. Belt adjustment. "V" belts of lengths usually used on water systems should be adjusted so that one side of the belt will push down about ½ inch with light finger pressure on it as indicated on the right.

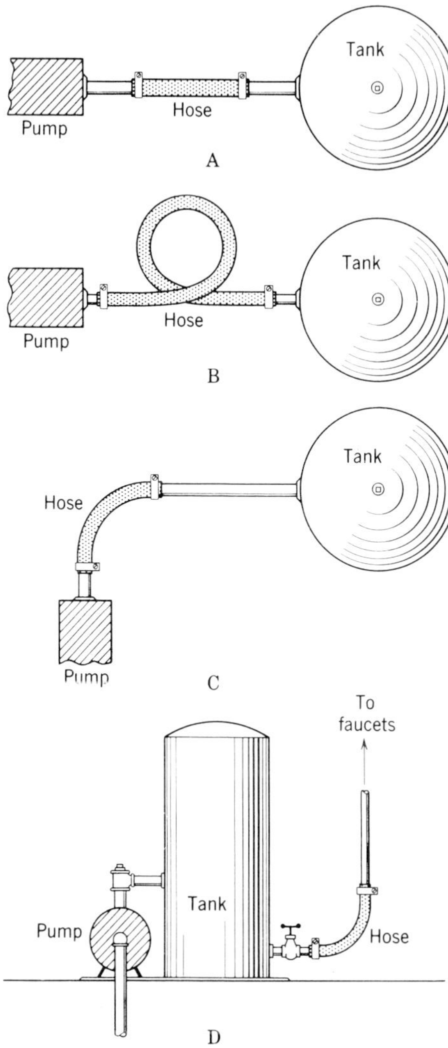

Fig. 9-4. A length of high-pressure rubber hose or plastic tubing inserted in a pipeline will reduce pump noises in the plumbing system. Where the pump and tank are mounted separately and far enough apart the hose should be placed between the pump and tank as shown at A, B, and C. A loop or bend in the hose as at B and C is most effective. If the pump and tank are close coupled or mounted on a common metal base the hose can be placed as at D.

Plumbing Systems for Homes and Farms 10

A complete plumbing system consists of the *supply plumbing* which carries the water from the source to all of the points of use, and the *waste plumbing* which carries the waste water, after use, to a disposal area.

Plumbing systems are of such a nature that they can be installed piecemeal if necessary — as might be the case when remodeling with limited funds. Before such a procedure is started a careful plan should be made of the ultimate completed project so that each successive step can be made as a permanent improvement. This should include the type and size of pump and tank which will eventually be needed.

The order of procedure for piecemeal installation is, of course, a matter of choice. The following order is offered as a logical one:

1. Install a kitchen sink with grease trap and disposal tile. See Fig. 10-1. This will eliminate the work of carrying wastes out by hand and will provide better sanitation. Later when a complete sewage disposal system is installed the discharge from the grease trap can be directed to the septic tank, as indicated in the inset of Fig. 10-2.
2. Install a pump to deliver a supply of cold water at the sink. This will eliminate the work of carrying water in. A hand pump, or preferably an automatic pressure system, can be used for this purpose.
3. Provide for a hot-water supply. See Figs. 10-1 and 10-2.
4. Install a bathroom and sewage disposal equipment to complete the system as indicated in Fig. 10-2.

SUPPLY PLUMBING

The supply plumbing consists of (1) the piping from the water source to the outlets, (2) the necessary fittings, valves, faucets, shower heads, drinking cups, etc., (3) the water heating equipment, and (4) water-conditioning equipment if any. See Chapter 4 for water-conditioning equipment.

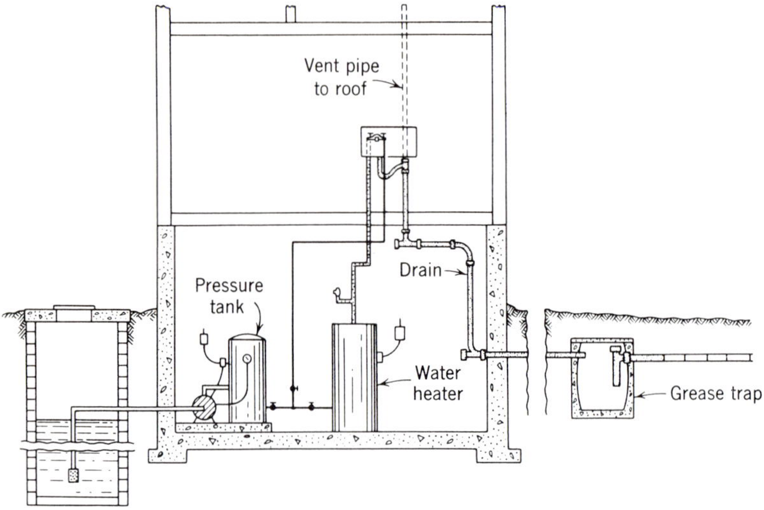

Fig. 10-1. Plumbing for a pressure type of water system, a hot-water supply, and waste disposal for a kitchen sink.

Supply Piping Materials

Three types of piping materials are commonly used for supply piping. They are (1) galvanized steel pipe and fittings, (2) hard and soft copper tubing and fittings, and (3) plastic tubing and fittings. See Fig. 10-3.

Galvanized steel.

Galvanized steel pipe is manufactured in 21-foot lengths threaded on both ends. A coupling is usually furnished on one end. A wide range of sizes is available. The fittings are factory threaded. Joints are made by screwing pipe and fittings together as shown at A in Fig. 10-3. Steel pipe is the strongest and most rigid of the piping materials. Its principal disadvantages are that it is susceptible to rusting and easily ruptured by freezing.

Copper tubing.

Copper tubing is noncorrosive with most waters. It is used extensively in better-grade houses and where ground water is highly corrosive to steel pipe. Two types of copper tubing are available, namely (1) hard-drawn tubing which is sold in 10-foot lengths in various diameters and is assembled with soldered fittings as illustrated at B in Fig. 10-3, and (2) soft tubing.

Hard-drawn tubing is used extensively in new structures where it can be installed before the inside finish is put on. It has a neater appearance than does soft copper. Soft copper is extensively used in

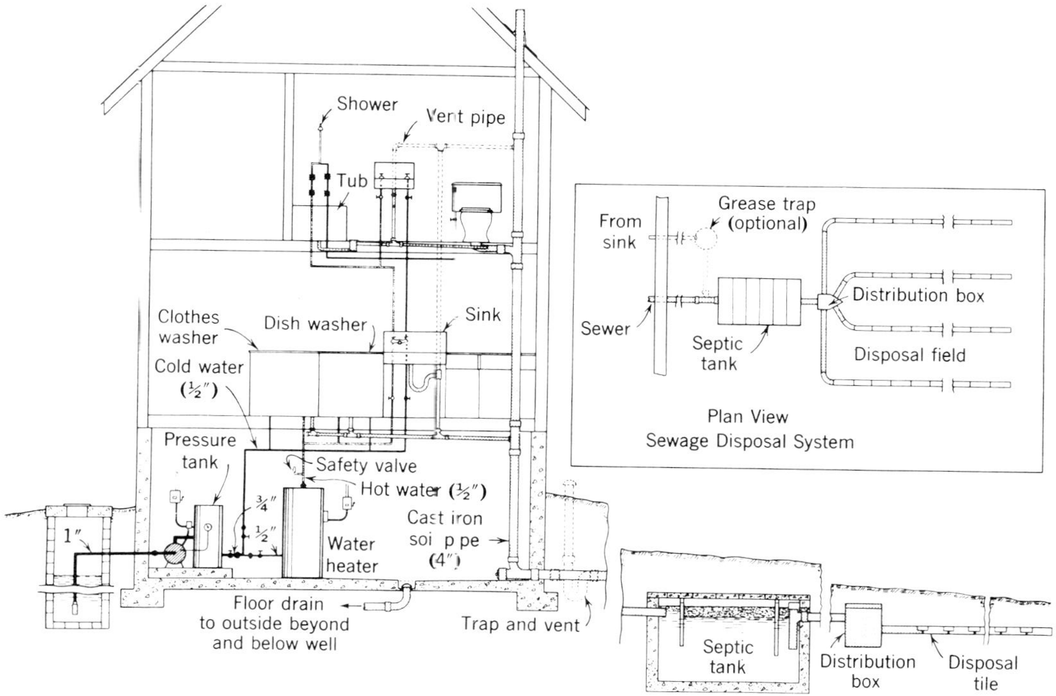

Fig. 10-2. A complete plumbing system for a house. Clotheswasher and dishwasher have built-in traps. The outside sewer trap and vent (shown in dotted lines) are required in some localities. Fig. 10-21 illustrates additions for a farmstead.

new and old buildings, for remodeling, etc., where it must be "fished" through partitions, ceilings, and floors. Soft copper is sold in coils of lengths up to 60 feet (18.3 m). For long runs this saves fittings and labor. Long sweeping turns can be made which offer less resistance to flow than do sharp turns with fittings.

Both hard and soft tubing are available in two grades. The standard grade, type L, is for use in indoor plumbing where pressures are moderate, and the heavy-duty grade, type K, is for underground use and for high-pressure lines. Both can be attached to steel pipe by means of adapters as shown at B and C of Fig. 10-3.

Copper, being softer than steel, will stretch to some extent and therefore is not as readily ruptured by freezing as is steel pipe. This is particularly true of the soft copper.

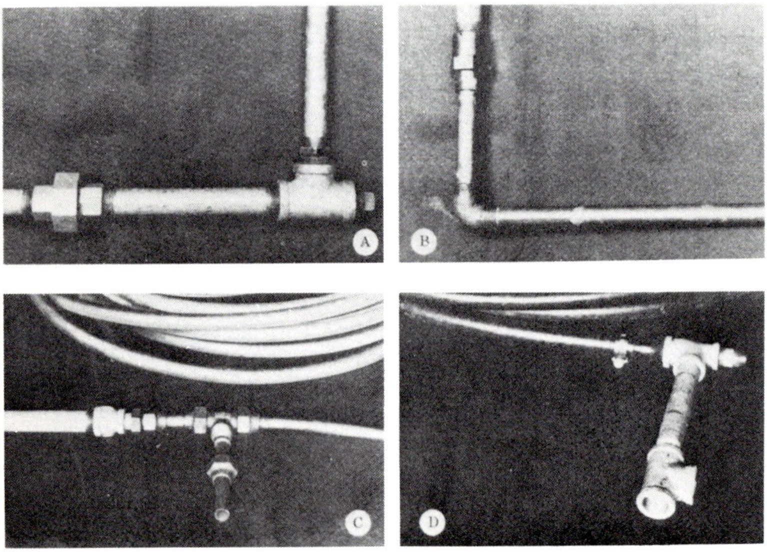

Fig. 10-3. Piping materials. A — Galvanized steel pipe and fittings. B — Hard-drawn copper tubing with soldered fittings and a copper-to-steel adapter. C — Soft copper tubing with flare-type fittings and a copper-to-steel adapter. Soldered fittings can and usually are used on soft tubing. D — Plastic tubing and a tubing-to-steel adapter. Note that the tubing is secured to the fitting with a clamp.

Plastic tubing.

Where not prohibited by plumbing codes, plastic tubing may be used both indoors and outdoors and for hot or cold water. It has a number of advantages over metal piping, namely, it is lower in cost, is non-corrosive, light in weight, can be installed with ordinary tools, does not require threading, is more resistant to lime and bacteria

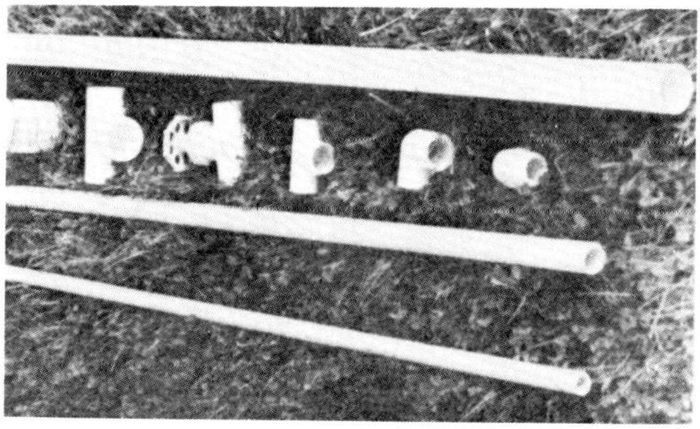

Fig. 10-4. Samples of hard plastic tubing. The larger 1" tubing at the top is of the PVC type used for cold water lines. It will withstand pressures up to 200 psi (14 kg/sq. cm.) and temperatures up to 73°F (22.8°C).

The smaller ½" and ¾" tubings and fittings are of the CPVC type used for hot water. Will withstand pressures up to 100 psi (7 kg/sq. cm.) and temperatures up to 180°F (82°C).

Tubings and fittings are joined together by means of special PVC and CPVC cements respectively.

No pipe cutters, No threading, No soldering, No torches. All you need is a hacksaw, screwdriver and an adjustable wrench. First cut Plastic Pipe to desired lengths with hacksaw.
Place loose stainless-steel clamps over pipe and push insert-fitting into pipe up to shoulder. (Insertion is easier if pipe-end is immersed in hot water for one minute.)
Position clamps over serrations on fitting; tighten securely with screwdriver.
See Fig. J-3-8 pg.

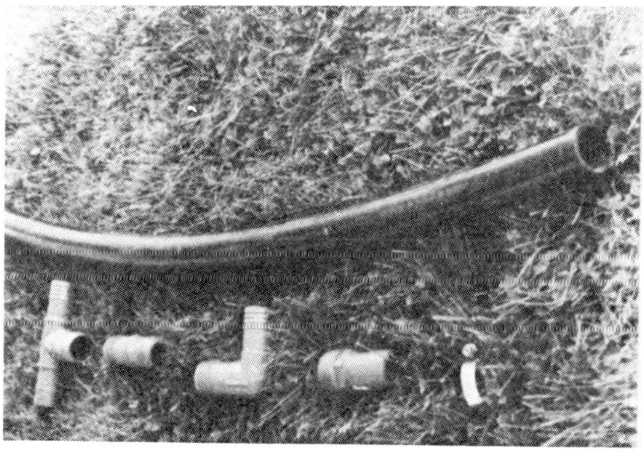

Fig. 10-5. A sample of PE type of flexible plastic tubing used for cold water lines, together with samples of fittings. The fittings and tubing are joined together by means of clamps.

scale, and has some insulating value.

Three general types of plastic tubing are available. See Figs. 10-4 and 10-5.

(1) A type used for hot water lines, designated as CPVC. It can also be used for cold water lines. It is semi-rigid and is sold in 10 foot (3m) lengths. Joints are made at fittings with a special CPVC solvent. It

withstands pressures up to 100 psi (7 kg/sq. cm.) and temperatures up to 180°F (82°C).

(2) A semi-rigid type for cold water only, designated as PVC. It is sold in 10 foot (3 m) lengths and joints are made at fittings with a special PVC solvent. Sizes ⅛″ to 1″ will withstand pressures up to 200 psi (14 kg/sq. cm.). *Not suitable for hot water lines.* Types CPVC and PVC should not be mixed in a water line.

(3) A soft, somewhat flexible type, designated as PE is used primarily for pump installations and outdoor cold water lines. It should not be used for hot water lines. Available for pressures up to 160 psi (11 kg/sq. cm.). It bends easily but will collapse on short bends. It has low resistance to puncture, therefore, when laid in a trench it should not be exposed to sharp stones. Rodents, particularly porcupines, will gnaw holes in it in exposed places. It is available in lengths up to 100 feet (30.5 m). Can be attached to fittings by means of clamps. Fittings are made of hard plastic.

VALVES

The following classes of valves are in general use on domestic water systems: (1) globe valves, (2) gate valves, (3) stop and waste valves, (4) hydrant valves, (5) check valves, (6) foot valves, and (7) safety valves. Most valves are made of brass; however, plastic valves are now available.

Globe valves and gate valves are used in pipelines for convenience in manually closing the pipes to control the flow of water.

Stop and waste valves are used as shutoff valves on lines that at times need to be drained. For example, they are used on the water service lines where they enter buildings and on the discharge lines from pressure tanks to shut off the pressure and drain the pipes in the buildings beyond the valves. They are also used on lines to sill cocks and out-of-door outlets which must be drained to prevent freezing.

Hydrant valves are used in cold climates as self-draining, underground valves for controlling the flow of water aboveground.

Check valves are installed in pipelines to prevent a backflow of water; i.e., they allow water to flow through the pipe in one direction only. Check valves are automatic in operation, being opened and closed by changes in direction of pressure and flow.

Foot valves are used on the lower end of pump suction pipes. They are really a form of check valve and are used to prevent loss of priming of pumps. They are automatic in operation.

Safety valves are used on pressure water systems, heating systems, compressed air lines, pressure cookers, and other places where excessive pressures might be built up. They function automatically to relieve excessive pressures.

The globe valve.

Figure 10-6 shows the construction of one type of globe valve. This valve should be installed with the water pressure under the valve seat as shown, and if installed in a line that must be drained, the stem should be in a horizontal position.

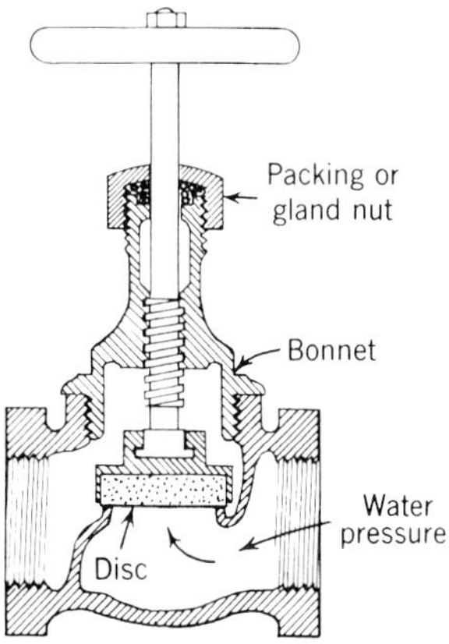

Fig. 10-6. Cross section of one type of globe valve. Note that the pressure should be under the seat.

The gate valve.

Figure 10-7 shows the construction of a common type of gate valve. Note that there are two seats and a wedge-shaped plunger that closes both seat openings. The seat openings are usually of the same diameter as the inside of the pipe for which the valve is made, and since they are in line with the axis of the pipe very little resistance is offered to the flow of water when the valve is completely open. The gate valve has an advantage over the globe valve in that it offers less

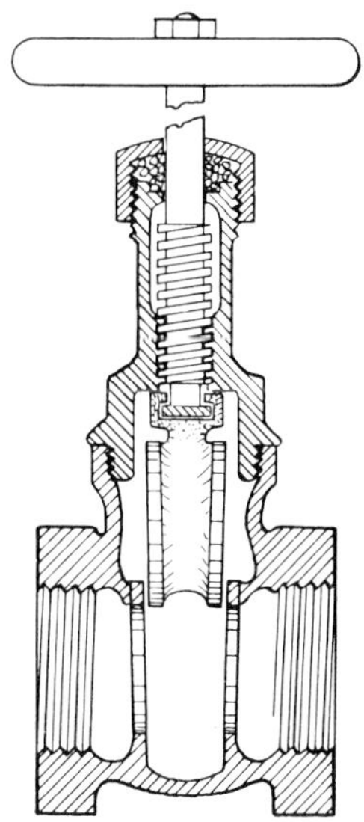

Fig. 10-7. Cross section of a gate valve.

resistance to flow. It is therefore used in preference to the globe valve where resistance to the flow of water is to be kept at a minimum. It will also control the flow equally well from either direction.

The globe valve has the advantage of quicker opening and closing, of longer life, and of being more easily repaired. Generally speaking, if the flow is in one direction only and if a valve is to be opened and closed frequently, the globe type is used; if opened and closed infrequently, if it is desired to keep friction at a minimum, or if it is desired to stop flow in either direction, the gate type is used.

Fig. 10-8. Method of installing a stop-and-waste valve. The waste valve should be on the outlet side as shown.

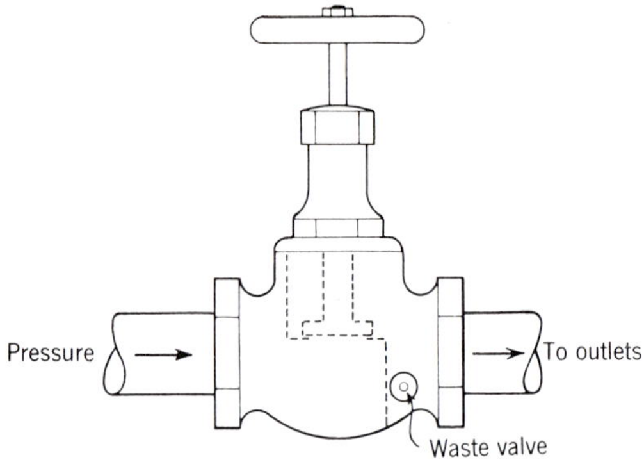

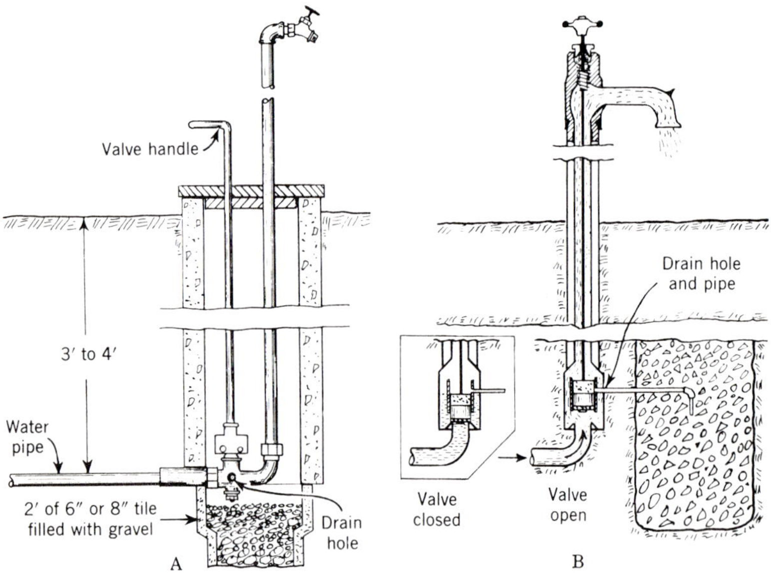

Fig. 10-9. Details of two types of frost-proof yard hydrant valves. When the valve is closed the water pressure is shut off from the left and the water in the pipe above the valve drains out into the gravel through the drain hole. As the valve is below frost line there is no danger of freezing. The type of valve shown at B is best where the hydrant is used frequently.

Stop-and-waste valve.

A stop-and-waste valve may be of the globe type or of the ground key type. It is used in a water line for shutting off the pressure and at the same time draining the pipes beyond the valve. On a farm water system it should be installed next to the tank on the faucet side or in the basement at the low point in the system. The valve must be installed with the drain opening on the house side of the plumbing, as shown in Fig. 10-8.

Hydrant valve.

A hydrant valve is very similar to a stop-and-waste valve except that it is designed for installation underground with a handle which may be extended to the surface as shown in Fig. 10-9. When the valve is closed the pipe to the surface is drained back to the valve.

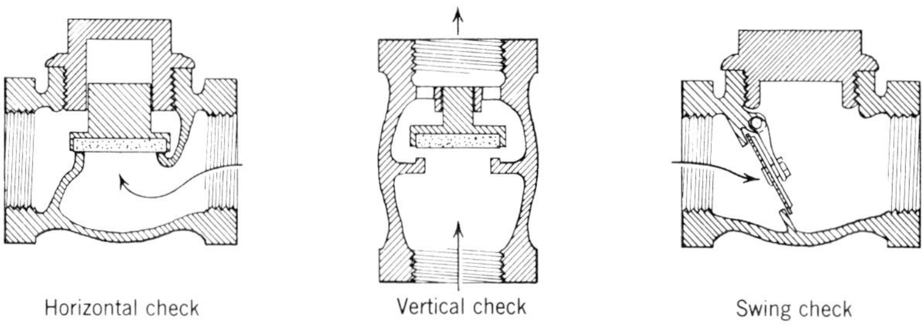

Fig. 10-10. Cross sections of three types of check valves. Available with or without spring-operated checks.

Check valves.

Figure 10-10 shows the construction of three types of check valves. The horizontal and swing checks must be installed in a horizontal position with the cap upward and with the flow in the direction of the arrows. The vertical check must be installed in a vertical position and the flow must be upward.

In all three of these check valves the water pressure under the seat will lift the check and let water pass through. If the pressure is reversed the check will be forced down on the seat and thus stop the flow.

Foot valves.

Figure 10-11 illustrates two types of foot valves for pump suction pipes.

Safety valves.

Figure 10-12 illustrates the pressure type of safety valve. The safety valve is held closed by a spring the tension of which can be adjusted over a wide range of pressures. When the pressure under the seat exceeds the pressure of the spring on top of the seat, the seat is lifted and the water flows through to relieve excessive pressure on the system. On automatic hot-water supply systems, such as a gas or electric heater, a safety valve with a temperature release as well as a pressure release should be used.

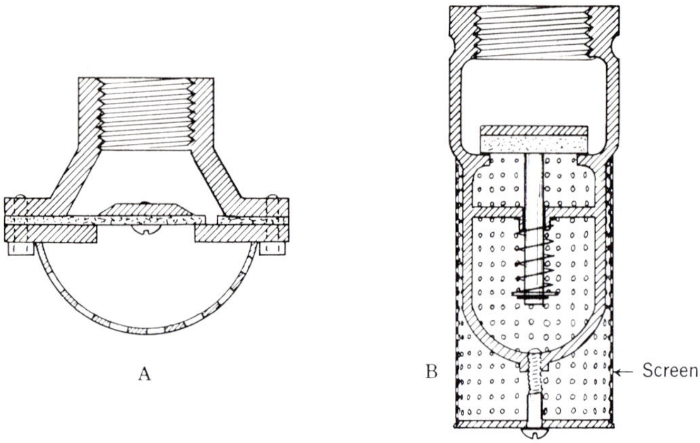

Fig. 10-11. Two types of foot valves. A shows an inexpensive type with the check made of a weighted piece of leather. B has a spring-loaded rubber check and is of much better quality.

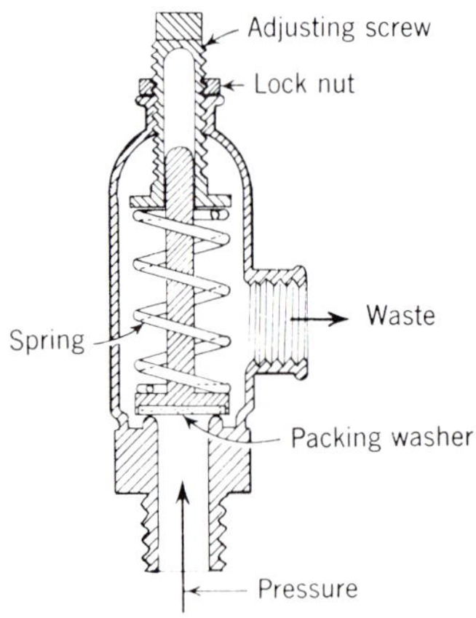

Fig. 10-12. One type of pressure-operated safety valve.

FAUCETS

All types of faucets illustrated here are available as singe or double ("mixing") faucets (see Fig. 10-13) and in various exterior designs to fit any standard plumbing fixtures. Most single faucets can be purchased with or without hose threads on the spout.

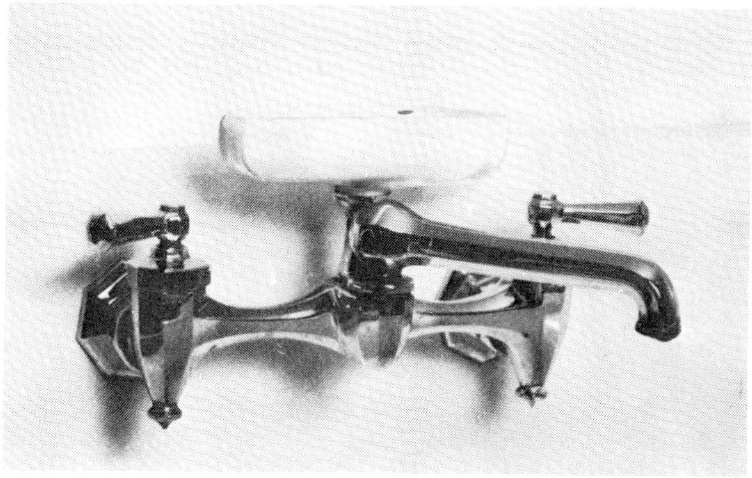

Fig. 10-13. A swing-spout mixing faucet on a kitchen sink. Mixing faucets with stationary spouts are available for lavatories, tubs, showers, and laundry tubs.

Compression faucets.

The common compression type of faucet closes *against* the pressure and has the washer held firmly in place with a screw. The washer is renewable on all compression faucets and on some the seat is also renewable. See Fig 10-15.

Figure 10-16 illustrates a more expensive type of compression faucet having a two-piece removable barrel. The lower part of the barrel has the seat and houses the threaded part of the stem and the washer. The whole lower barrel unit can be renewed. The washer can be renewed as with any compression faucet.

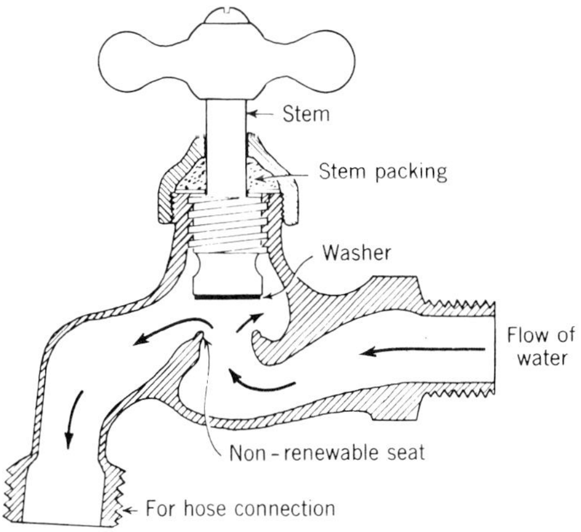

Fig. 10-14. Cross section of a compression type of faucet without renewable seat. Note that the faucet closes against the water pressure, and when open there is a relatively free passage for the water. The spout may or may not be threaded for hose connection.

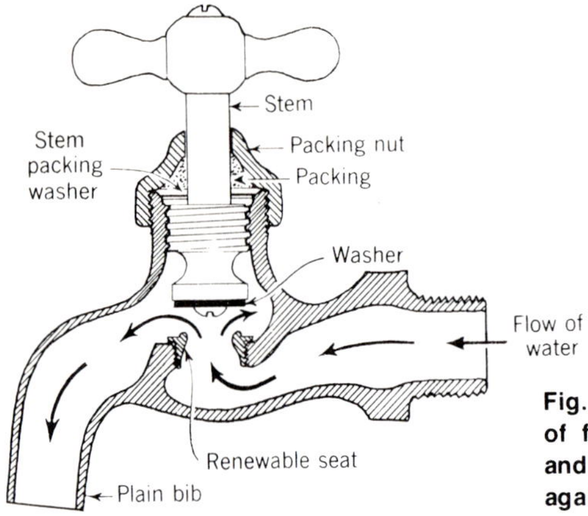

Fig. 10-15. A compression type of faucet with renewable seat and renewable washer. Closes against the water pressure.

In general the common compression type of faucets shown in Figs. 10-14 and 10-15, when used on a hot-water line, tend to loosen at the seat after closing because of contraction of the stem as the faucet cools. This accounts for the fact that they are sometimes found dripping even though they were closed driptight when last used.

Faucets which close *with* the pressure as indicated in Figs. 10-17 and 10-18 tend to tighten at the seat as they cool and the stem contracts.

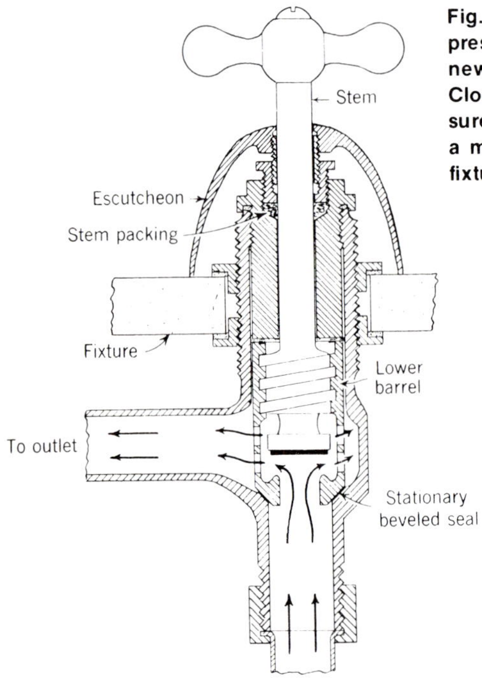

Fig. 10-16. A high-quality compression type of faucet with renewable seat and washer. Closes against the water pressure. Shown here as one-half of a mixing faucet mounted on a fixture.

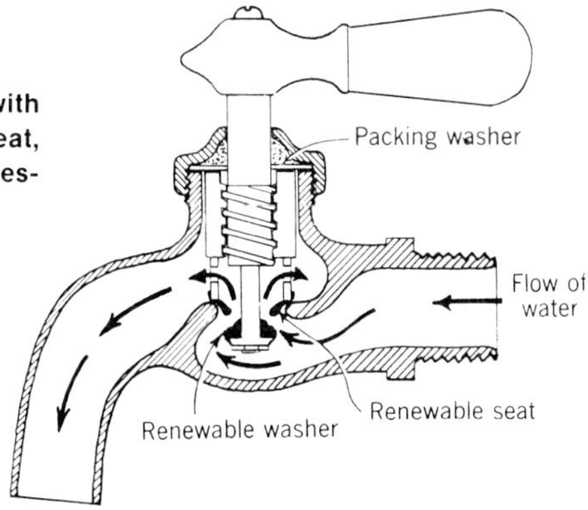

Fig. 10-17. A Chicago faucet with removable barrel, renewable seat, and washer. Closes with the pressure. Quick acting.

Single handle mixing faucets.

The single handle type of mixing faucet is now in general use on sinks and lavatories. There are a number of different designs on the market with a variety of features for controlling the flow of water. See Fig. 10-19. Some close with the pressure, some against the pressure. Some are opened by lifting the handle or a knob and some by pressing down on the handle. The temperature of the water drawn from the faucet is determined by swinging the handle to the right or to the left. With the handle all the way to the right only cold water is drawn. At positions in between various mixtures of hot and cold water can be drawn according to the need.

Most manufacturers of these faucets supply their dealers with repair kits which contain the necessary parts for making repairs.

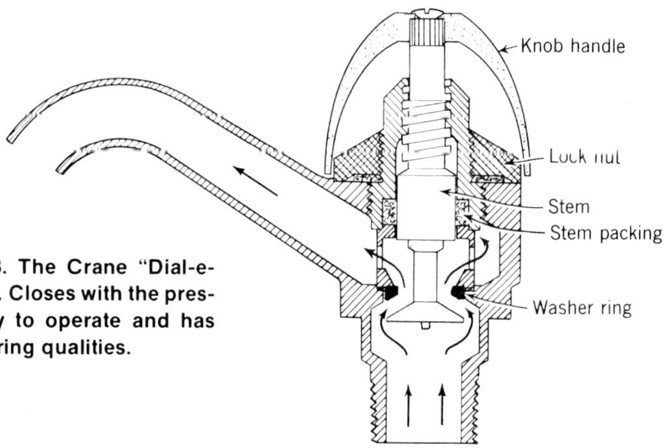

Fig. 10-18. The Crane "Dial-e-ze" faucet. Closes with the pressure. Easy to operate and has good wearing qualities.

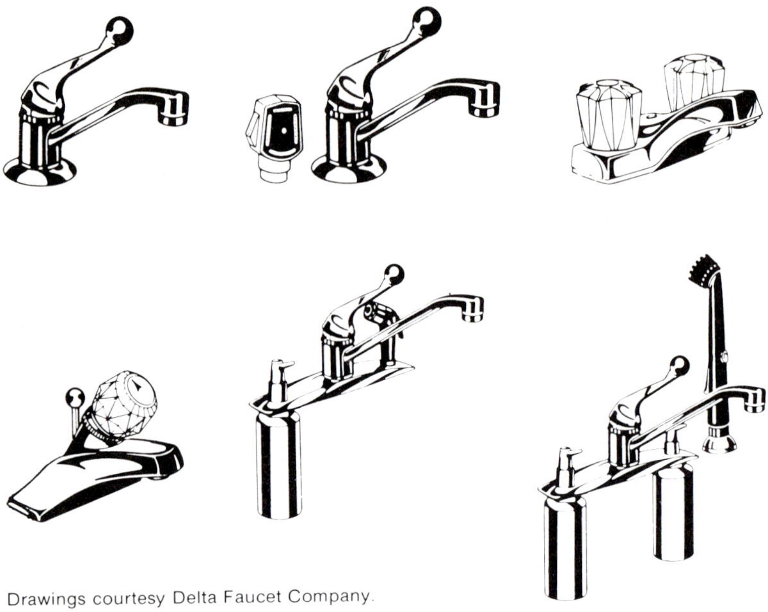

Drawings courtesy Delta Faucet Company.

Fig. 10-19. A variety of modern mixing faucets. The center faucet, top row, has a shampoo spray. At lower left is a faucet with a push-pull knob control. The knob can be turned clockwise or counter-clockwise to control the water temperature. At center, lower row, a faucet with a liquid soap, detergent, or shampoo liquid dispenser. At lower right the faucet has two dispensers, one for liquid soap and the other for hand lotion. It also has a dishwasher spray and brush.

Pipe Sizes

The size of pipe or tubing to use in any particular place depends upon the pressure available and the desired rate of flow. For a small house with short runs it is common practice to use ¾-inch size from the pressure tank or water meter to the points where the line to the water heater is tapped off. From that point to the outlets ½-inch size is recommended except on very short runs at fixtures. In the latter case ⅜-inch tubing is satisfactory. In large buildings and for long runs between buildings the size should be determined from friction tables as indicated in Job 6 and Chapter VIII.

It is sometimes recommended that one size smaller copper or plastic tubing be used than is required for steel pipe. Experience in the field indicates that this practice is not justified, especially for sizes up to and including 1 inch. It is therefore recommended that sizes for all three types of piping material through size 1 inch be calculated on the same basis and from the same friction table. For sizes over 1 inch the next size smaller plastic tubing can be used and where the friction table indicates a borderline choice, the next size smaller copper tubing can be used.

Pipe Joints

All joints in a plumbing system should be made permanently watertight. See Jobs 2 and 3 for instructions on procedures. Even a slow drip wastes water and may damage a building.

Protection from Freezing

Drainage provisions.

Where there is danger of the pipes freezing, drain plugs or valves should be installed at the low point or points for convenience in draining off the water. Lines to outside outlets such as sill cocks, garden outlets, and summer watering troughs should be provided with stop-and-waste shutoff valves as indicated in Fig. 10-9. If water is to be used out of doors or in unheated buildings in cold weather a frost-proof hydrant can be installed as indicated in Fig. 10-9, or electric heating cable can be used on the pipe as illustrated in Figs. 10-21 and 10-22.

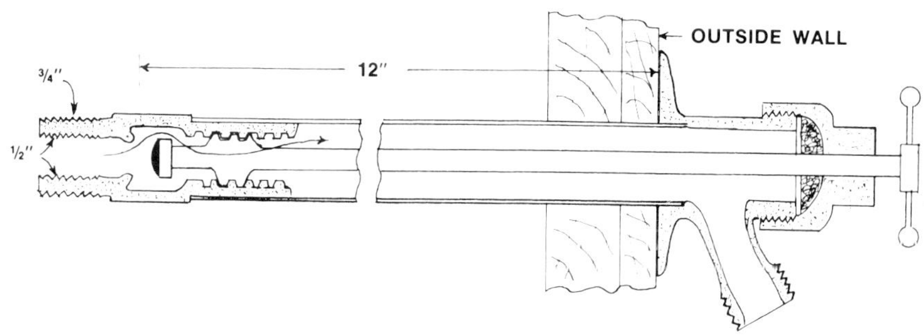

Fig. 10-20. A non-freezing sill faucet. This type of faucet is designed for use around the outside of heated buildings when there is a need to draw water during freezing weather. Note that the seat and washer are 12″ (30 cm.) back from the outside wall. When the faucet is closed the water in the 12″ tube drains out through the spout, provided the faucet is graded downward and there is no hose attached to the spout. That portion of the faucet beyond the seat must be kept at temperatures above freezing.

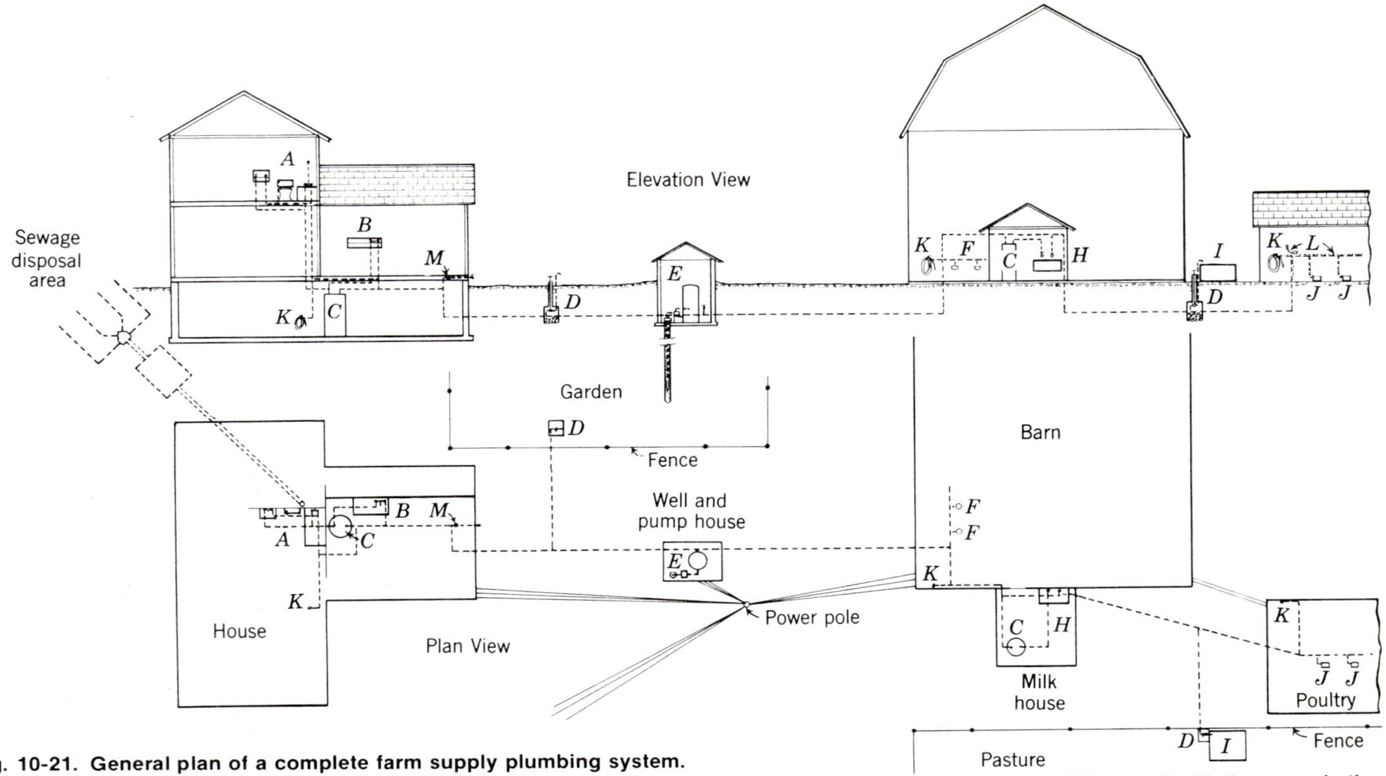

Fig. 10-21. General plan of a complete farm supply plumbing system.

Using a jet in the well, the pump and tank could be located in one of the buildings. A submersible pump could be used with the pump in the well and the tank in a building. They are shown here in a separate building with separate wiring from a power pole to illustrate a good arrangement for fire protection. Underground cables can be used instead of overhead wires. A — Bathroom; B — kitchen; C — water heater; D — hydrant cocks; E — pump house (could be aboveground even in cold climate, if heated); F — drinking cups for animals; H — milk house; I — watering trough; J — poultry watering fountains; K — emergency hose for fire protection; L — heating cable system to prevent pipes from freezing; M — stop-and-waste valve on line to sill cock. A frostproof sill cock can be used here. See Fig. 10-20.

The pipe sizes should be calculated from friction tables as indicated in Job 6.

Pipe and Tubing Installation

Regardless of the kind of piping material used, it should be installed in a workmanlike manner and where plumbing codes are in effect the work and materials should meet all code standards. A carefully made plan worked out on paper ahead of time will effect economies in materials and labor and result in a more satisfactory system when finished. Such plans can be provided by the architect or they can be made by the owner with the assistance of a good plumber.

In cold climates pipes should not be installed in outside walls unless thoroughly insulated. Pipes which *must* be run in exposed places can be protected by heavy insulation or by use of an electric heating cable under lighter insulation. See Fig. 10-22. The latter is used extensively on water systems in unheated farm buildings such as dairy barns and poultry houses.

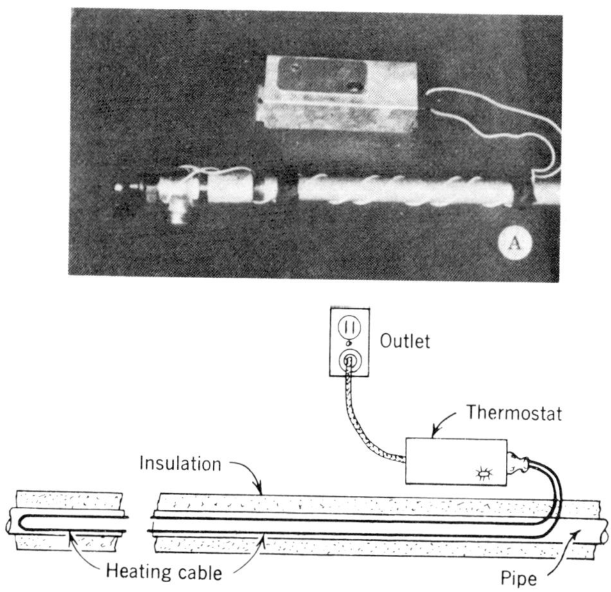

B

Fig. 10-22. Electric heating cable installed on an insulated water pipe to prevent freezing. The thermostat is set at about 35° F (1.7° C) so that the current is turned on only when there is danger of freezing. Just enough heat is supplied by the cable to keep the water from freezing. It is not a means of supplying hot water. The cable and pipe should be covered with insulation as shown at B.

Heating cables are available in various lengths and with ratings from 15 watts to 600 watts for application on various lengths and sizes of pipes.

Out-of-Door Outlets

Outlets around the outside of the house, around the garden, and at the garage for out-of-door sprinkling, washing vegetables, washing the car, etc., are a great convenience. If such outlets are used only in warm weather they can be drained in the winter. If they are to be used in freezing weather the supply pipes must be placed below the frost line and frostproof hydrants should be used.

Fire Protection

A little water on a little fire is as effective as a lot of water on a big fire. Ordinary ½-inch or ¾-inch outlets strategically located in a building and provided with a few feet of rubber or plastic hose *permanently attached to the outlet* provide an immediate source of water under pressure for fighting a fire before it gets a good start. See Figs. 10-21 and 10-23. One or two such outlets in the basement, in the barns, in a shop, or other hazardous locations are good fire insurance. Even if the fire is not put out it may be held in check until help arrives.

Where the water is provided by a pump it is important that there be no power interruption. For this reason, for fire-fighting purposes the pump should be isolated from the principal buildings and if possible wired directly from a metering pole, as indicated in Fig. 10-21.

If no rural fire-fighting equipment is available a special cistern filled from the roofs and equipped with a separate large-capacity pump and piping may be a good investment. See Figs. 3-32 and 10-24. Farm ponds, lakes, or streams, if nearby, can also be used as a source of water for such a fire-fighting system.

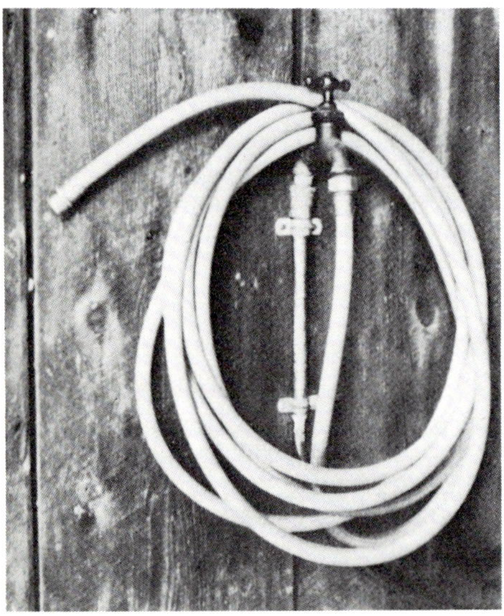

Fig. 10-23. A water outlet inside or outside of a building with hose attached at all times is an immediate source of water for fire fighting and for other purposes as well. The hose should be drained after each use if there is danger of freezing.

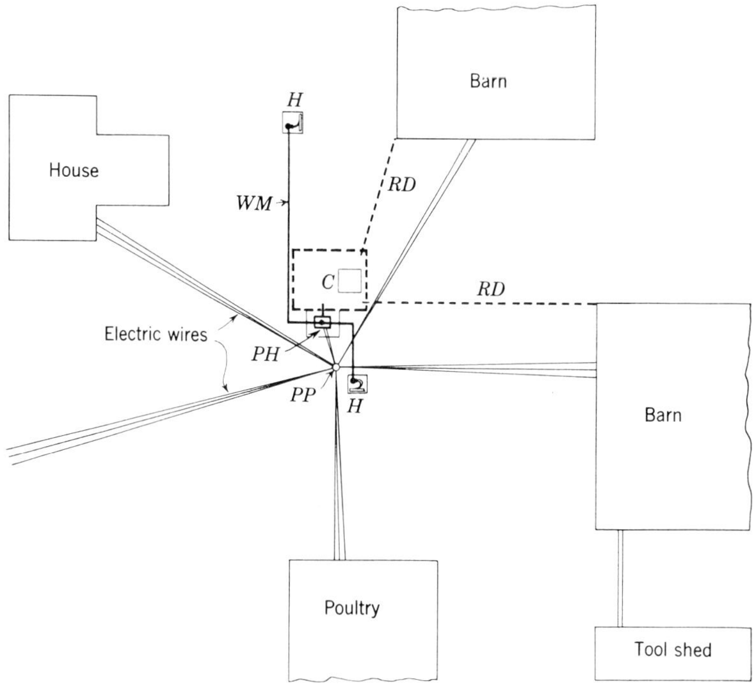

Fig. 10-24. Plan for special fire protection water system. In lieu of a cistern, a farm pond or nearby lake or stream can be used as a source of water. Although this system is intended to be independent of the regular water supply system, it can be used for spraying and irrigation if there is plenty of water at the source. The pump should be started periodically and the system flushed out to make sure it is in working order.
Key:

C = large cistern
RD = roof drains from barns to cistern
PH = pump house with large capacity pump
WM = 2-inch to 4-inch water main underground to hydrants
H = hydrants with fire hoses attached
PP = power pole (underground cables can be used from the power pole to the buildings instead of overhead wires)

Hot-Water Supply

Most homes supplied with running water, whether in a city or in the country, have some means of heating a hot-water supply. These range from a water front in the kitchen stove to completely automatic water heaters; see Fig. 10-25. Figure 10-26 illustrates the principle of operation of the *water heaters** shown in Fig. 10-25A, B, C, and D.

*Note that the term is *Water Heater,* not *Hot Water Heater.* There is no such device as a *hot* water heater on the market. If the water is hot we don't need to heat it.

Heating the water with the house-heating furnace or boiler.

It is erroneous to assume that the hot water supply can be heated with the house heating furnace or boiler without extra cost. Any heat that goes into the water comes from the fuel; therefore more fuel will be used. As a matter of fact, an installation such as shown at C in Fig. 10-25 where the water-heating coil is in the firebox may so interfere with the burning of the fuel, particularly coal, that the cost may be higher than for other methods of heating the water.

With a hot-water or steam house-heating boiler. The best practice for heating the hot-water supply with a boiler is to use a heat exchanger as shown at D in Fig. 10-25. With this method the water-heating coil is not in the firebox and therefore does not interfere with the fire. The fire heats the boiler water which in turn circulates by convection around the water-heating coil in the heat exchanger and thus heats the hot-water supply. As the boiler water temperatures are not as high as the temperatures in the firebox, the water-heating coil operates at lower temperatures, therefore there is less trouble with lime forming in the coil. The lime in hard water precipitates rapidly

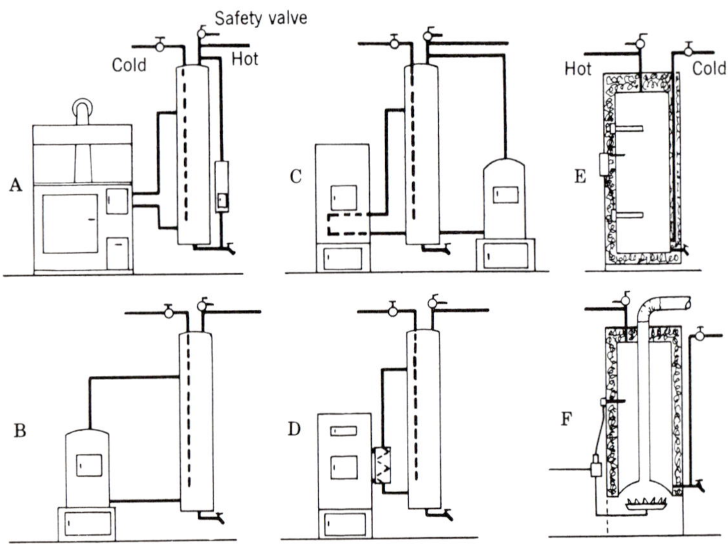

Fig. 10-25. Alternate arrangements for heating water. A — Heating with a water front in a kitchen range. A side-arm gas or oil heater is also shown which can be used when there is no fire in the range. B — Heating with a water heating stove. C — Heating with a coil or loop of pipe in the furnace. A water heating boiler can be used in the summertime, or a side-arm heater as shown at A. D — Heating with a heat exchanger on a steam or hot-water boiler. With forced-circulation, hot-water house-heating systems the boiler can be used year-round for heating the hot-water supply. Otherwise stand-by equipment as shown at A, C, E, and F can be used in the summer. E — Heating with an automatic electric heater. F — Heating with an automatic gas or oil heater.

when the water temperature exceeds 150° F. With a steam boiler or with gravity hot-water boilers a supplementary method of heating water is necessary in warm weather.

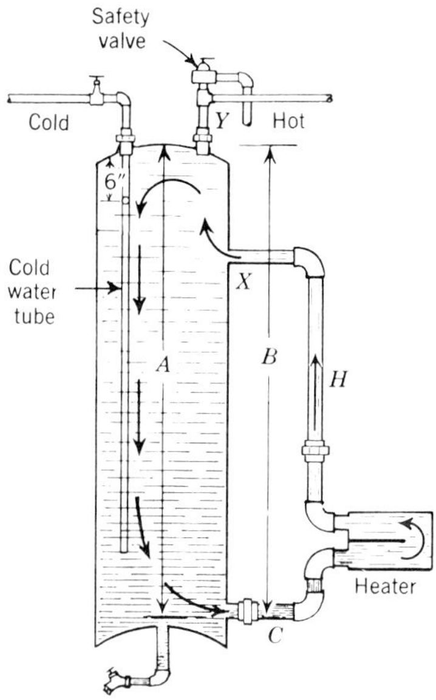

Fig. 10-26. Cross section of range boiler installation showing the circulation of water. The cold-water supply pipe should have a hand valve for quickly shutting off the water pressure in case of leaks. If the boiler is connected to a pressure type of water system, there should be a safety valve on the hot-water pipe as shown.

Automatic gas water heaters.

Automatic gas water heaters are used extensively where gas is available for fuel. The increasing use of liquid petroleum gas (bottled gas) makes the gas water heater popular in rural areas as well as in cities.

Gas water heater flues should be vented to a chimney or to the outside, as there is some hazard from fumes and/or escaping gas. See Fig. 10-27. Also, in burning the fuel a considerable amount of water vapor is formed as an end product of combustion. This water vapor will raise the relative humidity of the air in the space where the heater is located unless vented. Higher relative humidity adds to the discomfort in the summertime and if the heater is in a basement will tend to make the basement damp.

Modern gas heaters have a fairly high rate of recovery. For this reason the storage tank need not be large. This in turn makes the initial cost of the heater lower than for some other types. Tanks are available in almost any size but the 30-gallon size with a fast recovery burner is adequate for a household of four people. Larger tanks should be used for large families or for multifamily buildings. Gas companies usually are glad to advise customers on size and type of such equipment to install.

A safety valve should be installed on all automatic water heaters.

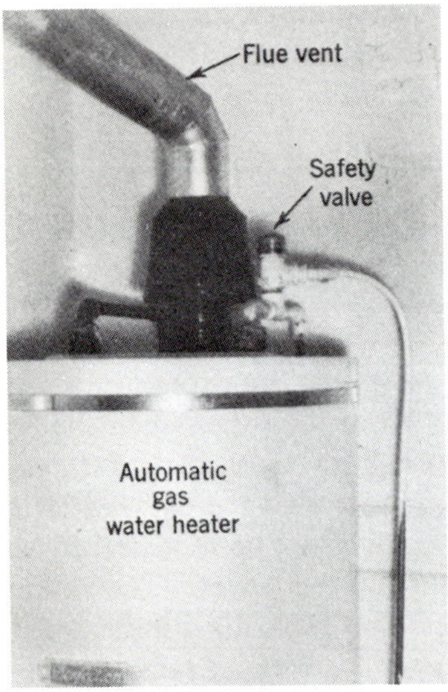

Courtesy Mr. Clay Chadwick, Sarasota, Fla.

Fig. 10-27. Gas water heater flues should be vented to the outside. A safety valve with a waste pipe to a drain or to the outside is also desirable. In some localities both are required by plumbing codes.

Automatic electric water heaters.

Where electric energy is available at favorable rates the automatic electric water heater provides one of the most satisfactory means of heating water. The efficiency is high, no venting is necessary as there is no danger from escaping fumes or gas, and no water vapor is formed. A well-insulated tank will add very little, if any, heat to a room; therefore it can be placed at any convenient place on a property. The principal disadvantage is the fact that power interruptions may deprive a family of hot water for short periods. In most communities power interruptions are becoming less common and are usually not of long duration; therefore this is of diminishing importance. In many localities, particularly in cities, the cost of electric energy for heating water is higher than for gas. Comparable costs with the two forms of energy can readily be obtained by investigation in the community.

Electric water heaters are availabel in a number of sizes. The minimum size to install depends upon two factors: the need for hot water, and the manner of metering the electric energy. If the heater has a good recovery rate and is energized at all times a 30- to 50-U.S. gallon tank is satisfactory for an average family. On the other hand, if the metering is of the "off-peak" or "night-rate" type where the heater is turned on only during the nighttime hours, then an 80-U.S. gallon tank is the recommended minimum size for an average family of three or four people. Where the heater serves a larger family or where for some reason the demands for hot water are above average, then a 100- or 120-U.S. gallon (83 to 100 Imp. gals.) tank is advisable. The size of tank will have practically no effect upon the cost of heating the water except for a slightly higher initial cost of tank.

Some power companies discourage the use of high-wattage, fast-recovery electric water heaters on their lines as they tend to cause low-voltage conditions. For this reason the low-wattage, large-capacity off-peak metered type of heater is now being used extensively.

Automatic oil heaters.

When gas or electricity is not available for automatic heater operation, automatic oil heaters are sometimes used. These heaters have a high recovery rate as do gas heaters. The flue must be vented to the outside and a fuel tank must be provided. They usually require more attention for refueling and for cleaning than do the gas or electric heaters. The installation is similar to the gas installation of Fig. 10-25, except for the fuel tank and controls. With the advent of "bottled" gas this type of heater has become less common in rural areas.

TABLE 10-I

WASTED WATER AND HEAT IN HOT-WATER PIPES

Size of Pipe,	Length of Pipe,		Volume of Water Drawn off to Obtain Hot Water at Faucet,		Heat Wasted at Each Draw. Pipe and Water Cold (70°F.-21°C) at Start, Hot (120 F-49 C.) at Faucet,	Equivalent of Heat Wasted
Inches	Feet	Meters	U.S. Units	Metric Units	Btu.	Kw-Hrs.
1	10	3.00	1 gals.	0.833 Imp. gals.	415 Btu.	0.120
	25	7.60	2-2/5 gals.	2.00 Imp. gals.	996 Btu.	0.290
	50	15.00	4-3/5 gals.	3.83 Imp. gals.	1971 Btu.	0.580
3/4	10	3.00	2-1/5 gals.	1.83 Liters	228 Btu.	0.060
	25	7.60	5-3/5 Qts.	5.29 Liters	580 Btu.	0.170
	50	15.00	11-1/5 Qts.	10.60 Liters	1159 Btu.	0.340
1/2	10	3.00	1-1/5 Qts.	1.15 Liters	124 Btu.	0.036
	25	7.60	3 Qts.	2.84 Liters	310 But.	0.090
	50	15.00	6 Qts.	5.67 Liters	620 Btu.	0.180
3/8	10	3.00	1-4/5 Pts.	0.85 Liters	94 Btu.	0.027
	25	7.60	4-1/2 Pts.	2.13 Liters	234 Btu.	0.068
	50	15.00	9 Pts.	4.26 Liters	468 Btu.	0.137

Piping and Insulation for Hot Water

Hot-water pipes should be as short as possible. This means that the hot-water tank should be near the place where the most hot water is used.

Use the smallest size of piping that will provide a satisfactory flow. Short, small-sized pipes are less expensive and they waste less heat and less water. Between the times when the hot water is used, the water standing in the pipes cools off; thus the heat in it is lost. The next time hot water is needed the cool water in the pipes must be drawn off and the pipe must be reheated by the water before hot water can be obtained at the faucet. The volume of water standing in the pipes is also lost. Table 10-I indicates the amount of water and heat wasted for several sizes of pipe and tubing.

As ⅜-inch copper tubing will, if not too long, provide full flow for one faucet, that is the most economical size to use for short runs under sinks, lavatories, etc. Copper tubing absorbs less heat than steel pipe and because of the small volume of water it holds it is unnecessary to insulate it.

Good insulation on the hot-water tank and on large-sized pipes will materially reduce heat losses. In cold areas insulation may be necessary on all pipes to prevent freezing. Hot water pipes usually freeze before the cold water pipes in the same location.

Corrosion Prevention

Some waters are highly corrosive to metals, particularly when heated. Water containing high concentrations of dissolved oxygen and/or carbon dioxide is in this class. Corrosion destroys pipes and tanks and frequently causes a discoloration of the water with iron rust. Corrosion is accelerated by heat, therefore the hot-water side of the plumbing system corrodes faster than the cold-water side. Water-heating coils, the hot-water supply tank, and the discharge pipe adjacent to the tank are the most affected because there the highest temperatures occur.

Corrosion is often caused by electrolytic action between different metals or different parts of the same metal in contact with water. Some metals and some parts of the same metal are more active chemically than others. When electrolytic action sets in, the more active metal is corroded away, forming a pit with a nodule or "blister" over the pit. If this action continues long enough, a hole will eventually be eaten through the wall of the tank or pipe causing a leak. Figure 4-1A shows a portion of the inside of a tank destroyed in this manner.

Once pitting has started the corrosive action tends to become localized which may result in holes corroded through the wall at one or two places long before the remainder of the metal is seriously damaged. Corrosion prevention involves protecting the metals from electrolytic action. This is at least partially accomplished by several different methods.

By water treatment.

One method is to treat highly corrosive waters to free them of oxygen and carbon dioxide. This can be done for municipal water supplies but is rarely practiced for private domestic supplies.

By protective coatings.

Where the water contains certain minerals such as calcium or silicon in rather high concentration, the water will, under favorable conditions, precipitate a protective coating of the minerals on the metals. However, such a coating, to be effective, must be formed before pitting occurs. As the formation of this coating is extremely uncertain it is not safe to rely upon it unless former experience with the same water has proved its success.

One of the most successful methods for protection of steel hot-water tanks is to use a tank having a precast protective lining. A form of glass, bonded to the steel, is a good example. If such a lining is flawless the water does not come in contact with the metal, therefore the electrolytic action does not occur and corrosion is prevented. Such tanks are slightly higher in cost.

Effects of temperature.

As previously stated, corrosion is accelerated by heat. There is evidence that electrolytic action reaches its maximum when the water is at temperatures above 160° F (71.1° C). For this reason corrosion can be reduced by keeping the water temperature as low as the demands for hot water will allow. It is common practice to set the thermostat on automatic water heaters at 145° F (62.2° C). Water at that temperature is hot enough for most domestic purposes except for dishwashers and sterilizing milking equipment. For the latter purposes the thermostat should be set at 180° F (82.2° C) or higher, and it is for this kind of operation that corrosion prevention methods are most important.

In rare instances ground water is corrosive to copper. This is usually in regions where the water is exceptionally soft. Where this type of corrosion occurs the use of copper tubing and copper tanks should be avoided.

Suggestions for Economy in Heating Water

The cost of a hot-water supply is dependent upon:

1. The hot-water demands.
2. The efficiency of the water heating and distributing system.
3. The price of the energy used.

Hot-water demands.

Hot-water demands vary widely even between families of the same size. Some modes of living demand more hot water than others, and in many instances a great deal of hot water is wasted. To reduce the demands, and hence the cost of heating water, less hot water must be used, the wastage must be reduced, or both. The easiest economy is to prevent wastage. The following are common causes of wastages:

a. Leaky faucets. A faucet dripping at the rate of only 60 drops per minute will waste 113 U.S. gallons (94 Imp. gals.) per month. See Fig. J-4-1. Assuming the temperature is raised 100°F (37.8°C) by the water heater, the loss in heat would be 94,000 Btu. Two leaky faucets could easily double this loss. If the water heater were electrically operated this wastage would represent approximately 37 kilowatt-hours.

b. Drawing from the hot-water faucet when cold water would do just as well. In fact, very often the water drawn from the hot-water faucet is cold anyway, having stood in the pipes and cooled off. Perhaps because of habit or because of the greater convenience of opening the hot-water faucet with the left hand, many people regularly use the hot-water faucet unless they specifically want cold water. For economy the practice should be just the reverse, i.e., use the hot-water faucet *only when hot water is specifically needed.*

c. Such practices as filling a bathtub to overflow and letting a shower run when not in use flush a lot of heat down the drainpipes. Generally speaking a shower, if used with economy, requires less hot water than does a tub bath.

Efficiency of the hot-water supply system.

Radiation from heater, tank, and pipes, incomplete combustion of the fuel, and heat losses through the flue are factors affecting the efficiency of a hot-water supply system. Radiation losses can be reduced to a minimum by use of short, small-diameter pipes, and by good insulation. Incomplete combustion is a matter of draft and burner adjustment, and flue losses are affected by the conditions of the chimney, the smoke pipe, the draft controls, and the amount of lime scale in the heater.

Price of energy.

The price of energy used for heating water varies somewhat from time to time and with the location. Near natural gas fields gas may be the cheapest fuel. Near coal fields coal may be the cheapest. In rural areas electrical energy may be the cheapest. Comparable costs in a particular location at a specific time can usually be obtained from a local utility or a dealer in water-heating equipment.

WASTE PLUMBING

The waste plumbing consists of (1) the fixtures, such as sink, lavatories, tubs, showers, and toilets, and (2) the waste or sewer pipes, including traps, vents, clean-outs, etc., which carry the waste from the fixtures to the disposal system. See Figs. 10-2, 10-28, 11-1 and 11-2.

There should never be any water pipe connections between the waste plumbing and supply plumbing.

Plumbing Fixtures

These are available in a wide range of design, color, and quality to suit almost any need, taste, or price range. Most house plumbing systems have one or more of the following plumbing fixtures: kitchen sink (available with a dishwasher and a garbage disposal); bathroom lavatory; bathtub; shower stall; toilet; and laundry tubs. (The increasing use of automatic laundry equipment is rapidly making the laundry tub obsolete.)

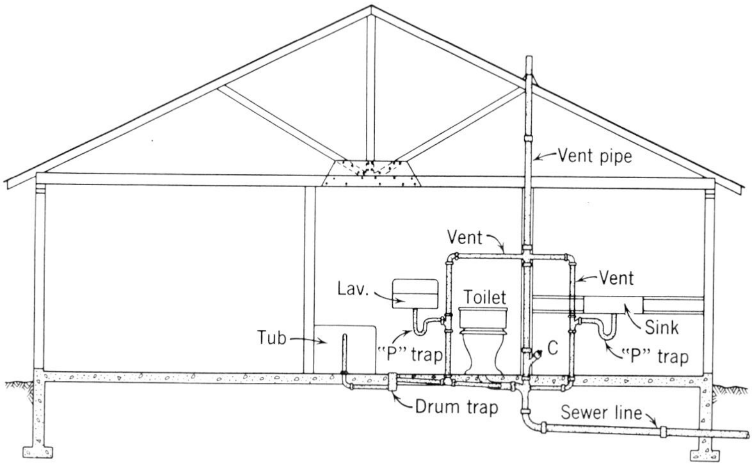

Fig. 10-28. Waste plumbing for a one-story building. The vent pipes for traps would normally be inside of partitions. C indicates a clean-out plug. The out-of-door sewage disposal system can be the same as for any other building.

Materials for Waste Plumbing

For many years cast-iron soil pipe was the standard material for waste plumbing in all localities. It is still the standard material in some cities where plumbing codes are in effect. However, since the development of suitable plastic materials, cast-iron is seldom used in rural areas unless specifically required by local plumbing codes.

Plastic piping materials have several advantages over cast-iron and steel piping. They are lower in cost, light in weight (weighs ⅛ as much as cast-iron and ½ as much as copper tubing), easy to install with ordinary tools, corrosion resistant, and won't lime up. For these reasons plastic materials are being used more and more in rural areas and in cities. However, in no case should they be used where prohibited by local plumbing codes.

Cast-iron pipe, plastic pipe, or vitrous tile can be used underground outside of building foundations (if not prohibited by code regulations). Such pipe or tile should be watertight to the sewer or private disposal area.

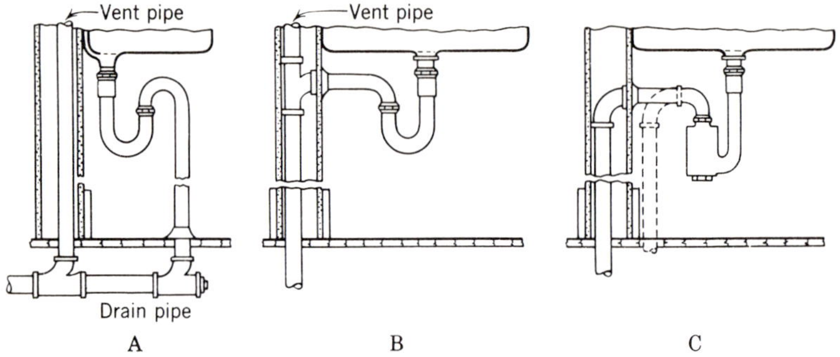

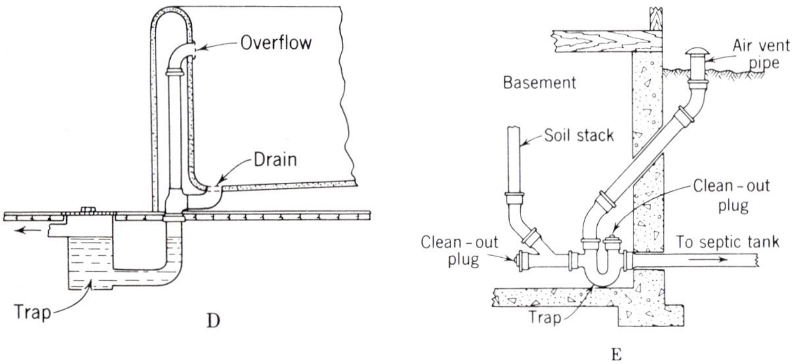

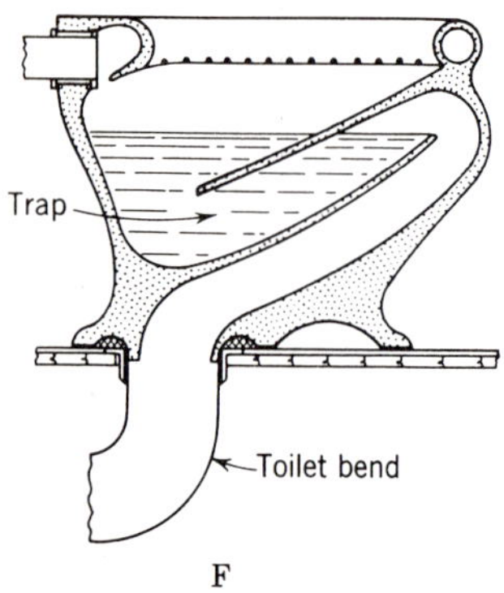

Fig. 10-29. Traps for waste plumbing. A — An S trap for use on lavatories or sinks drained through the floor. B — A P trap for use on lavatories or sinks drained through the wall. C — A "drum" or non-siphoning trap for use where venting is impractical; the drainpipe can be either inside or outside of the wall. D — A drum trap for bathtub or shower. E — A running trap in a sewer line; usually required on city sewer systems; is often omitted in rural homes. F — A built-in trap in a toilet.

Drain and sewer pipes should be graded downward to facilitate flow and adequate clean-out plugs should be provided. The pipe should be substantially supported in the building to prevent settling or sagging.

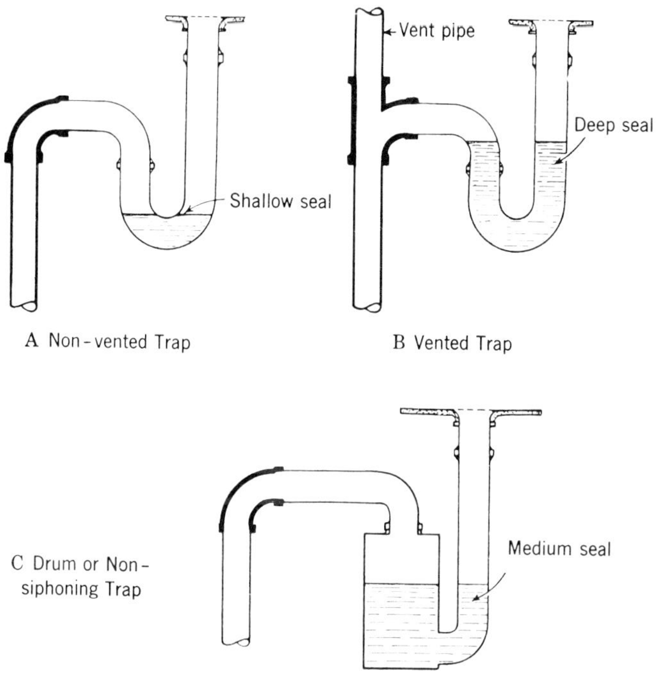

Fig. 10-30. Trap seals. A illustrates the shallow seal left in an unvented ordinary trap. B shows the deep seal in the same type of trap if correctly vented. C illustrates the seal in a nonvented drum or nonsiphoning trap. The enlargement or drum in the trap retains a considerable volume of water after the siphoning action is broken. This large volume of water will, without dropping appreciably, raise the level in the small pipe high enough to provide a satisfactory seal as shown. However, it may make a gurgling noise if not vented.

Traps

All plumbing fixtures should be equipped with a trap. It is the function of the trap to hold enough water to prevent sewer gases from escaping into the building. Figure 10-29 illustrates some of the modern traps.

Ordinary traps must be vented to prevent siphoning of the water seal. When venting is not possible or practical, nonsiphoning traps, Fig. 10-29C and D, should be used. Figure 10-30A illustrates how a nonvented ordinary trap will be unsealed by siphoning the water out of the trap. The low water level will allow sewer gases to escape into the building. Also, an unvented trap will make a gurgling noise after flushing water through it. The nonsiphoning trap will retain an adequate seal as indicated at C and D but may gurgle if not vented.

Sewage and Garbage Disposal 11

REASONS FOR SANITARY DISPOSAL

To safeguard health, and for convenience, all homes should have some sanitary means of sewage disposal. This includes the disposal of kitchen and laundry waste as well as human excrement.

Many communicable human diseases can be spread from person to person through contact with human excrement or through the medium of animals, flies, and insects which carry the diseases to food and clothing. Also, improper sewage disposal may cause contamination of the drinking-water supply and thus spread disease.

A safe and sanitary sewage disposal system is one which absolutely prevents contact with human feces, either by persons, animals, or insects, and which does not in any way contaminate the water supply.

SEWAGE DISPOSAL SYSTEMS FOR RURAL HOMES

The best method of sewage disposal is by means of an underground collecting sewer system which terminates in a sewage treatment plant. Unfortunately the cost of such systems limits their use to densely populated areas such as cities, towns, and villages. In rural areas not served by such a system the sewage must be disposed of by private means and on the individual property concerned.

The most common type of private sewage disposal system for individual homes is a *septic tank with an underground disposal area.* Unfortunately in some areas it is difficult and sometimes expensive to make such a system function satisfactorily. Heavy and impervious soil, a high water table, lack of adequate land area for the load, and danger of contamination of the water supply are the principal limiting factors.

Anyone considering building a new home should first investigate thoroughly the possibilities of adequate sewage disposal as well as an adequate and safe water supply. In fact, the two should be considered in relation to each other. The best method of determining the suitability of a soil for a disposal area is (1) to make a percolation test and (2) to determine the level of the water table in wet weather. Methods of procedure are explained later. From these tests one can determine if an absorption field can be made to work and if so how much area will be required. If the soil is unsuitable or if such a system cannot be used without contaminating the water supply, then another building site should be chosen.

For existing buildings already on unsuitable soil some alternate method of disposal may have to be used. The most commonly used alternate methods are (1) a septic tank with seepage pit, (2) a septic tank with underdrained sand filter, and (3) cesspools. Where there is no indoor plumbing the outdoor privy or chemical toilet can be used for disposal of human excrement.

A new method of aerating sewage in especially designed septic tanks is worth considering where disposal fields are impractical. Figure 11-10 illustrates this system. The motor drives an agitator and at the same time pumps air into the sewage. The agitation and the added air hastens the septic action which will, according to claims of the manufacturer, produce an effluent pure enough to be safely discharged directly into a stream, or even onto the surface of the ground, therefore no disposal field is needed. Before purchasing such a system one should check with the local health department to be sure it is acceptable locally.

Many states have sanitary regulations with respect to any or all of these methods of disposal. Such regulations have two purposes: one is to protect the health of the general public and the other is to protect the individual property owner by setting up minimum standards which will insure satisfaction for the money invested. The regulations are published and can be obtained through local health offices or by writing to the State Health Department. These regulations should be studied before construction is started and in some states it is required by law that the construction be inspected by a health officer before it is covered and put into use.

The Federal Housing Administration and the Veterans Administration have minimum requirements for homes on which they make loans. These requirements must be met in order to obtain a loan.

The above-mentioned methods of disposal are described in more detail on the following pages. The recommendations presented here are of a general nature only and are based upon the latest available state regulations and experimental data.

The principal causes of failure of private disposal systems stem from (1) inadequate capacities, (2) poor construction, and (3) lack of adequate care. The recommendations presented here are intended to eliminate these troubles.

Septic Tank and Disposal Tile Field Systems

This type of system is similar in operation to a municipal system except it is on a very small scale and usually no chlorination takes place. Without chlorination the waste at final disposal is not purified, but is covered and away from contact by humans, animals, and insects. If such a system is well designed, carefully constructed, well cared for, and is located at a safe distance from the source of water it provides a minimum of danger of contamination of the ground-water supply.

It is possible to chlorinate the effluent from a septic tank to kill the disease organisms before the effluent is discharged into the soil or elsewhere. This, however, should be done only with the approval and the supervision of the local health department.

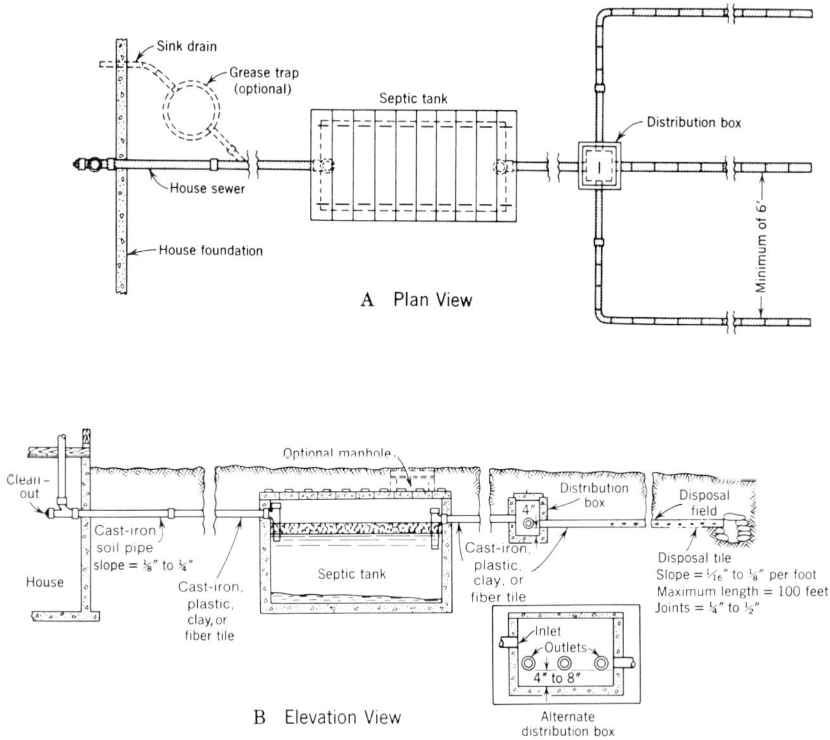

Fig. 11-1. Plan for domestic sewage disposal system where the ground is fairly level. Figures 11-13 through 11-16 illustrate alternate systems for uneven ground. The sewer line from the house to the septic tank and from the septic tank to the distribution box, or boxes, should be made of plastic pipe, (if permitted by the local health department) cast-iron soil pipe, or bituminized fiber tile. In any case all joints should be water tight. There should be at least two lines of disposal tile of equal length out of the distribution boxes.

A concrete septic tank is indicated but others are satisfactory if large enough.

A small seepage pit at the end of the disposal tile as shown at B permits solids to be flushed out of the tile during peak discharge periods and provides additional capacity for temporary overloads.

The essential features of a complete septic tank and disposal field are illustrated in Figs. 10-2, 11-1, and 11-2, and include:

1. The sewer line from the house.
2. The septic tank; in some cases also a grease trap as indicated by the dash lines in Fig. 11-1A.
3. The sewer line to the distribution box. (In the case of Fig. 11-2 a pump is used on the effluent.)
4. One or more distribution boxes (except for Fig. 11-2.)
5. The disposal area.
6. A disposal tile field for final disposal of the liquids.

For all types of sewer pipe the trench should be carefully graded and the pipe should have a firm support *throughout its length* to prevent sagging or shifting.

Sewer line from the house.

The sewer line from the house carries both solid and liquid wastes to the septic tank. It should be made of plastic tile, bituminized fiber tile, or cast-iron soil pipe. Cast-iron is rarely used except in some cities where it is required by plumbing codes. Plastic tile is quite generally used in rural areas, both for the sewer lines and for the disposal field. In any case the tile should be installed underground and *all joints should be watertight.* See Fig. 11-3 and 11-4. It should slope towards the septic tank on a uniform grade of approximately ¼-inch (0.635 cm.) per foot and should have as few bends as possible. No bend should exceed 45 degrees. The line should be at least 50 feet (15.24 m.) away and downhill from a well or spring.

The septic tank.

It is the function of the septic tank to provide a place:

1. For sewage solids to separate out of the liquids.
2. For bacterial action to decompose or "digest" the major portion of the solids.
3. For storage of residual solids.

It is sometimes referred to as the "stomach" of the sewage disposal system.

When correctly installed and in operation the incoming sewage stratifies as shown in Fig. 11-5. The lighter portions rise to the top and together with a foam formed by gas bubbles form a thick scum which acts as a seal. The heavier portions settle to the bottom while the liquid remains in the middle section until flushed out to a disposal area.

The *bacteria* which decompose sewage are called anaerobic bacteria because they thrive best without air and in a dark place. As a rule the entering sewage carries enough of such bacteria to inoculate the tank. Under the favorable conditions for growth provided by the tank, namely lack of air, darkness, and plenty of food, the bacteria

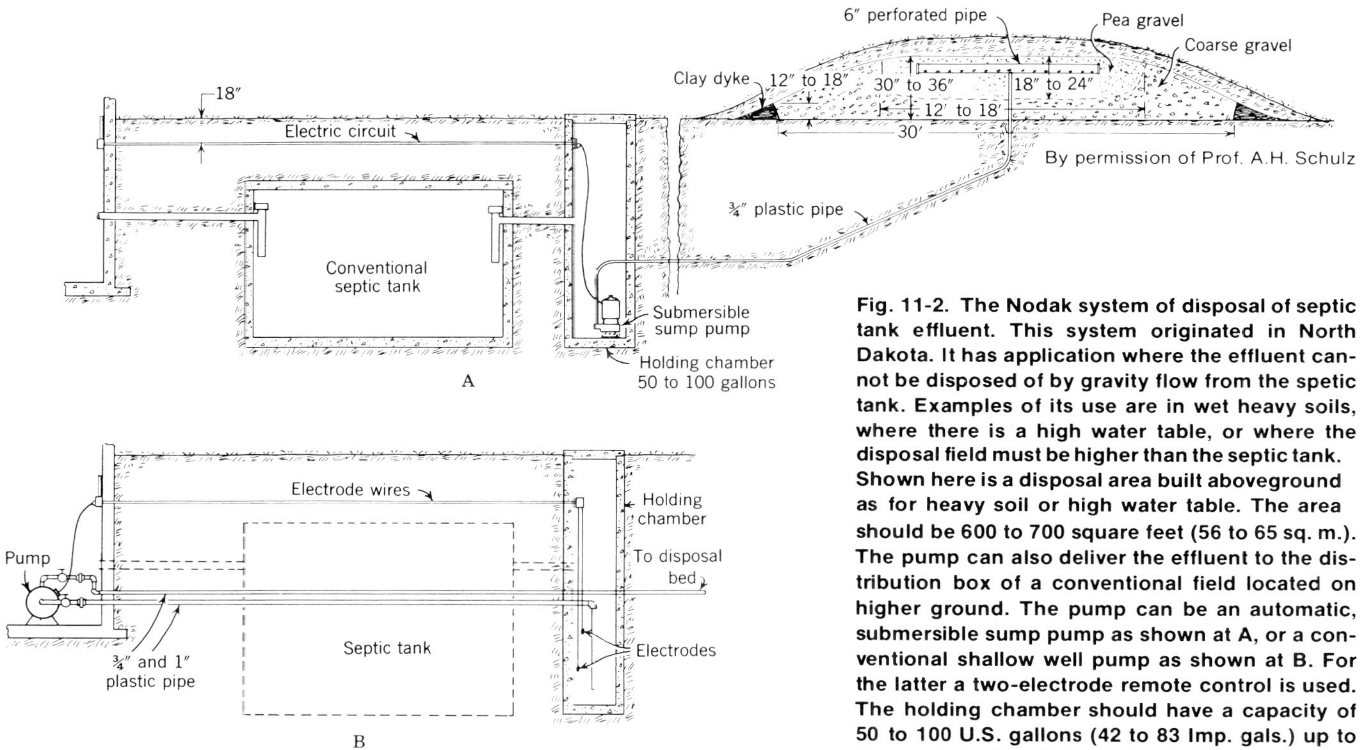

Fig. 11-2. The Nodak system of disposal of septic tank effluent. This system originated in North Dakota. It has application where the effluent cannot be disposed of by gravity flow from the spetic tank. Examples of its use are in wet heavy soils, where there is a high water table, or where the disposal field must be higher than the septic tank. Shown here is a disposal area built aboveground as for heavy soil or high water table. The area should be 600 to 700 square feet (56 to 65 sq. m.). The pump can also deliver the effluent to the distribution box of a conventional field located on higher ground. The pump can be an automatic, submersible sump pump as shown at A, or a conventional shallow well pump as shown at B. For the latter a two-electrode remote control is used. The holding chamber should have a capacity of 50 to 100 U.S. gallons (42 to 83 Imp. gals.) up to the septic tank outlet and should be watertight.

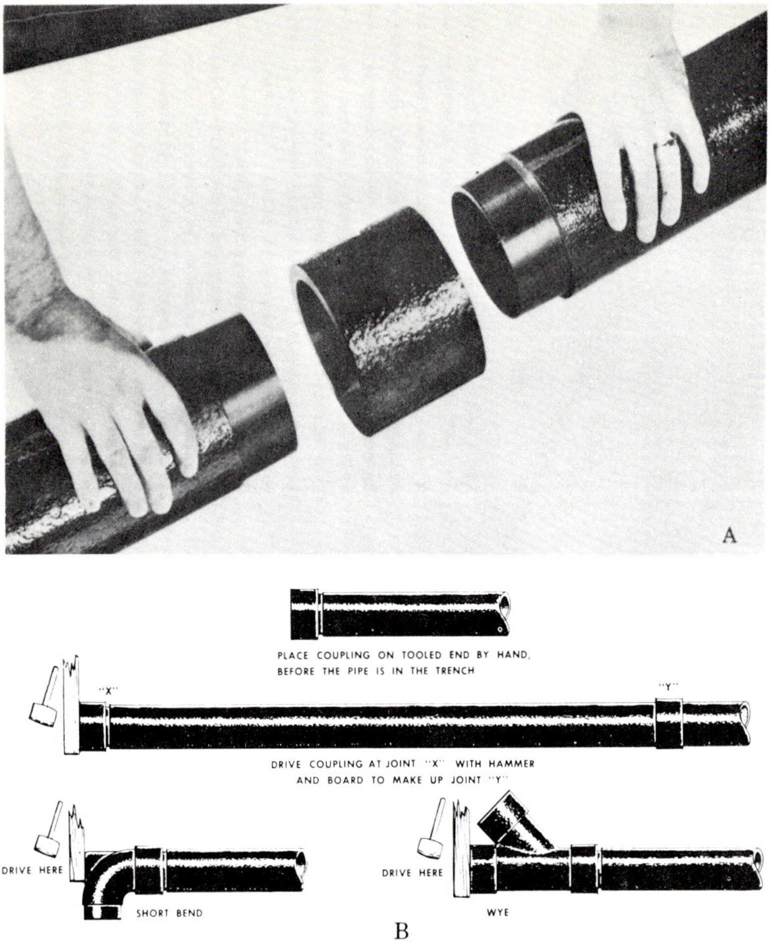

Courtesy Orangeburg Manufacturing Co., New York, N.Y.

Fig. 11-3. Method of assembling bituminized fiber sewer tile. A shows the tapered ends on the tile and the tapered coupling ready for assembly. B illustrates other fittings and the method of assembly.

will multiply rapidly. The more they multiply the more rapidly they will decompose the sewage.

In the process of decomposing or "digesting" the sewage the solids are converted to liquids, gases, and a small residue of undigestible solids usually referred to as sludge. The gases escape through vents and/or through the soil, and the liquids flow out to the disposal area where they are taken up by the soil. The residual solids settle to the bottom of the tank and eventually must be cleaned out. Even under the most favorable conditions a minimum of 24 hours is required for settling. For this reason the tank should be at least large enough to hold all of the sewage discharge over a 24-hour period.

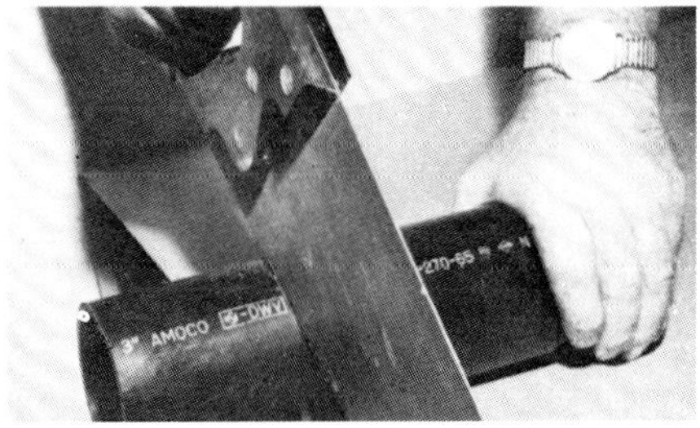

Cut pipe to length desired.

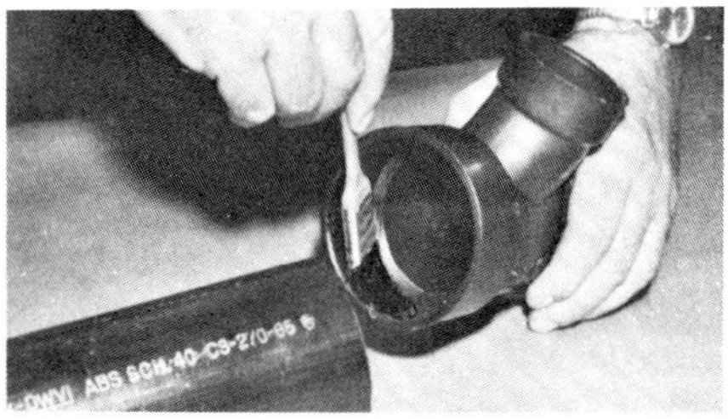

Brush on Amoco solvent cement to fitting socket.

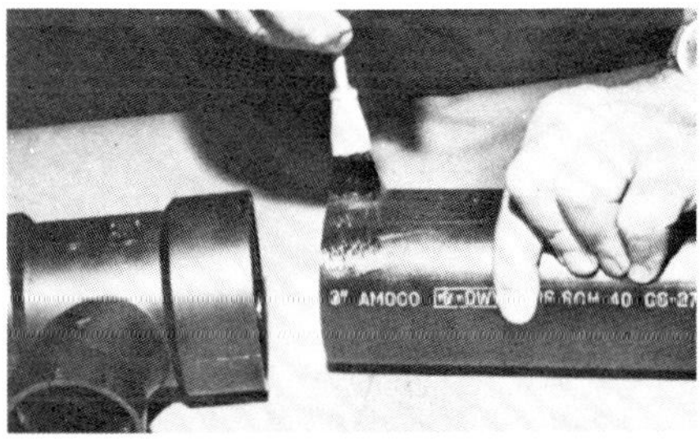

Do the same to pipe end.

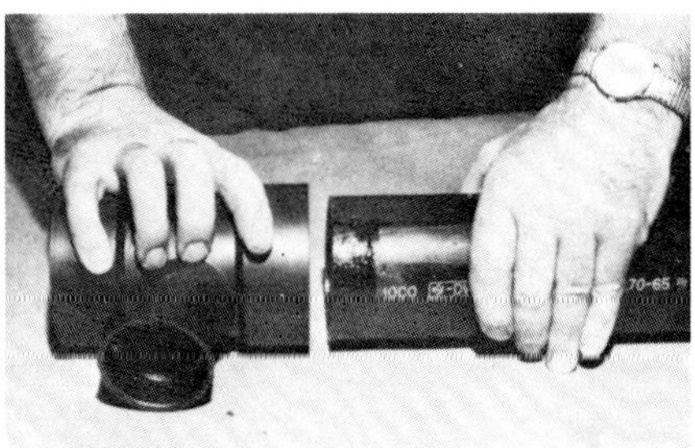

Join fitting and pipe. (Wait about fifteen minutes and joint will be ready to pressure test.)

Fig. 11-4. Method of assembling plastic tile. Tools needed are a measuring rule, a saw, and a paint brush. This same method applies to the white plastic tile. It is important that the cement used be of a type recommended by the manufacturer of the tile being used.

Courtesy Amco Chemicals Corp.

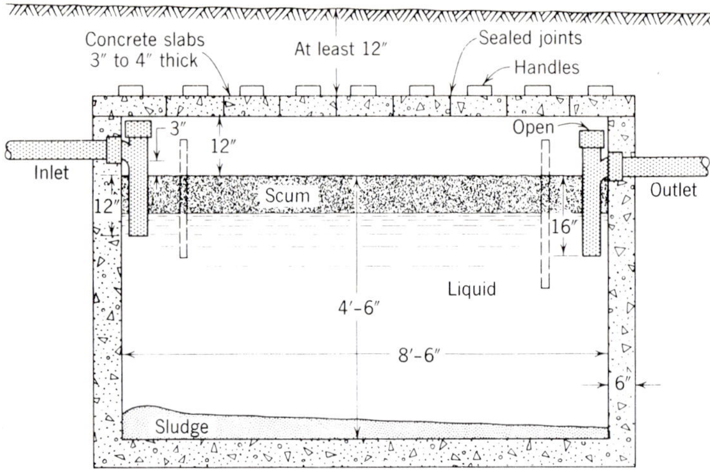

Fig. 11-5. Cross section of a septic tank. The raw sewage enters at the left. The grease and lighter solids rise to the top to form a scum. The heavy solids sink to the bottom and the liquid remains in between. The entering sewage is deflected downward by either a pipe or baffle (position of baffles indicated by dashed lines) to prevent disturbance of the tank contents. An outlet pipe or baffle tends to prevent solids from leaving the tank. The liquids flow out at the right to the distribution box and disposal field. The residue of solids or "sludge" must eventually be cleaned out.

The *size of tank* should be calculated on the basis of the maximum number of people who might use the system rather than on the minimum number who use it at the time of installation. If a family frequently has extra guests for week ends or several days, or if the family is expected to increase, these extra persons should be included in the calculations. It is during periods of overload with a house full of guests that the tank is most likely to develop trouble. The extra cost of the large tank is negligible in comparison to the service rendered. Figure 11-6 illustrates one advantage of a large tank.

The best indication of the potential load on a tank is the residence capacity of the house. The number of bedrooms, counting two people per bedroom, is a basic indication of residence capacity. If some other room such as a living room is used also for sleeping, it should be counted as a bedroom. This method of estimating the load allows for week-end guests and for a change of occupancy in the future. If there are plans for enlarging the house in the foreseeable future the proposed enlargement should be included in the calculations. For these reasons the recommendations given here are based upon the number of bedrooms rather than the older method of the number of people actually in residence.

If a garbage disposal unit is used, the size of the tank should be increased by 50% because of the extra solids to be decomposed. If

TABLE 11-I.
RECOMMENDED LIQUID CAPACITIES FOR HOUSEHOLD SEPTIC TANKS, BASED UPON CLEANING INTERVALS OF 5 TO 10 YEARS*.

No. of Bedrooms in Home	Minimum Liquid, Capacity, Gallons			
	Without Garbage Disposal Unit		With Garbage Disposal Unit	
	U.S. Gals.	Imp. Gals.	U.S. Gals.	Imp. Gals.
2 or less	500	400	750	625
3	600	500	900	800
4	650	550	1000	900
Over 4	160/Bed R.	135/Bed R.	250/Bed R.	208/Bed R.

*From S.R. Weibel of Robert Taft Sanitary Engineering Center, Cincinnati, Ohio.

large amounts of grease are to be disposed of, or if the water is quite hard, a grease trap on the sink and/or laundry drain is recommended, especially if a small-sized septic tank is used. See. Fig. 11-1A.

Talbe 11-I indicates recommended tank sizes for various numbers of bedrooms, with and without garbage disposal units. The table is based upon average performance with a time interval of 5 to 10 years between cleanings. In no case should the tank be smaller than 500 U.S. gallons' (400 Imp. gals.) liquid capacity.

Larger sizes are in general more satisfactory because they allow more time for solids to settle out and be digested and they have more tolerance for temporary overloads, disinfectants, and other harmful chemicals which might be flushed into them. In view of the cost of having a tank cleaned a larger tank requiring less frequent cleaning can effect a considerable saving over a period of years.

The shape of the tank — rectangular, oval or round — has little or no effect upon performance at the same capacity.

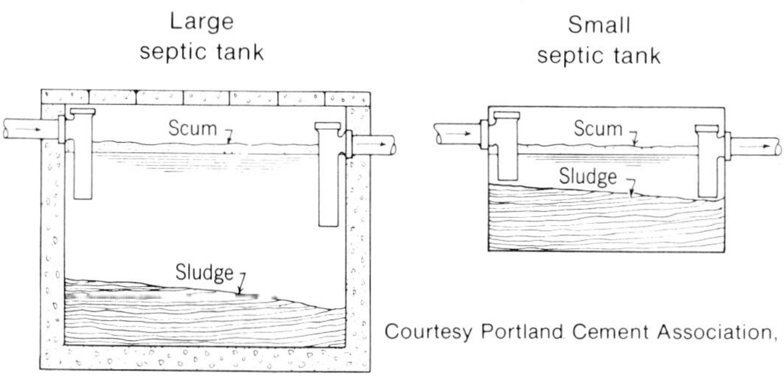

Courtesy Portland Cement Association, Chicago, Ill.

Fig. 11-6. The inside of a large and of a small septic tank after 2 years' operation by an average family. About 180 U.S. gallons of sludge collect at the bottom of the tanks. Sludge in the large tank is well below the outlet level, whereas sludge in the smaller tank is dangerously near the outlet and can easily pass off into disposal lines, ruining the entire system.

For best results the tank should hold at least 500 U.S. gallons (400 Imp. gals.) for an average farm family. Table 11-1 gives recommended size tank to build.

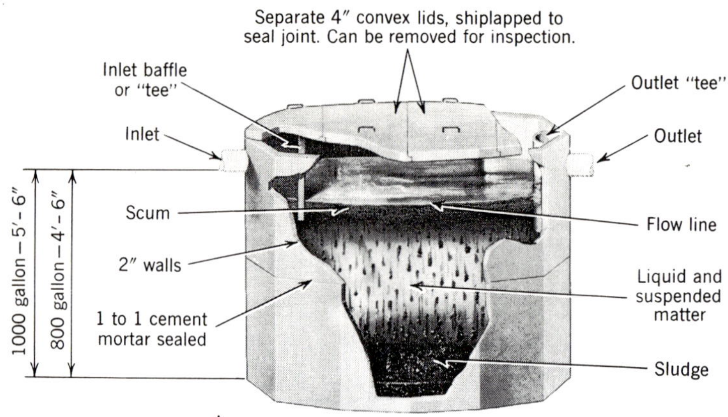

A

A, courtesy Phillip Sitton Septic Tank Co., Dayton, O.

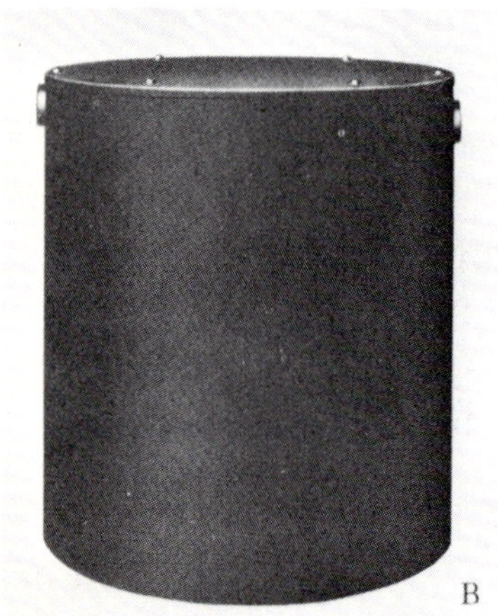

B

Fig. 11-7. Prefabricated septic tanks. A — Precast concrete, showing section through tank when in operation. B — A vertical steel tank. C — Horizontal steel tank. Full partition forms separate treatment and effluent chambers. Available in sizes up to 5000 gallons.

Concrete tanks can be installed in series as shown in Fig. 11-8 to increase capacity.

B and C, courtesy San Equip. Co., Syracuse, N.Y.

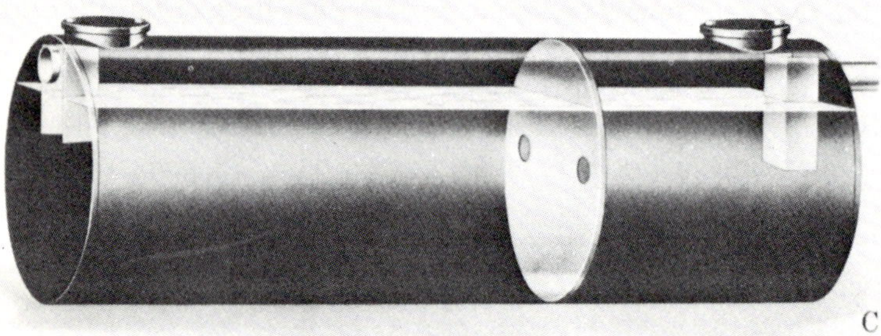

C

Types of tank

The cast-in-place concrete tank is satisfactory if good quality concrete is used. It can be built to any desired size. However, the pre-cast or pre-fabricated tanks now on the market are quite generally preferred and may be cheaper when labor costs are high.

Factory built tanks of pre-cast concrete, vitrified tile, or asphalt coated steel are readily available throughout the United States and are used extensively. See Fig. 11-7. These are satisfactory if large enough, if correctly installed, and if not cracked or damaged in handling. Asphalt-coated steel tanks should meet the minimum standard requirements for construction as set up by the U.S. Department of Commerce. Tanks which are manufactured according to these requirements will carry the stamp of approval of the Department of Commerce.

All steel tanks should be carefully inspected for scratches just before lowering into the hole. Any exposed metal should be covered with asphalt. The manufacturer usually supplies a small can of asphalt for this purpose. The tank should be lowered vertically into the hole to avoid scratching the asphalt coating.

Septic tanks are sometimes built on the premises with concrete block or construction tile layed up with cement mortar and waterproofed on the inside. This type of construction is not favored in most localities because the tanks are more likely to leak, thus endangering the water supply.

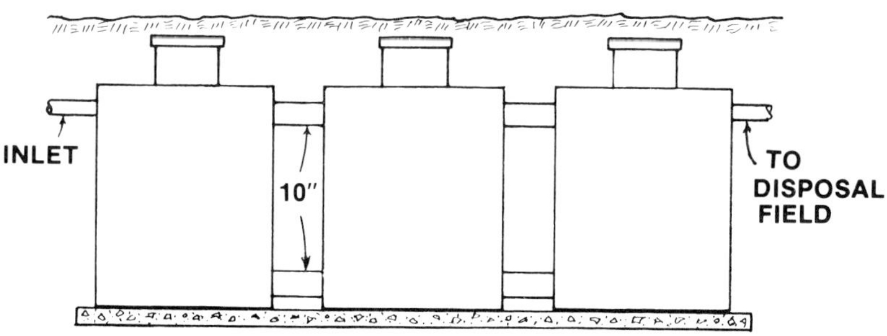

Fig. 11-8. Precast concrete septic tanks arranged in series to increase capacity. Can be used where needed capacities range from 1,500 U.S. gallons (1250 Imp. gals.) to 5,000 U.S. gallons (4160 Imp. gals.). Suitable for rural schools, hospitals, motels, mobile home parks, etc. Secondary treatment tanks and/or siphon tanks can be added at the end.

The tanks should be installed on a level concrete base as shown. The sewage drifts from inlet end to outlet end passing from tank to tank through the 10" connecting tile at top and bottom.

The single-compartment tank is the most generally used and is quite satisfactory for average household purposes. However, two or more compartment tanks (see Figs. 11-7C and 11-8) are recommended in sizes above 1500-gallon capacity. A siphon chamber tank, illustrated in Fig. 11-9 is recommended for large volumes of sewage where the tile field exceeds 500 linear feet (152 m.) or where the disposal field is in heavy soil or is over a sand filter. It is used principally for schools, camps, etc. The siphon chamber should have two-thirds of the total tile capacity. The Nodak system of Fig. 11-2 can be used in lieu of the siphon chamber tank.

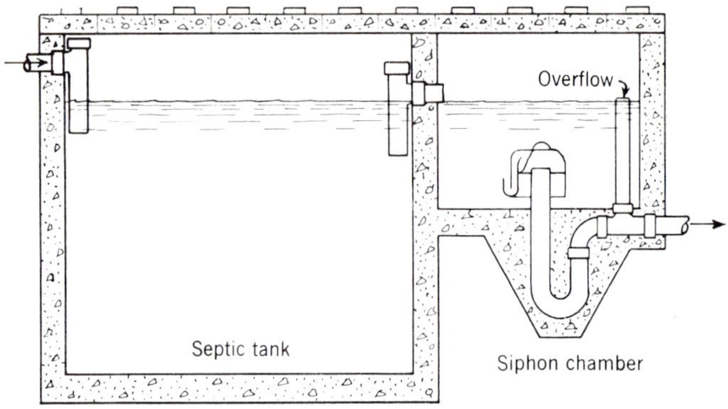

Fig. 11-9. A siphon chamber septic tank.

A new type of sewage treatment plant for individual homes is shown in Fig. 11-10. The operation of the plant is as follows:

1. The raw sewage from the house enters the primary treatment compartment (A) where settling and anerobic action takes place as in the conventional type of septic tank.

2. The overflow from compartment (A) flows into the aeration chamber (B) where it is mixed with activated sludge and is aerated by means of the motor driven aerator and at the same time is thoroughly mixed by the agitator driven by the same motor. The aerator injects tiny bubbles of air into the sewage for maximum contact of air and sewage. This supplys extra oxygen for the aerobic bacteria which further digests the sewage and converts it to odorless liquids and gasses.

3. From the aeration compartment (B) the sewage passes into the settling and clarifying compartment (C). In this compartment are tubes or baffles which prevent currents thus hastening the settling of the finely divided particles remaining in the sewage. The finely divided particles are returned to the aeration chamber via the sloping end wall where they are further aerated and further digested. Any remaining floating material is hydrolically skimmed off and returned to the aeration chamber. The remaining odorless and colorless liquid passes through the outlet of compartment (C) to the disposal area.

The total capacity of the tank is 1200 U.S. gallons (1000 Imp. gals.) (A) has a capacity of 475 U.S. gallons (396 Imp. gals.) Compartment

(B) 600 U.S. gallons (500 Imp. gals.) and compartment (C) 125 U.S. gallons. (396 Imp. gals.)

The system is automatic in operation. The fractional horsepower motor runs only a part of the time, therefore is not expensive to operate. The manufacturer claims that installation costs are comparable to the cost of conventional septic tank and disposal tile installations.

Where necessary or desirable chlorination treatment can be added to the system. Also, tertiary treatment can be added by means of a special upflow filter.

Although most of the solids are digested there is a small residue which must eventually be cleaned out. It is claimed that this system will operate five times as long between cleanings as will the conventional septic tank. In some areas less disposal tile can be used. Disposal tile do not become clogged with solids as often happens with the conventional tanks.

As this is a new type of tank, it may be that some local health departments have not yet approved its use. It would be well to consult the local health department before purchasing.

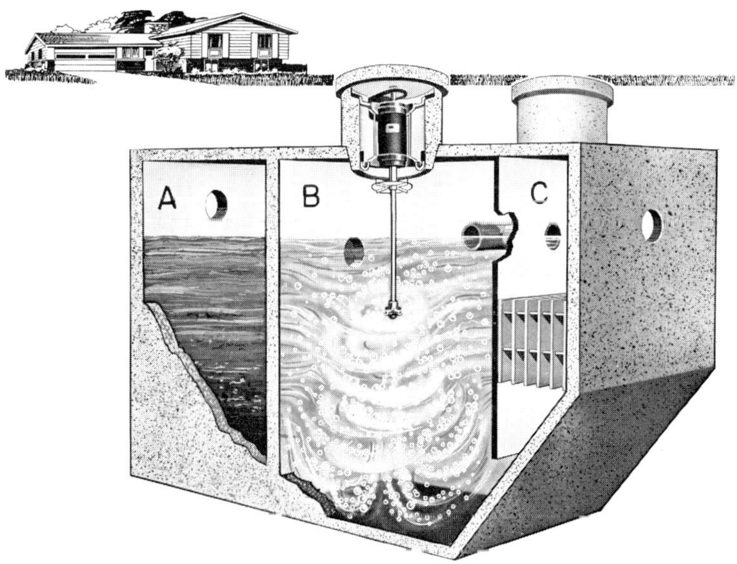

Courtesy of Jet Areation Co. of Cleveland, O.

Fig. 11-10. A new type of sewage treatment plant for individual homes designed to be used in lieu of the conventional septic tanks. It has a total capacity of 1,200 U.S. gallons (1000 Imp. gals.) and will handle the sewage from all domestic fixtures and appliances, including garbage grinders. The manufacturer claims that this system will, in just 24 hours, reduce all household sewage to an odorless, colorless liquid which is easy to dispose of.

Location of tank. The septic tank should be located at a safe distance from the water source, at least 50 feet away, and on the downhill side. This is to insure against contamination of the water supply in case of a leak. If possible, locate the tank on the side of the house nearest the bathroom and in the general direction of the disposal field. It can be located near the house but there is less danger of odors if located 20 to 30 feet (6 to 10 m.) away.

For the best operation the tank must be low enough in the ground so that the sewer pipe from the house can have a grade of ¼-inch per foot. A grade less than that will not maintain a rate of flow high enough to carry the solids and the sewer may become plugged. A grade of more than that may produce such a high velocity of discharge into the tank that turbulence may occur, causing solids to be carried out the outlet to plug up the disposal tile.

The tank should not be located under driveways, walks, flower beds, or other areas which would be spoiled by excavation at cleaning time. If cleaning is to be done by pumping into a tank truck, consideration should be given to accessibility by the truck. Where a pump

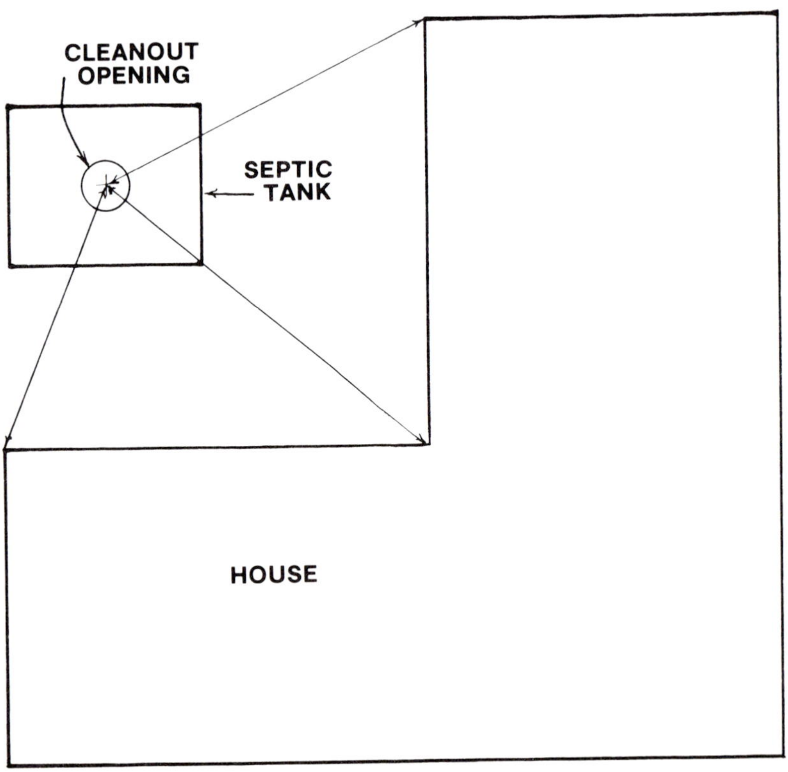

Fig. 11-11. Locate the septic tank clean-out opening with reference to permanent cations such as corners of buildings as shown. A map with dimensions on it should filed for future reference.

cleaning service is readily available an extension manhole to the surface, as indicated in Fig. 11-12 makes inspection and cleaning possible without excavation.

Before backfilling over a tank make a chart showing the exact location of clean-out openings with respect to some perminent land marks such as corners of buildings. See Fig. 11-11. Such a chart may save considerable searching and digging years later when the tank has to be cleaned.

If the land slopes steeply away from the house it is best to locate the tank close to the house and let the steep grade come *after* the tank rather than before. Figures 11-13 through 11-16 illustrate various

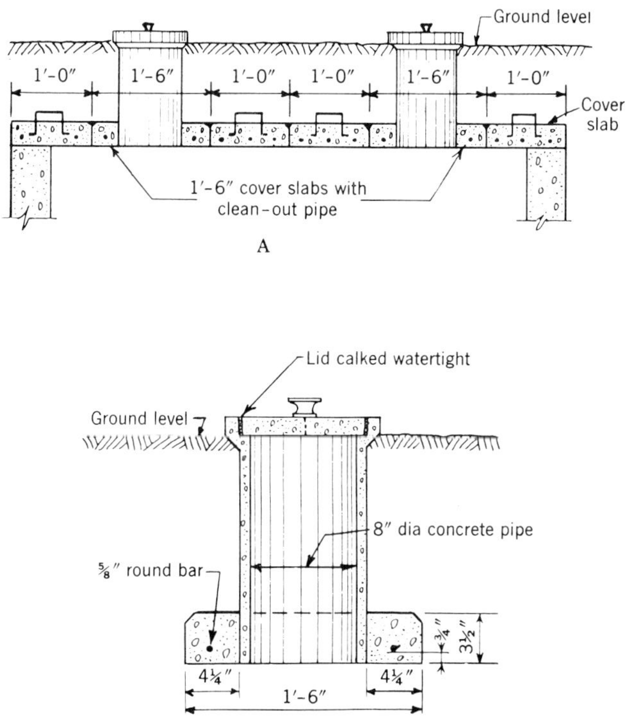

Courtesy Portland Cement Association

Fig. 11-12. Optional clean-out openings for a septic tank. A — Top of septic tank showing location of clean-out pipes. B — Close-up of clean-out pipe.

methods of handling the effluent on steep grades. The top of the tank should be at least 1 foot underground for frost protection and to provide enough soil for sod to grow over it.

In special cases where the tank must be lower than the disposal field the Nodak system of Fig. 11-2 can be used.

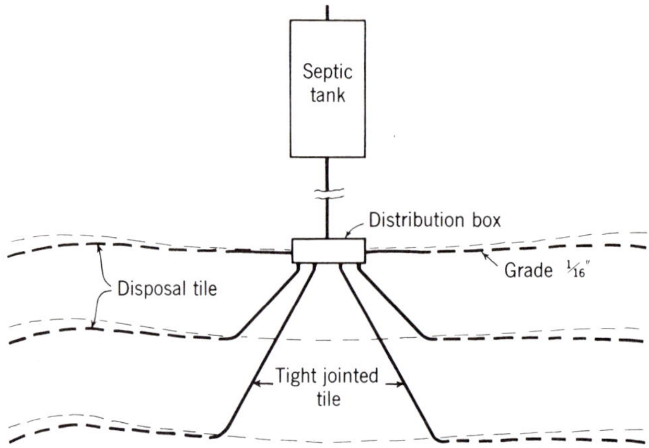

Fig. 11-13. Tile field plan for fairly steep grade with wide space available for tile. Tile outlets in distribution box must be at exactly the same level to insure even distribution.

Limitations of a septic tank. A septic tank provides a place for decomposing or digesting sewage of human excrement and kitchen and laundry waste. Other materials, such as cloth of *any kind,* paper other than toilet paper, metals, plastics, etc., are not readily decomposed; therefore they should not be flushed into the tank. Furthermore, such objects frequently lodge in the pipes and cause stoppage. *Many kinds of objects and chemicals which can safely be flushed into a city sewage system should not be flushed into a septic tank system.*

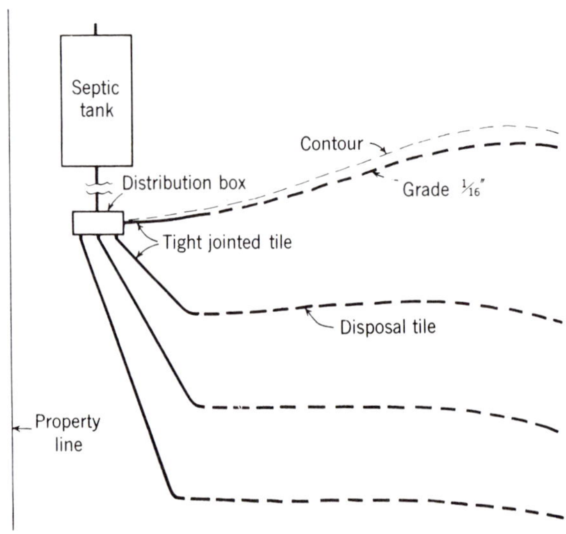

Fig. 11-14. Tile field plan for steep grade where tank is at one side of a property.

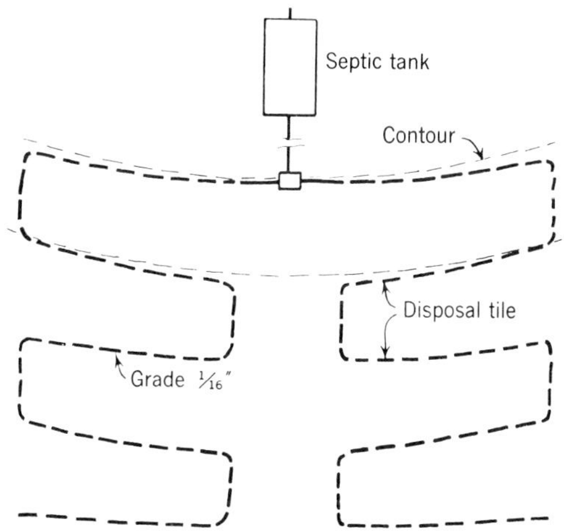

Fig. 11-15. Tile field plan for steep grade with porous soil and plenty of space. Upper reaches of tile receive greatest load; therefore this plan is not as good as those of Figs. 11-13 and 11-14.

As the septic action in the tank is dependent upon bacterial growth nothing should be flushed into the tank which will kill or seriously retard the growth of bacteria. A limited amount of chlorine bleaching agent, drain solvent, strong soap, salt solutions, and disinfectants will cause no trouble if the tank is large enough. However, *frequent use* of such chemicals should be avoided. Waste from the kitchen sink and laundry, where hard water is used and where there is considerable soap and grease, should be diverted to a grease trap before entering the septic tank. Soap and hard water form an insoluble precipitate which is not readily decomposed in the tank; therefore the tank will fill with sludge more quickly. Grease tends to fill the pipe and is not readily decomposed.

Waste from milkrooms, backwashing water filters, and water softeners should be disposed of otherwise than in the septic tank. *Floor drains and down spouts from the roof should not be led into the septic tank.*

Cleaning the septic tank. A septic tank should always be cleaned before the solids or scum begin to discharge into the disposal tile. Failure to do so usually means digging up and cleaning the tile as well as the tank.

The frequency at which a tank needs cleaning depends upon:

1. Size of tank in relation to the daily volume of sewage.
2. The kind and quantity of solids and chemicals flushed into the tank.

Under normal operating conditions a tank should serve from 5 to 10 years between cleanings. For a new tank, inspection should be made once a year until experience indicates the frequency of cleaning. *Never use matches or other open flames for inspection of a tank* as the gases may ignite causing a serious explosion. Use a flashlight if a light is needed. No one should be allowed to enter a large tank until it is aired out as there is danger of being overcome by gases.

Solids will leave the tank through the effluent opening when either the sludge or the scum builds up too close to the outlet. The velocity of flow through a small tank is greater than through a large tank for the same amount of sewage. The greater the velocity of flow the greater the carrying capacity of the liquid for solids, and the more likely are solids to be carried out to the disposal field. For this reason the sludge should not be built up as close to the outlet in a small tank as is permissible in a large tank. In small tanks the top of the sludge should not be less than 18 inches (46 cm.) from the bottom of the outlet and in large tanks, 1000 U.S. gallons (833 Imp. gals.) or more, not less than 6 inches. (15 cm.)

The bottom of the scum should be at least 3 inches (7.5 cm.) *above* the outlet opening. When ground garbage is discharged into a tank the scum builds up faster than without garbage.

Cleaning can be accomplished by removing a part or all of the cover and bailing or pumping out the sludge and scum. It is not necessary to remove all of the liquid. In no case should the tank be completely emptied. A residue of the old sewage will serve to reinocculate the tank with bacteria after cleaning.

If the waste removed by cleaning is to be disposed of on the premises, it should be burried in a pit or trench and covered with 12 to 18 inches of soil. In no case should these wastes be buried where they might contaminate the water supply.

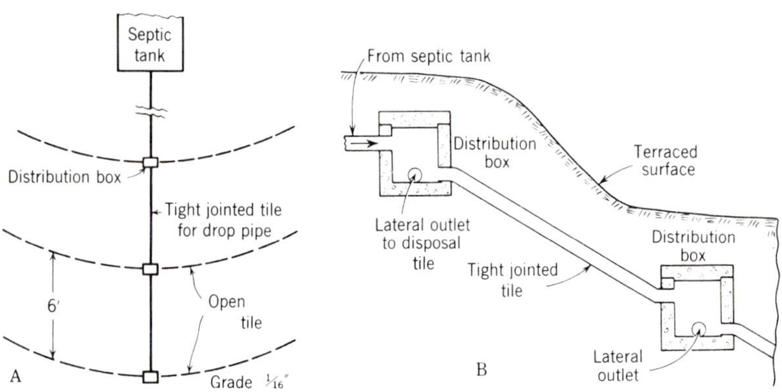

Fig. 11-16. Tile field plan for steep grade with long narrow space. Distribution is uneven. Upper laterals take most of load. Not recommended except for unusually steep grades. B is an elevation view of the distribution boxes shown in A; sometimes called drop boxes.

Once the frequency of cleaning has been established a record should be kept as a guide for future cleaning.

Sewer line from septic tank to distribution box.

This sewer line functions to carry the liquid effluent from the septic tank to the disposal area (except in the Nodak system). It can be made of cast iron, vitrified clay tile, cement tile, plastic tile, or bituminized fiber tile with watertight joints. The line should have a grade of ⅛-inch per running foot and should not have sharp bends. The ends of the tile should be sealed into the septic tank and into the distribution box with watertight joints. Trenching, grading, and backfilling for this line is the same as for the house sewer except for the grade.

Distribution boxes.

It is the function of the distribution box to divide the liquid effluent equally to all of the disposal lines. To do this, all of the outlets must be at *exactly the same level.* If this is not done some disposal lines will be overloaded while others may receive no liquid. This, of course, will reduce the effectiveness of the field.

Distribution boxes are usua-ly made of pre-cast concrete or steel; see Fig. 11-17. In any case the box should be watertight and should have a removable cover for cleaning.

The disposal area.

The correct design and location of the effluent disposal system is just as important as is the septic tank. It is the function of the effluent disposal system to receive the liquid effluent from the septic tank and allow it to leach away into the soil. *It must therefore have the capacity to absorb the entire liquid output of the septic tank.* The capacity of the ground to take up liquids varies widely with the character of the soil and the level of the water table. These factors must be taken into consideration in the design of a satisfactory disposal area. The best method of disposal of liquid effluent is by means of an absorption tile field fed by gravity flow from the septic tank. If the topsoil is too heavy, or the water table is too close to the surface, or the topography will not permit gravity flow, the pumped system of Fig. 11-2 can be used. Where space is too limited for a disposal tile field, seepage pits, sand filters, or underdrained tile may have to be used as indicated later. All disposal areas should be at least 100 feet (30 m.) from and on the downhill side of a water source.

Disposal tile system.

Figures 10-2, 11-1, and 11-13 through 11-16 illustrate various arrangements of disposal tile lines for different topography situations. It is the function of the disposal tile to distribute the liquid effluent from the septic tank over such an area that it will *all* be taken up by the soil. This means that the size of the field is very important.

The *size of the field* should be determined by (1) the volume of sewage to be disposed of, (2) the character of the soil in which the tile is to be installed, and (3) the manner of construction, i.e., width and depth of trench, amount of gravel used, etc.

The volume of septic tank effluent to be disposed of will vary considerably with the residence capacity of the house and the water habits of the occupants. According to metered flow in a number of installations as reported by Weibel, the range was from 8 to 150 gallons per person per day with an average of 39 U.S. gallons (32.5 Imp. gals.) per persons per day. The recommendations given in this book are based upon 40 U.S. gallons (33 Imp. gals.) per person per day. If it is known that the water consumption exceeds this figure the disposal area should be enlarged accordingly.

Automatic dishwashers and garbage grinders add only a small amount to the liquid volume, although the garbage grinders add considerably to the load of solids on the septic tank. Automatic clothes washers add roughly 50% on the average to the waste volume. These values are reflected in the recommendations in Tables 11-II and 11-III.

TABLE 11-II.
ABSORPTION TRENCH AREAS PER BEDROOM FOR FOUR USAGE COMBINATIONS*

Percolation Rate (Time Required for Water to Fall 1 Inch (2½ cm.).	Required Area (Square Feet of Absorption Trench Bottom per Bedroom)							
	Without Garbage Grinder or Automatic Washer		With Garbage Grinder		With Automatic Washer		With both Garbage Grinder & Automatic Washer	
Minutes	Sq. Ft.	Sq. M.	Sq. Ft.	Sq. M.	Sq. Ft.	Sq. M.	Sq. Ft.	Sq. M.
2 or less	50	4.65	65	6.04	75	6.97	85	7.90
3	60	5.57	75	6.97	85	7.90	100	9.29
4	70	6.50	85	7.90	95	8.83	115	10.69
5	75	6.97	90	8.36	105	9.76	125	11.62
10	100	9.29	120	11.15	135	12.55	165	15.33
15	115	10.69	140	13.01	160	14.87	190	17.66
30	150	13.94	180	16.73	205	19.05	250	23.23
45	180	16.73	215	19.98	245	22.77	300	27.88
60	200	18.59	240	22.30	275	25.55	330	30.67
Over60	Unsuitable for shallow absorption system. Investigate for seepage pit, subsurface filter arrangement, or Nordak system.							

*From S.R. Weibel, Robert A. Taft Sanitary Engineering Center, Cincinnati, Ohio.

The water-absorbing character of soils varies widely. In coarse gravelly soil where the liquid is readily taken up, less tile is needed than in heavy soil. The best method of determining the capacity of the soil to absorb the liquids is by means of a percolation test.

It is recommended that the location and size of the disposal field, and the percolation test be made under the supervision of a local health officer.

Percolation test.

Briefly a percolation test involves the digging of holes in the proposed disposal area and then measuring the rate of percolation of

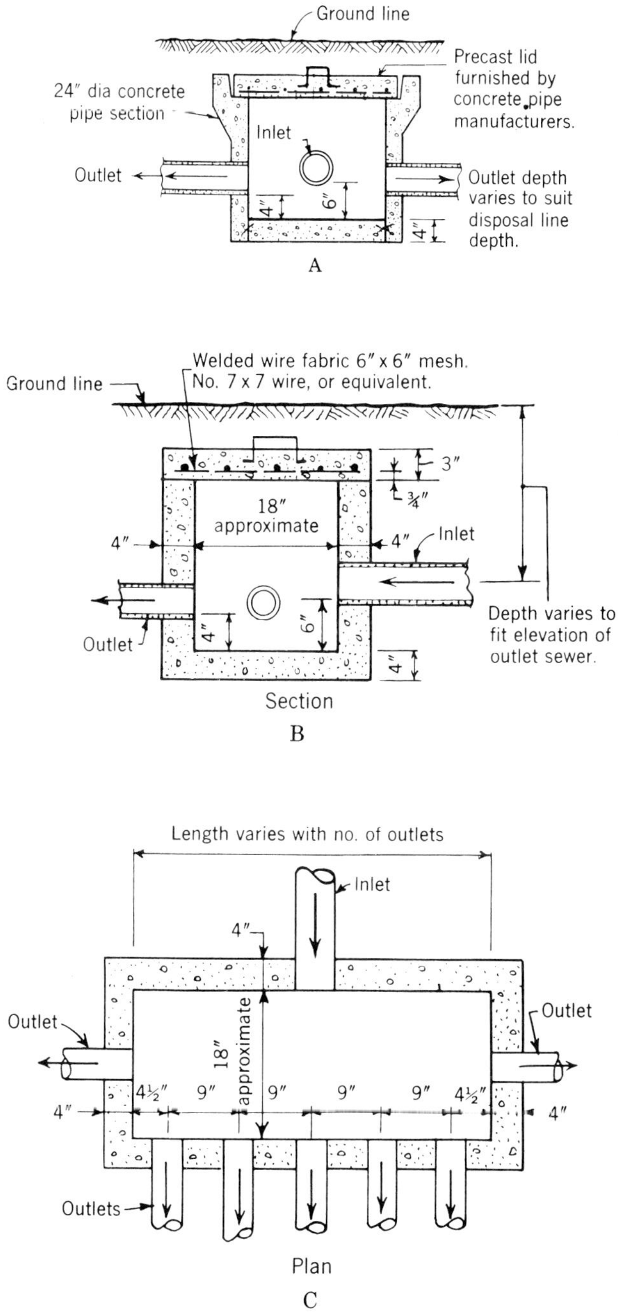

Ground line
Precast lid furnished by concrete pipe manufacturers.
24″ dia concrete pipe section
Inlet
Outlet
Outlet depth varies to suit disposal line depth.
4″
6″
4″
A
Welded wire fabric 6″ x 6″ mesh. No. 7 x 7 wire, or equivalent.
Ground line
3″
¾″
18″ approximate
4″
4″
Inlet
Outlet
Depth varies to fit elevation of outlet sewer.
4″
6″
4″
Section
B
Length varies with no. of outlets
Inlet
4″
Outlet
Outlet
18″ approximate
4½″
9″
9″
9″
9″
4½″
4″
4″
Outlets
Plan
C

Fig. 11-17

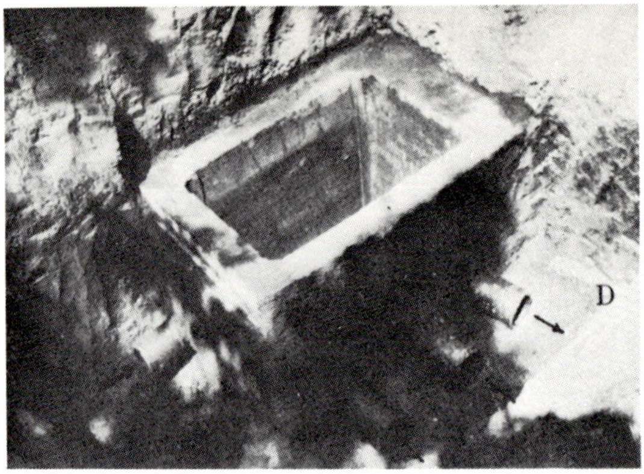

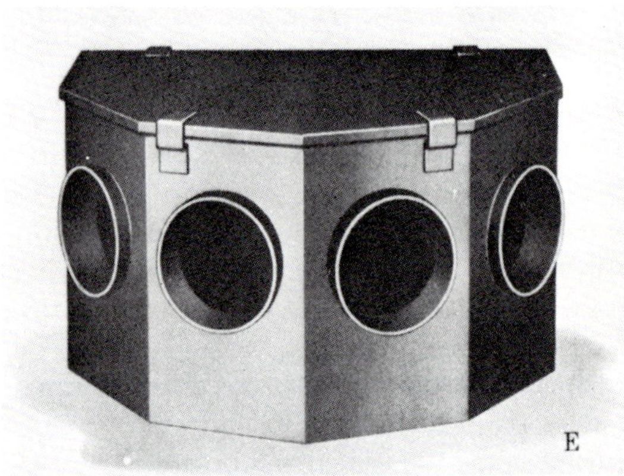

Fig. 11-17. Distribution boxes. A — Distribution box with three outlets or less. B — Distribution box with four or more outlets. C — Top view of distribution box with seven outlets. D — Distribution box installation with three outlets. A, B, C, and D show precast concrete boxes. E — Steel box.

A. B, C, and D courtesy Portland Cement Association
E and F courtesy San-Equip Co., Syracuse, N.Y.

water from these holes over a period of time. The following is an outline of the procedure.

1. Dig five or six holes uniformly spaced over the proposed disposal area. The holes should be about 1-foot in diameter with vertical sides and as deep as the tile trench will be, usually 20 to 24 inches.

2. Carefully scratch any "slicks" left by digging tools and remove all loose soil from the bottom. Add 2 inches of fine gravel or coarse sand to the bottom of the hole to protect the bottom from puddling when water is poured in.

3. Carefully fill the hole with clean water and keep it filled for an hour or two to insure thorough moistening of the soil. In heavy clay soil soak the soil for at least 4 hours.

4. While the hole is still moist from doing step 3, fill the holes with clear water to a depth of 6 inches above the gravel and observe the time required for the water level to drop 1 inch in each hole. Measurement can be made from a board laid across the top of the hole. Use the average of all holes as the percolation value for the area being tested. Table 11-II indicates the number of square feet of trench bottom required per bedroom with various percolation rates.

TABLE 11-III.

LENGTH OF 4-INCH DISPOSAL TILE PER BEDROOM FOR THREE WIDTHS OF TRENCHES UNDER VARIOUS PERCOLATION RATES AND TYPES OF USES.

			Length of 4-Inch Tile per Bedroom							
Percolation Rate (Time Required for Water Level to Drop 1-Inch)	Trench Width		Sewage Without Ground Garbage or Automatic Washer		Sewage With Ground Garbage		Sewage With Automatic Clothes Washer		Sewage With Both Ground Garbage and Automatic Clothes Washer	
Minutes	Inches	Cm.	Feet	Meters	Feet	Meters	Feet	Meters	Feet	Meters
2 or less	12	30	50	15	65	20	75	23	85	26
	18	46	34	10	44	13	50	15	57	17
	24	61	25	8	33	10	38	12	43	13
3	12	30	60	18	75	23	85	26	100	30
	18	46	40	12	50	15	57	17	67	20
	24	61	30	9	38	12	43	13	50	15
4	12	30	70	21	85	26	95	29	115	35
	18	46	47	14	57	17	64	20	77	23
	24	61	35	11	43	13	48	15	58	18
5	12	30	75	23	90	27	105	32	125	38
	18	46	50	15	60	18	70	21	84	26
	24	61	38	12	45	14	53	16	63	19
10	12	30	100	30	120	37	135	41	165	50
	18	46	67	20	80	24	90	27	110	34
	24	61	50	15	60	18	68	21	83	25
15	12	30	115	35	140	43	160	49	190	58
	18	46	77	23	94	29	107	33	127	39
	24	61	58	18	70	21	80	24	95	29
30	12	30	150	46	180	55	205	62	250	76
	18	46	100	30	120	37	137	42	167	51
	24	51	75	23	90	27	103	31	125	38
45	12	30	180	55	215	66	245	75	300	91
	18	46	120	37	144	44	164	50	200	61
	24	61	90	27	108	33	123	37	150	46
60	12	30	200	61	240	73	275	84	330	101
	18	46	134	41	160	49	180	55	220	67
	24	61	100	30	120	37	138	42	165	50
Over 60	Unsuitable for Shallow Absorption Tile. Use Seepage Pit, Sand Filter, or Underdrained Tile System, or if Approved by Health Department, One of the Newer Systems Shown in Figures II-10 and II-37.									

As the square-foot area of the bottom of a trench varies with the width as well as the length, it is obvious that a wide trench need not be as long as a narrow trench. Table 11-III indicates the length of tile needed per bedroom under various percolation rates and from different widths and usage conditions.

In addition to the percolation test the soil should be examined for high water table, and the presence of hardpan, bedrock, or other impervious layers within the upper 4 feet of soil. These checks can be made by digging or boring a hole to a depth of at least 4 feet. (1.2 m.) Depths of 5 or 6 feet (1.5 to 1.83 m.) are better. The hole can be made with a soil auger or with a post hole digger. If standing water or impervious layers are encountered within 4 feet (1.2 m.) of the surface, the functioning of the tile field will be materially impaired and more tile will have to be used, or a more suitable location chosen, or another method of disposal considered.

As an example for determining the size of a disposal tile field, the following conditions are assumed:

1. A house with three bedrooms.
2. Load to be sewage with automatic clothes washer. (No garbage disposal.)
3. A land area 50 feet by 50 feet (15 m. by 15 m.) at a safe distance from the well where the tile field can be located.
4. A percolation time, as determined by a percolation test, of 1 inch (2.54 cm.) in 4 minutes.

Table 11-III indicates that with a percolation time of 1 inch in 4 minutes and for sewage with an automatic clothes washer either 95, 64, or 48 feet (29, 20 or 15 m.) of tile per bedroom could be used depending upon the width of the trench. As there are three bedrooms in the house the total length of tile would be respectively 285, 193 or 144 feet. (87, 60 or 45 m.) Because of the limitations of the available land space no tile run can be more than 50 feet (15 m.) long; therefore the logical choice would be three lines of tile 48 feet (14.6 m.) long and in a 24-inch-wide (61 cm.) trench.

If in the example given the percolation time were 15 minutes the minimum length of tile would be 3 times 80 or 240 feet. (3 × 24m. or 72 m.) Using 24-inch-wide trenches in a 50-foot by 50-foot space it would be necessary to have five lines 48 feet (14.6 m.) long. Spacing the tile lines 8 feet (2.44 m.) apart the entire system would fit nicely in the available space.

Construction of the tile field.

There should be at least two runs of tile about equal in length. No single run should exceed 100 feet (30 m.) in length. The minimum total lenght should be approximately 100 feet (30 m.) unless the soil is exceptionally porous. In heavy soils or where space is somewhat limited, wide deep trenches with deep gravel beds are recommended. See Fig. 11-18C.

The effluent from an ordinary septic tank is by no means purified; therefore a disposal tile field is a likely source of contamination of a water supply. For this reason the tile field should be located at least 100 feet (30 m.) [200 feet (60 m.) in gravelly soil] away and downgrade from a well or other source of water. The filtering action of the soil tends to purify the liquid *if the liquid passes through enough soil.* Chlorination under controlled conditions gives added assurance of purification.

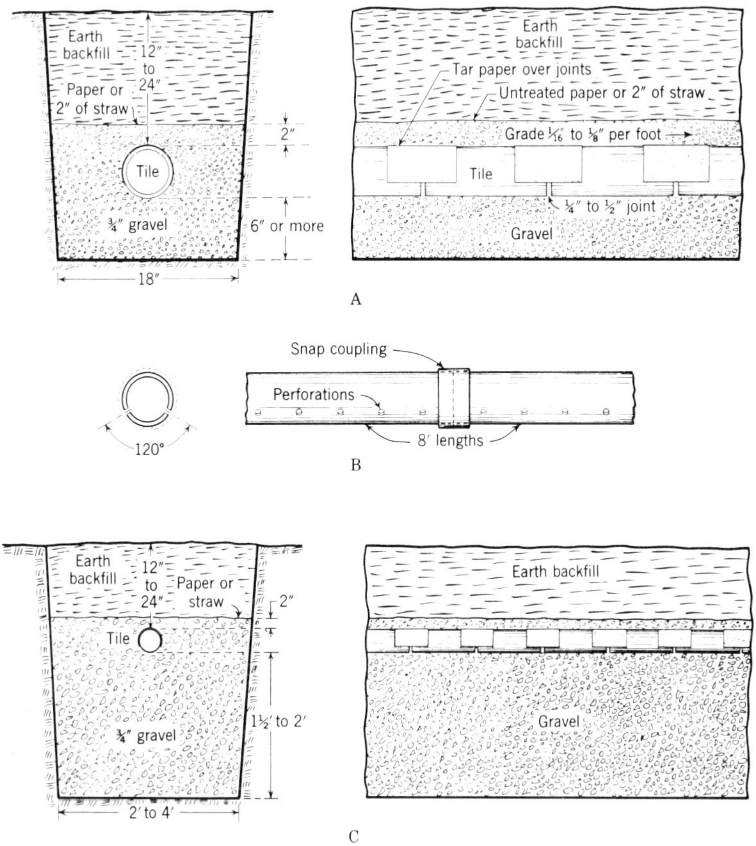

Fig. 11-18. Construction of disposal trenches. A — Construction for porous to medium heavy soils. B — Perforated disposal pipe which can be used in place of the drainage tile shown at A. C — Trench construction for heavy soils, and for a location where space is a limiting factor or where tree roots are encountered. The larger trench provides more absorption area per lineal foot of trench. Do not use tar paper between the gravel and the earth backfill as it will prevent moisture from moving upward to the surface and grass may not grow over the trench. Also, the tar paper will reduce the capacity of the tile field to dispose of the liquid.

The tile should always be placed within the upper 36 inches (1 m.) of the soil. The usual depth is 18 to 24 inches (46 to 61 cm.) (8 to 10 inches can be used over a high water table). This places the liquid where much of it can rise to the surface by capillary action to be evaporated or taken up by plant roots. What does not rise toward the surface percolates downward and is, under favorable conditions, more or less purified by the filtering action of the soil. If the soil surface is uneven it may be necessary in some places to go deeper than 24 inches or even 36 inches in order to maintain grade, but such depths should be limited to a very small portion of the entire field. The deeper the trench the wider it should be in order to provide more percolation capacity. Shallow tile functions best under sod. Lawn grass will take up much of the moisture and give it off to the air by transpiration yet the roots do not go deep enough to plug the tile.

If it can be avoided the tile lines should not be laid under driveways, walks, plowed areas, or near trees or other large plants with deep roots. Deep roots will grow toward water and the hair roots will grow into the tile causing a stoppage. If the tile must be laid in rooted areas it is recommended that a deep bed of gravel (1½ to 2 feet), 1/2 m. to 2/3 m. deep) be placed under the tile. See Fig. 11-18C. There is some evidence that a deep bed of gravel under the tile tends to prevent root stoppage. The deep gravel allows the water to drop quickly below tile level and the hair roots which follow the water grow toward the lower part of the gravel instead of into the tile.

For best results the discharge into the disposal tile should be intermittent. With the average household sizes of tanks the discharge is intermittent. For very large tanks such as might be used for schools, motels, hotels, hospitals, etc., the discharge may be almost constant. The siphon chamber type of tank, the pumped system, or two absorption fields can be used for these latter purposes. With two absorption fields a switch is provided in the effluent line so that the sewage can be diverted alternately from one field to the other.

The disposal tile trenches should be dug from the distribution box and to a grade of about 1/16 inch per running foot. The trench should be dug deep enough to allow for the necessary gravel or crushed stone under the tile.

The gravel bed should be carefully graded on the surface to a uniform slope of 1/16 inch per running foot before the tile is laid in place. If the slope is too steep, or if the grading is not uniform, the liquids will tend to concentrate in localized areas and thus reduce the capacity of the field and may break out on the surface. When the topography is steep, one of the plans shown in Figs. 11-13 through 11-16 can be used for maintaining grades.

Kind of tile

The tile may be ordinary clay or cement drainage tile as indicated in Fig. 11-19, or perforated clay, cement, plastic, or bituminized fiber tile as shown at B in Figs. 11-18 and 11-20. It should be at least 4 inches (10.6 cm.) in diameter. Plastic tile is most commonly used.

Laying the tile

Clay or cement drainage tiles should be laid end to end with ¼- to ½-inch (0.64 to 1.27 cm.) spacing at the joints. Over each joint place a piece of tar paper about two-thirds of the way around the outside of the tile. See Figs. 11-18 and 11-19.

Place gravel along the sides of the tile as shown in Fig. 11-19 to hold the paper in position. Joints in perforated tile are usually made with a bell or a coupling. Cover the tile to a depth of 2 inches (5 cm.) with gravel. Over the gravel fill, place a layer of *untreated* porous building paper or 2 inches (5 cm.) of straw to prevent soil from filtering into the gravel and the tile. Do not use tarred paper as it will act as a barrier to the movement of water toward the surface. Backfill the trench with soil, mounding the soil 4 to 6 inches (10 to 15 cm.) to allow for settling. When the soil is settled replace the sod, or seed.

If the natural excavated soil is heavy impervious clay or adobe, or if *very* rocky, a selected porous soil should be brought in for a backfill. Loam, sandy loam, and gravelly soil are suitable for this.

There is little danger of either septic tanks or disposal tile freezing. Exceptions may occur where tile is laid under driveways, walks, or other areas where snow is cleared.

A well-designed and carefully constructed disposal field should serve for 20 years or longer *provided the septic tank is large enough and is cleaned at the correct intervals.* However, with the best systems some solids are likely to enter the tiles and will eventually fill them up. When this happens, regardless of the length of time the tile has been in service, the lines must be dug up, cleaned, and relaid or abandoned in favor of a new disposal field.

Table 11-IV summarizes the general recommendations for minimum standards for a septic tank and disposal tile field installation.

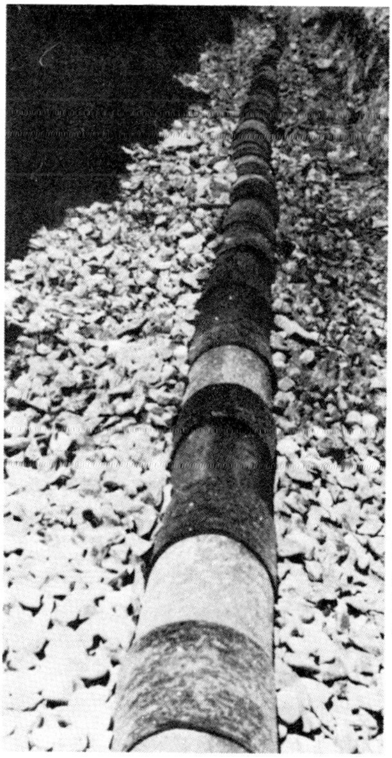

Fig. 11-19. A disposal lateral made of drainage tile. Must be covered with 2 inches of gravel, straw or porous paper and earth backfill.

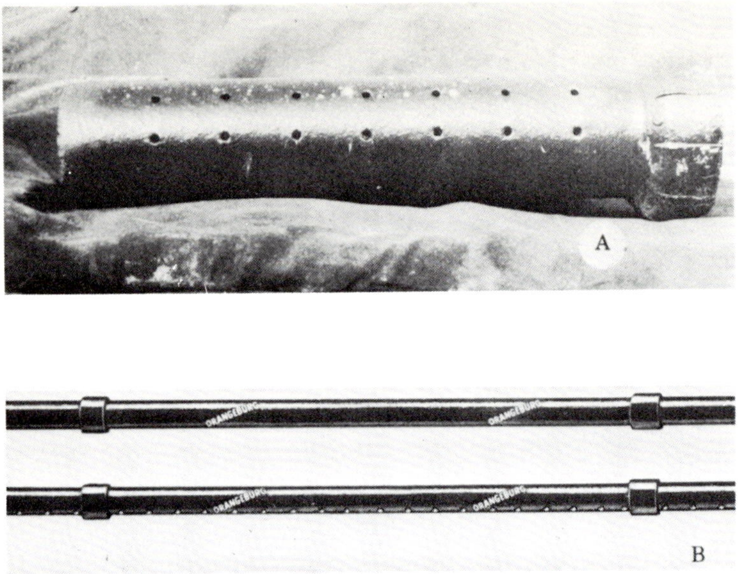

Fig. 11-20. Perforated vitrified clay tile at A. Bituminized fiber tile at B; top is sewer tile and bottom is perforated drain tile. Slotted flexible drain tile is available in lengths up to 250 ft.

Seepage Pits, Drain Pools, and Underdrained Filters

When conditions are such that a disposal tile field cannot be made to work, some other method of septic tank effluent disposal must be used. The commonly accepted alternate methods are by means of (1) one or more seepage pits, (2) a drain pool, (3) an underdrained filter bed, or (4) the new Aerating system.

A health officer should be consulted on the use and construction of any of these alternate methods before materials are purchased or construction is started.

Seepage pit.

This consists of a hole in the ground walled up with unmortered blocks or bricks, or pre-cast concrete pits may be used. and covered with earth. See Fig. 11-22, and 11-23. The most common application is in areas where there is an impervious layer of clay or hardpan close to the surface with a porous layer of soil beneath. *A seepage pit should not be used if the water table is less than 8 feet (2.5 m.) below the surface or if there is danger of contaminating a water supply.* Seepage pits, drain pools, and cesspools are a greater hazard to the ground-water supply than are disposal tile fields because they are deeper and seepage downward is more concentrated. They should be located at least 150 feet (46 m.) away and downgrade from a water source.

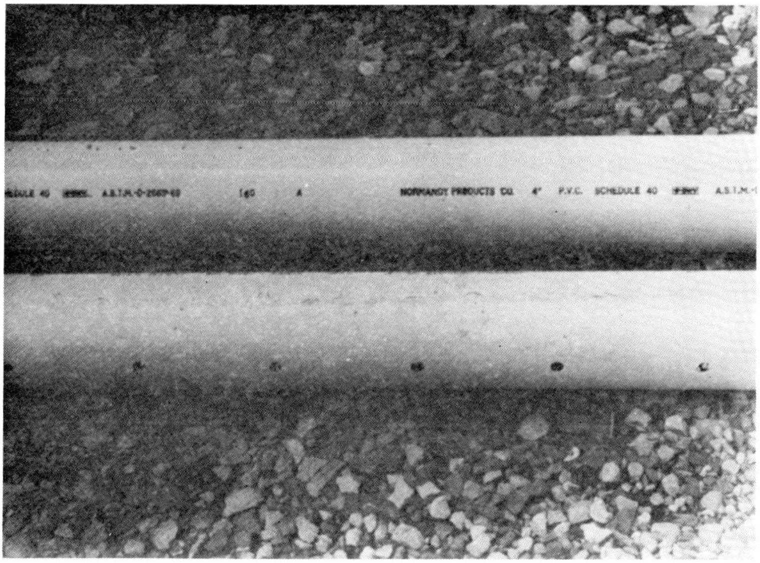

A

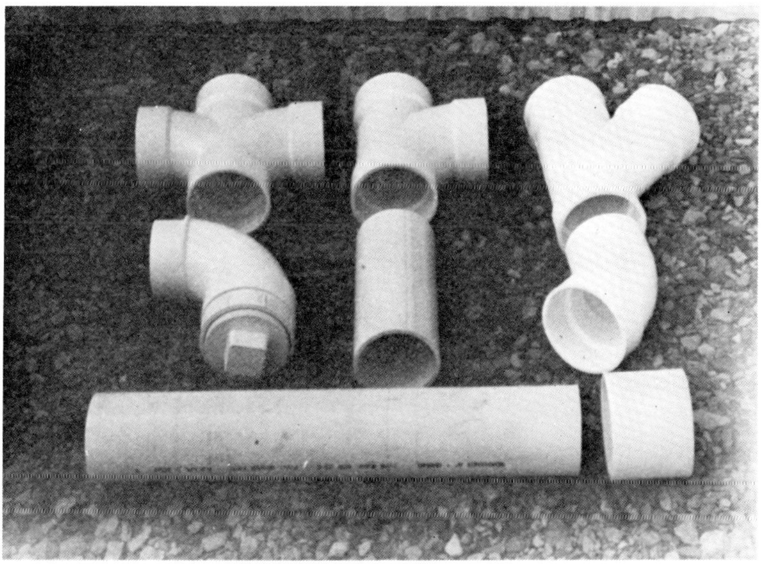

B

Fig. 11-21. Plastic sewer pipe and fittings. At A the top pipe is the nonperforated type used for the sewer lines from the house to the distribution boxes. The lower pipe is the perforated type used for the distribution lines in the disposal field.

At B is an assortment of plastic fittings. They are joined to the pipes by means of special solvent cement.

TABLE 11-IV.
MINIMUM STANDARDS FOR SEPTIC TANK AND DISPOSAL TILE FIELD INSTALLATION.*

Item	Material	Minimum Size	Grade	Governing Distance** To Building or Property Line Ft.	M.	To Water Source Ft.	M.
Sewer Line: house to septic tank	Cast iron to at least 5 feet beyond foundation. Cast iron, cement, plastic, or bituminized fiber with watertight joints optional from there on.	4 inches	¼ inch per foot	10	3	50	15
Septic tank	Concrete, metal, vitrous tile	500 U.S. gallons	—	10	3	50	15
Sewer Line: septic tank to distribution box	Cast iron, vitrous tile, cement, plastic, or bituminized fiber. Watertight joints.	4 inches	⅛ inch per foot	10	3	50	15
Distribution box	Concrete or steel. Waterproofed slab cover.	Adequate for no. of outlets.	All outlets at same level and at least 4 inches above bottom of box.	10	3	50	15
Disposal tile field trench	---------	12 to 24 inches wide. Depth according to soil.	1/16 inch per foot at least 2 feet above rock, hardpan, or water table.	10	3	100 (200, gravelly soil)	30 (60 gravelly soil)
Tile	Drainage tile or perforated tile.	4 inches. Joints ¼ to ½ inch or perforations downward.	1/16 inch per foot.	10	3	100 (200 gravelly soil)	30 (60 gravelly soil)

*Data largely from Mr. F.R. Ligouri, Ithaca, N.Y.
**1 inch = 2.54 cm.
1 foot = 30.48 cm. = 0.3048 m.
Imp. gals. = U.S. gals./1.2

Drain pool.

This consists of a specially constructed, open-bottom steel dome, placed over a bed of gravel as indicated in Fig. 11-24. The principal use of a drain pool is where there is porous soil but not enough room for a disposal tile field. It is easier to install than is a seepage pit. Drain pools or seepage pits can also be used at the ends of disposal tile runs as indicated in Fig. 11-24C to increase the capacity of an existing field or to take care of temporary overloads.

Underdrained filters.

These are generally used only as a last resort where a high water table or other unfavorable soil conditions preclude the use of any of

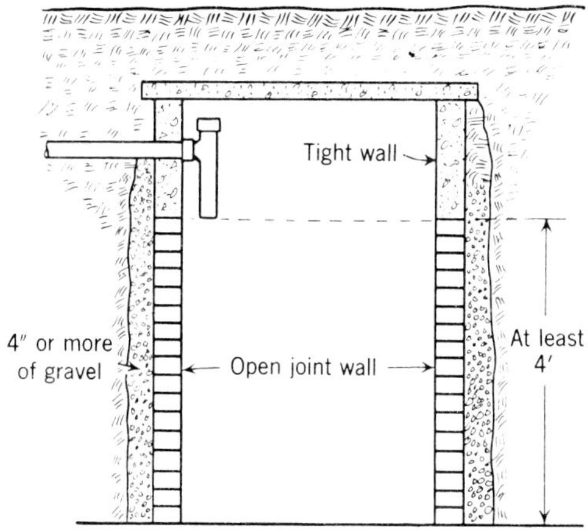

A

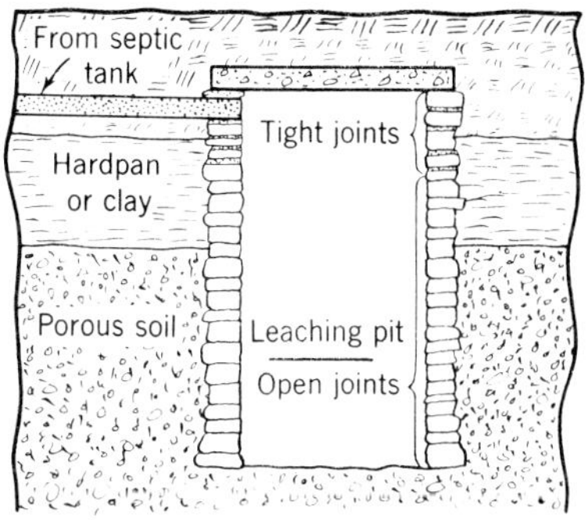

B

Fig. 11-22. Plans for seepage pits as a means of liquid effluent disposal. A bed of gravel around the outside of the open-jointed wall will improve the performance. B is a plan for a seepage pit where impervious layers close to the surface are underlain by porous layers.

the preceding methods. They are expensive to build and to maintain. As indicated in Fig. 11-25 such a filter consists of a bed of sand and gravel with disposal tile on top and drain tile underneath. The liquid effluent filters downward through the sand which removes solids, leaving a clear liquid discharge through the underdrained tile. This liquid must be disposed of in a sanitary manner. It should never be discharged into a stream, lake or pond unless chlorinated under controlled conditions. In any case such a system should be installed under the supervision of a health officer.

Figure 11-26 illustrates a variation of the sand filter principle. It is sometimes used: (1) to increase the capacity of a limited disposal area, (2) where bedrock is close to the surface (less than 4 feet), or (3) where the water table is at times too high. Its use is contingent upon sanitary disposal of the underdrained effluent. To insure intermittent dosing of the filter a siphon chamber septic tank is usually employed ahead of the filter.

When a sand filter becomes clogged with solids the top soil should be removed and the clogged portion of the filter taken out. Any sand and gravel thus removed should be replaced with an equal amount of fresh material. If the filter becomes deeply clogged it may be better to abandon it and construct a new one.

If the area available for a disposal field or a sand filter is wet because of underground drainage from higher levels, it is sometimes practical to intercept this underground water with a line or two of drainage tile placed uphill from the disposal area as illustrated in Fig. 11-27. The discharge from such a drainage tile is not likely to be badly contaminated; therefore it can be discharged on the surface at a lower level.

Cesspools

A *cesspool* differs from a seepage pit in that the cesspool receives the entire sewage while the seepage pit receives only the liquid part, usually the liquid effluent from a septic tank. When the soil is quite porous and *there is no danger of pollution of the drinking water,* a

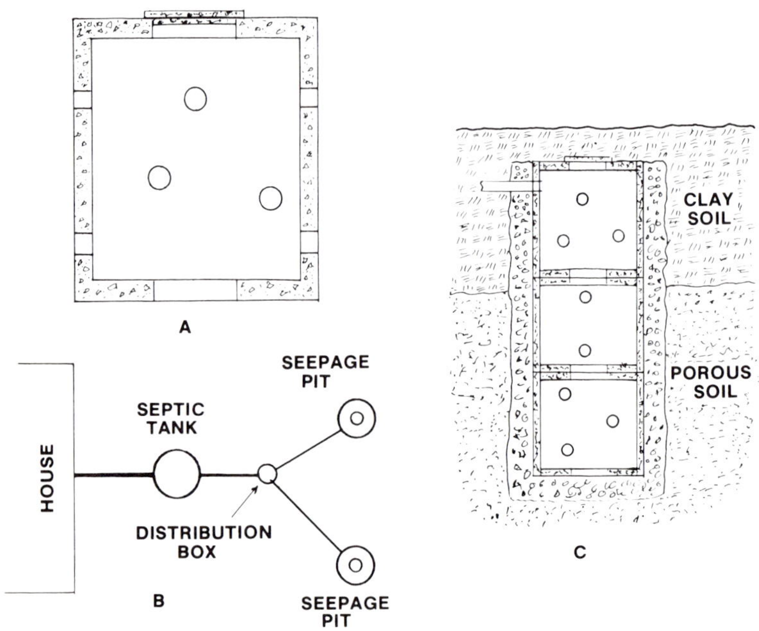

Fig. 11-23. The use of pre-cast concrete seepage pits. At A, a cross section of a pre-cast concrete seepage pit. At B, seepage pits used in place of a disposal tile field. At C, a cross section of stacked seepage pits to reach porous soil beneath impervious soil. A generous portion of coarse gravel around the pits increases the absorption area.

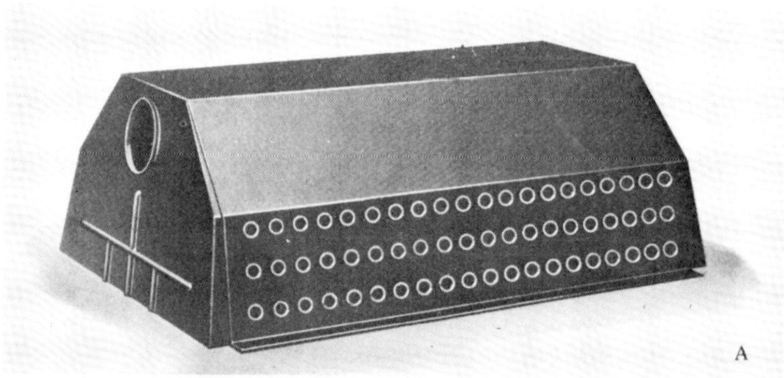

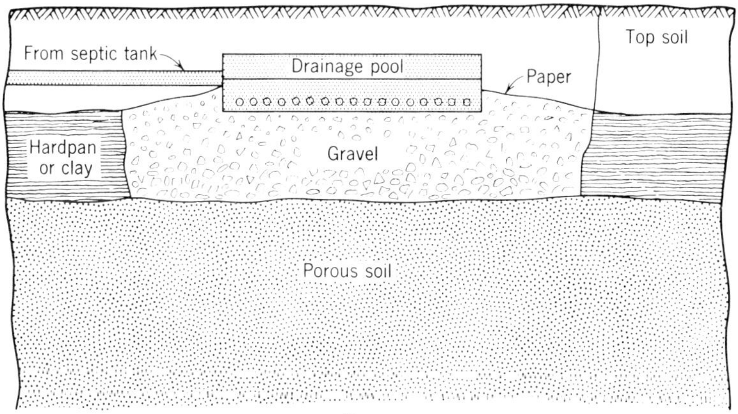

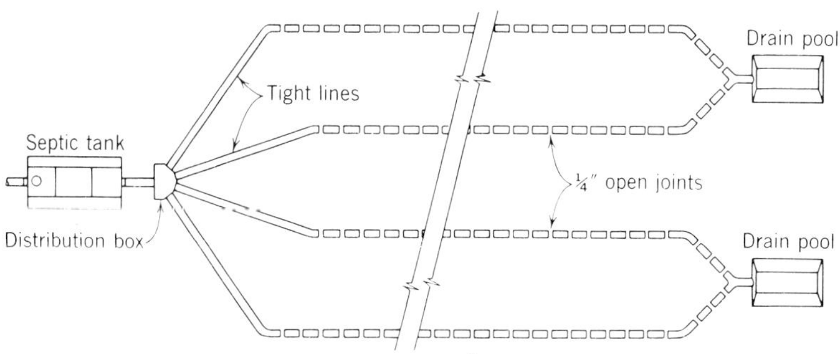

Fig. 11-24A courtesy San-Equip Co., Syracuse, N.Y.

Fig. 11-24. Drainage pools. A — A steel prefabricated dome for drainage pool. B — Cross section of installation. C — Use at ends of drain tile.

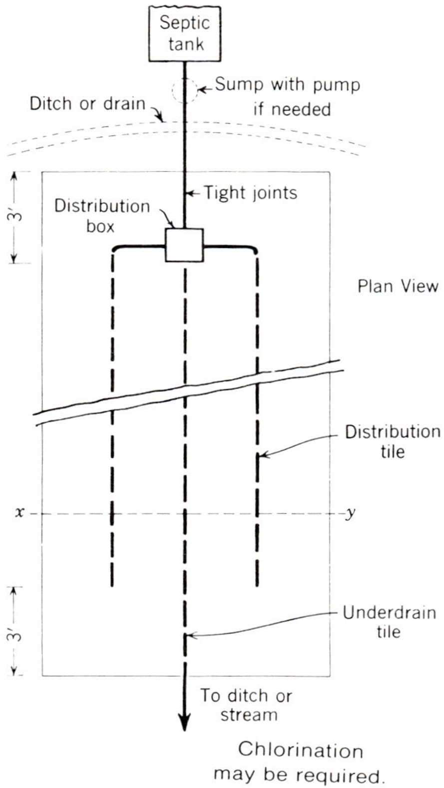

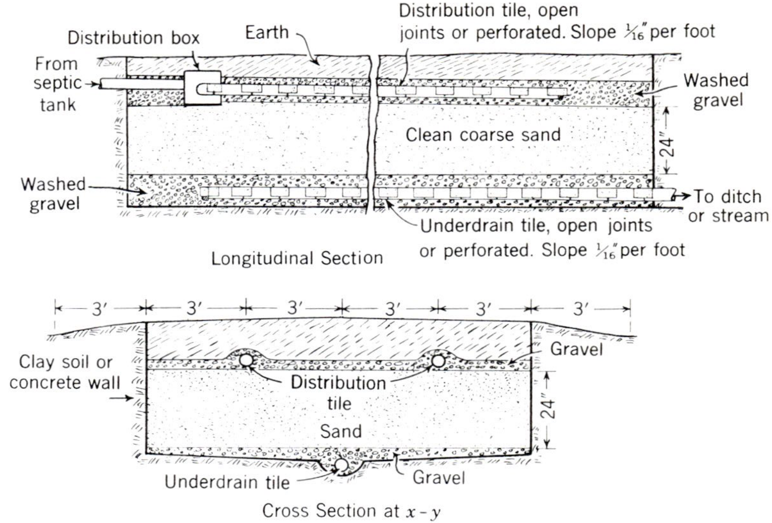

Courtesy Mr. F.R. Ligouri, Ithaca, N.Y.

Fig. 11-25. Plan of an underdrained sand filter for individual home. An alternate method is to use only one line of distribution tile with the underdrain tile directly below it. In any case allow 6 feet (1.8 m.) of width of filter bed for each line of distribution tile. Underground and surface water should be diverted from the filter bed area. See Fig. 11-27. The discharge from the underdrain tile should be disposed of in an approved sanitary manner. Health authorities should be consulted on plans before construction is undertaken.

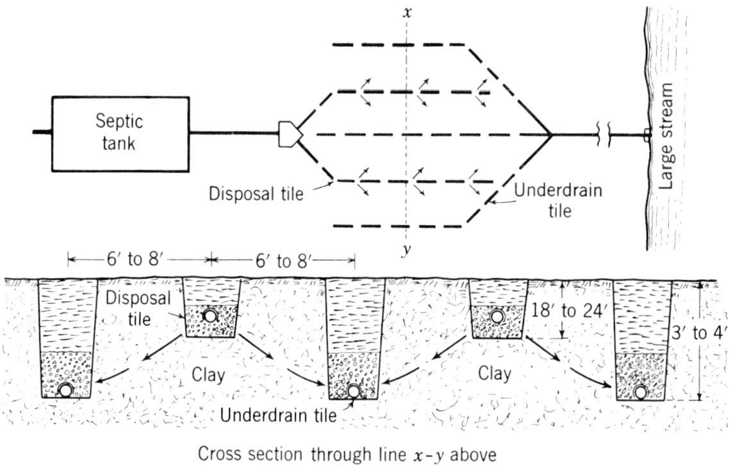

Fig. 11-26. Plan of an underdrained disposal field suitable for soils open enough to provide some seepage or where there is a shallow water table. Effluent must be disposed of in a sanitary manner.

cesspool alone can be used to dispose of the sewage. As shown in Fig. 11-28, a cesspool is essentially a walled-up hole in the ground into which the house sewer pipe empties and from which the liquids seep away through the soil. *A cesspool is an especially dangerous source of contamination of drinking water* and should be used only after careful investigation to make sure that it will be safe.

The inside diameter of a cesspool should not be greater than 6 feet and in no case should the bottom extend below the level of the water table. See Fig. 11-28. The wall should be laid up with stones, brick, or building blocks, and without mortar. The top of the wall should be drawn in so that a cover can be placed over the top. A large flat stone or a concrete slab may be used for a cover. The cover should be at least 12 inches (30 cm.) below the surface of the ground so that grass will grow over the top to conceal it. The wall should be carefully laid to prevent collapse.

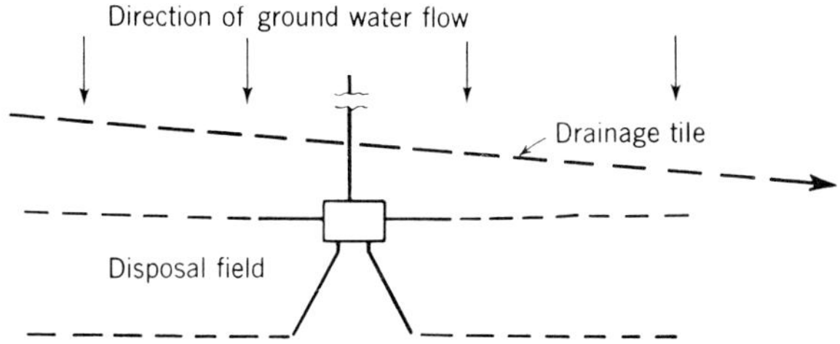

Fig. 11-27. Plan for intercepting natural ground water with drainage tile before it enters a disposal area.

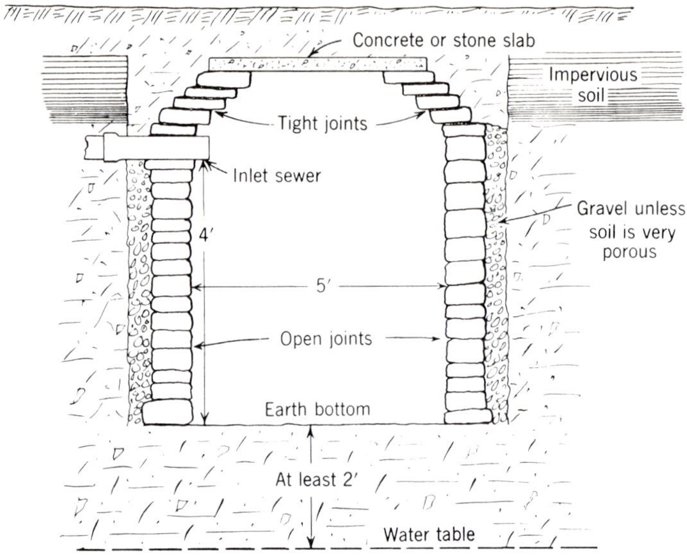

Courtesy N.Y. State Department of Health

Fig. 11-28. Cross section of one type of cesspool. The walls are laid up without mortar. The single pool is satisfactory in porous soil if large enough for the load.

Size.

The size of a cesspool is determined by (1) the volume of sewage to be disposed of, and (2) the type of soil in which it is located. The effective leaching area is that of the vertical wall up to the sewer. The bottom is not effective for long as the solids soon clog it. To calculate the effective leaching area, multiply the diameter by three times the height of the vertical wall to the sewer. The effective leaching area of the cesspool shown in Fig. 11-28 would be 5 feet times [3 times 4 feet] or 60 square feet. Layers of heavy clay or hardpan will effectively reduce the leaching capacity; therefore allowances should be made for such formations.

Table 11-V may be used as a rough guide to the required leaching area under different soil conditions. Larger areas can best be obtained by two or more cesspools.

In a cesspool, solids will accumulate as in a septic tank. Therefore, the cesspool should be cleaned occasionally and the solids disposed of in a safe place, preferably underground. In time the soil around the pool may become clogged with solids in spite of periodic cleaning. In such a case the best remedy is to abandon the old pool and construct a new one.

Privies

Where indoor plumbing has not been installed the outdoor toilet or privy is most commonly used for the disposal of human excrement.

Even in the United States where the percentage of flush toilets is probably the highest in the world, there are still many thousands of homes, cottages, and camps where a privy is the only means of disposal of human excrement.

A carefully designed and well-constructed privy can be a fairly safe method of disposal, although it is definitely inferior to a good underground disposal system. A poorly designed and poorly constructed privy can be a nuisance and a distinct health hazard. Unfortunately this is rather common.

A building set on the ground without a sanitary receptacle under it and open so that flies and animals have access to the feces can be a focal point for the spread of a number of human diseases. Foul odors from such a structure can be a nuisance.

Privies should be of good tight construction with screened ventilators to keep out flies, animals, and birds. They should be located not less than 50 feet (15 m.) away from a well and downgrade from it. On porous soil a distance of 100 feet (30 m.) is recommended. A location 50 to 100 feet (15 to 30 m.) from the house and out of line with prevailing winds or air drainage toward the house will reduce the odor nuisance to a minimum. A good walk, windbreaks, and shrub screening, although not necessary for sanitary reasons, are added conveniences.

The following types of outdoor privies are suggested as acceptable designs:

1. Sanitary pit privy.
2. Concrete vault privy.
3. Septic privy.
4. Removable receptacle privy.

TABLE 11-V.
LEACHING AREA OF CESSPOOL UNDER VARIOUS SOIL CONDITIONS.

Character of the Soil	No. of Bedrooms	Required Effective Leaching Area Sq. Ft.	Sq. M.
Clean, coarse sand or gravel	1	36	3.3
	2	60	5.6
	3	90	8.3
	4	120	11.1
Fine sand or light loam	1	55	5.1
	2	90	8.3
	3	135	12.5
	4	180	16.7
Fine sand with some clay or loam	1	80	7.4
	2	130	12.1
	3	195	18.1
	4	260	24.1
Clay with some sand or gravel	1	140	13.0
	2	240	22.3
	3	350	32.5
	4	480	44.6
Clay with little or no sand or gravel	Generally unsuitable		

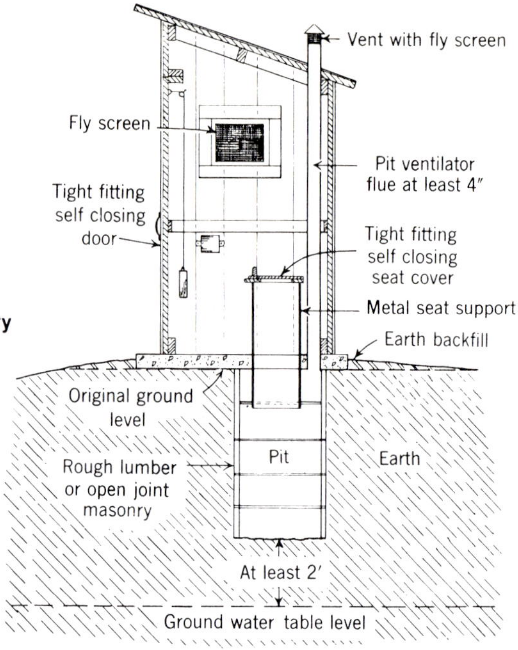

Fig. 11-29. Plan for a sanitary pit privy with concrete floor.

Courtesy N.Y. State Department of Health

Sanitary pit privy.

The sanitary, or earth pit, privy is the easiest to build and is probably the most commonly used of the accepted designs. That of Fig. 11-29 with a concrete slab floor is suitable for home or farm use where it can remain in one location for a long period of time. That of Fig. 11-30 with a wood floor is suitable for camps where the volume of sewage necessitates frequent movement of the structure. The urinal is a desirable and sometimes required feature for camp use.

This type of privy is especially dangerous to the water supply. If possible it should be located at least 100 feet from a well and on the downgrade side.

The pit should be about 5 feet (1.5 m.) deep and, if possible, the bottom should be at least 2 feet (61 cm.) above the ground water table. A pit capacity of 50 cubic feet (1.4 cu. m.) is considered adequate for four or five people for a period of 8 to 10 years. The pit should be lined with masonry or boards to prevent cave-in. The structure over the pit should be well constructed and made flyproof. A counterweight or some other means should be provided for keeping the door closed and the seat covers should be chocked so that they cannot be left open. Both the building and the pit should be ventilated as indicated.

When the accumulated solids in the pit are within 1½ feet (½ m.)

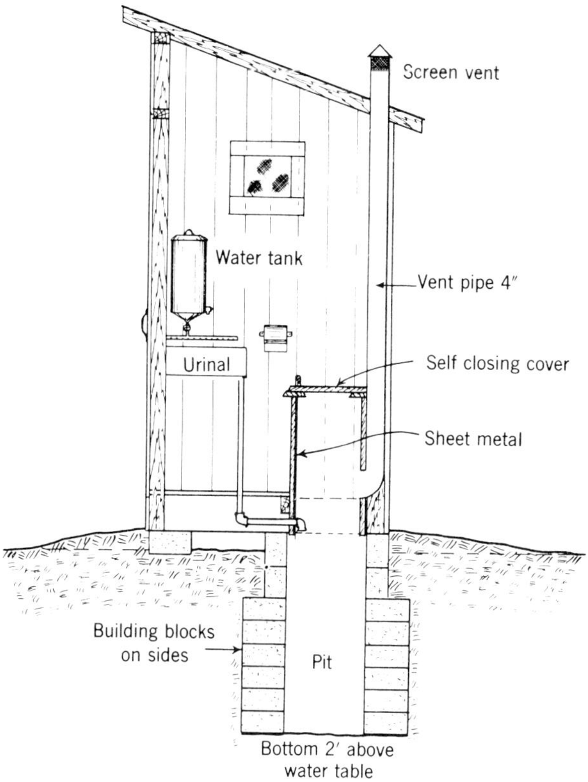

Fig. 11-30. Plan for a wood floor sanitary pit privy designed as a movable structure for use in summer camps, parks, etc. The urinal and water tank are required in some localities but may be omitted for home use.

of the top of the pit they should be removed and buried in a safe place or the building should be placed over a new pit. The new location should be chosen carefully, as has already been suggested. The old pit should be covered with about 2 feet (61 cm.) of earth.

To reduce odors a frequent application of chloride of lime or a mixture of lime and dry soil, ashes, or sawdust to the pit is effective. Commercial deodorants are also available on the market. A quantity of these deodorants should be kept in the building at all times.

In warm weather fly and mosquito eggs can be destroyed by pouring a mixture of borax and water (1 pound of borax to 10 U.S. gallons (8.3 Imp. gals.) of water) or some of the nonflammable commercial preparations over the contents. Seats should be scrubbed weekly with a soap and disinfectant solution such as chlorox. An occasional scrubbing of the floor with the same solution is recommended.

The concrete vault privy.

In locations where the soil is heavy and impervious or where there is not room to establish the sanitary pit type of privy at a safe distance from the water supply, the concrete vault privy may be used. However, because of the possibility of leaks, the vault should be at least 50 feet (15 m.) distant from the water source and should be on ground which slopes away from the water source.

The vault should be constructed of reinforced concrete, as shown in Fig. 11-31 and should have a capacity of 3 cubic feet (.84 cu. m.) per person served. The top of the vault should extend 5 to 8 inches (85 to 200 cm.) above the ground level and should be banked to divert surface water away from the vault. The structure over the vault should be of the same type suggested for the sanitary pit privy. The contents of the vault should be frequently sprinkled with lime to reduce odors. The vault should be cleaned when about two-thirds full. Usually such a vault can be pumped out the same as a septic tank. In fact precast concrete septic tanks make good pits. The contents of the vault should be buried at a safe distance from the water source.

The septic privy.

The septic privy is similar in construction to the concrete vault privy except that a drain tile is provided to carry liquids off into porous soil. Owing to the nature of the drain from the vault it is a very dangerous source of pollution of water sources and for this reason should be located with extreme care.

No chemicals such as lime are added to the contents of the vault as they would interfere with the bacterial action on the solids. The bacterial action is necessary to reduce the solids to a minimum as in the case of the septic tank. It is from this bacterial action that the name "septic" privy is derived.

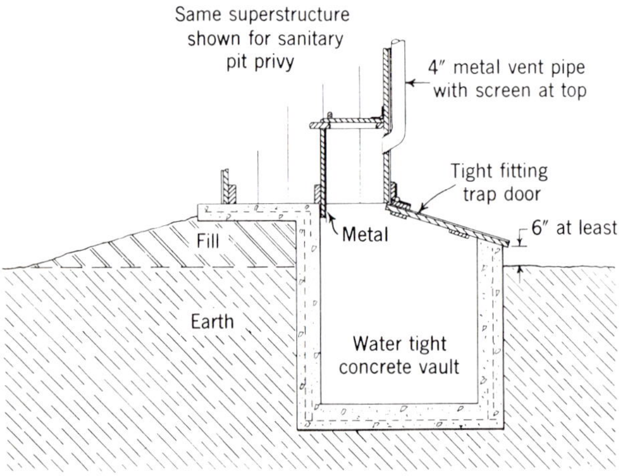

Fig. 11-31. A concrete vault privy.

Courtesy N.Y. State Department of Health

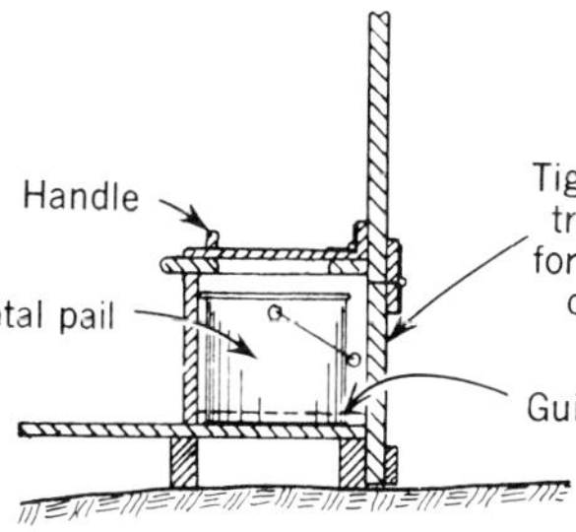

Courtesy N.Y. State Department of Health

Fig. 11-32. Seat details of removable receptacle privy.

Water must be added to the contents of the vault of the septic privy to make up for evaporation losses and to insure a flow through the drain tile. About 2 gallons a day should be sufficient.

Because of the danger of water pollution and the unpleasant odor of a septic privy, it is perhaps the least desirable of all the outdoor toilets described here.

The removable receptacle privy.

The removable receptacle privy consists of a building having a seat under which a metal receptacle is placed as shown in Fig. 11-32. The receptacle is emptied at frequent intervals, the contents being buried at a safe distance from the water supply. This type of privy is sometimes used in camps, at summer cottages, and at other places of *temporary residence.*

Chemical toilets.

Chemical toilets can be used either outdoors or indoors. However, because of the cost of the necessary chemicals and the daily care required, they are seldom used out of doors where other types of toilets are acceptable. Their chief application is indoors for elderly or infirm people. Unless cared for exactly according to manufacturers' instructions they are not sanitary and soon become a nuisance. In some areas they are prohibited by health regulations.

GARBAGE DISPOSAL

Disposal of household garbage in a sanitary manner is important from a health point of view. Careless handling of garbage attracts rats and other rodents and provides breeding places for flies and sometimes mosquitoes. In addition, foul odors and unsightly garbage areas are a nuisance.

In cities garbage is collected at regular intervals and hauled away to a disposal point. In rural areas the problem is one for the individual family to work out. Even in cities there is the problem of containing the garbage on the premises between collections.

Grinders

For disposal of food scraps a garbage grinding unit mounted under the kitchen sink is very satisfactory for both city and country homes. Private sewage disposal systems should have 50% more capacity to take care of the extra solids from these grinders. See Tables 11-I and 11-II.

Burning

Burning, as ordinarily practiced, is seldom satisfactory except for papers and other combustible materials. Wet garbage such as food scraps and refuse from dressed meat will not burn satisfactory unless first dried.

Burning of papers and other combustible garbage in suitable enclosures greatly reduces the volume to be buried or otherwise disposed of. Figure 11-33 illustrates an incinerator for burning combustible garbage. Figure 11-34 illustrates portable trash burners. Such devices should be placed at a safe distance from buildings and on the lee side if possible.

Calcinators

Meat and other wet food scraps can readily be burned if dried. Calcinators (drier and burner combinations) are relatively expensive and are not always justified for a small home. However, when large quantities of wet garbage are to be disposed of, as on farms where meat is dressed for market or where dead birds have to be disposed of, the calcinator may be a good investment. Figure 11-35 illustrates the principle of operation. Heat is applied to the wet garbage until dehydrated; then the remains are burned. The ash makes good garden fertilizer.

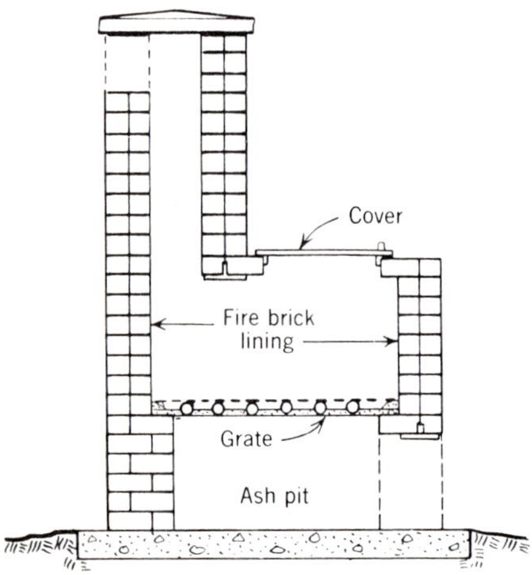

Fig. 11-33. An incinerator constructed of masonry. The firebox and chimney should be lined with firebricks. The outside can be of bricks, stone, or building blocks. The grate is made of heavy expanded metal resting on lengths of old pipe or rods set in a thin layer of mortar at the ends. A wire basket can be hung on the inside for drying and eventually burning wet garbage.

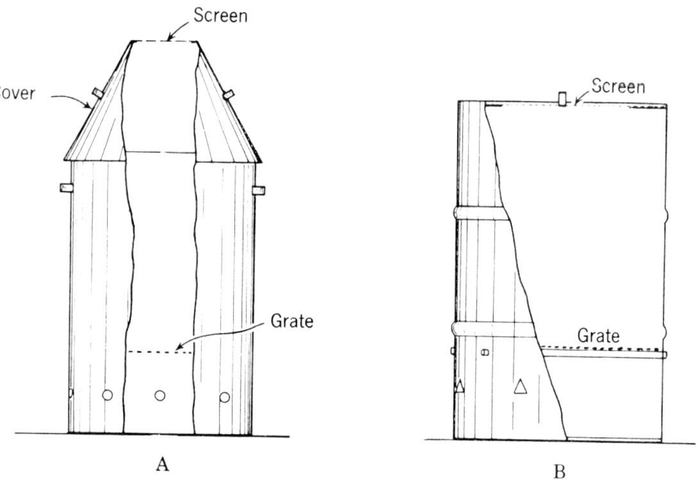

Fig. 11-34. Trash burners. Type A can be purchased ready-made. Type B can be made from an oil drum.

Burying

Burying of wet garbage under several inches of soil is one of the most satisfactory and least expensive methods of disposal for rural homes provided it can be done at a safe distance (50 feet or more) (15 m.) from the water supply. However, a suitable space is not always available, and in areas where the ground freezes it may be difficult in the wintertime. Garbage should never be disposed of on the surface. Garbage fed to swine should be cooked first. In some states this is required by law.

Pits

Covered pits provide a safe means of wet garbage disposal if correctly located and properly constructed. Figure 11-36 illustrates a garbage pit suitable for disposal of all types of wet garbage. No lime or other chemicals are necessary for decomposition or odor control.

For convenience the pit should be located as near to the buildings as is possible without endangering the water supply. It should be at least 100 feet (30 m.) away from the well and downgrade from it. If covered with at least 12 inches (30 cm.) of dirt and equipped with a tight lid on the tile, odors will not be a nuisance.

The earth over the pit should be graded upward toward the center and good surface drainage should be provided for the area around the pit. If located on a slope, a diversion ditch should be made above the pit.

The size of the pit should be determined by the amount of material to be disposed of and the length of life desired. The larger the pit the longer it will function before it must be abandoned. The deeper the pit the more rapid the decomposition, particularly where severe winters occur. Low temperatures retard decomposition by bacterial action. For a long narrow pit two or more tiles should be installed through the top in order to distribute the garbage more evenly on the bottom.

Water in the pit does not interfere with the anaerobic bacteria which cause decomposition as in a septic tank, but water tends to cause cave-ins. Surface water should not be allowed to enter as it

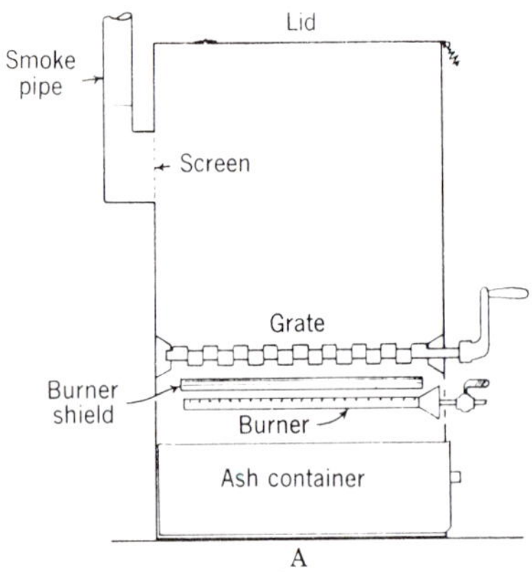

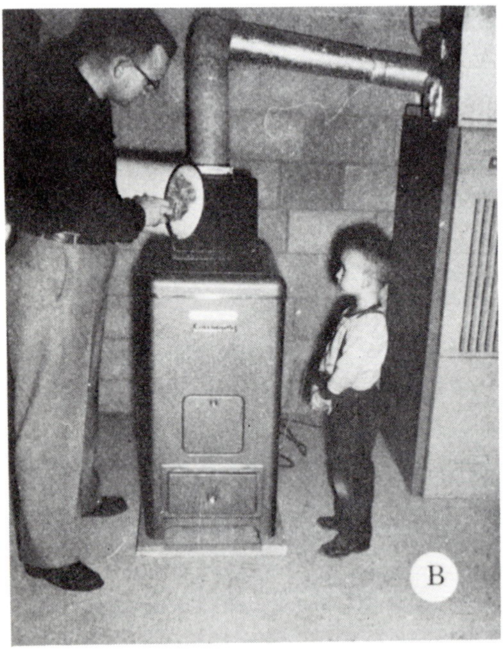

Fig. 11-35. A calcinator for wet garbage. Heat applied to the garbage dries it to the point where it will readily burn. A gas-burner type is shown at A and an electrically operated type at B. Oil-fired burners are also satisfactory. Any other convenient source of heat can be used. An advantage of gas, electric, or oil units is the fact that they can be controlled automatically. They can be used indoors if vented to a chimney as shown at B.

Fig. 11-35B courtesy E.O. Eaton

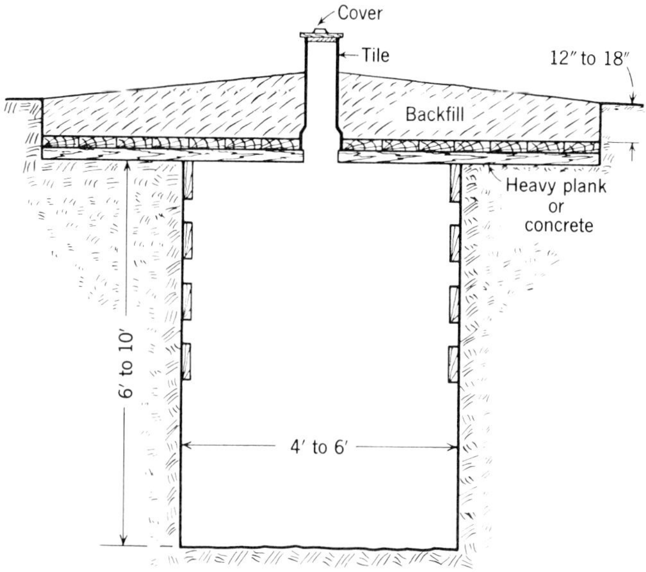

Courtesy Department of Poultry Husbandry, Cornell University

Fig. 11-36. A garbage pit suitable for disposal of all types of wet garbage, including dead birds. If the soil is of such a nature that it will cave in, the walls of the pit should be supported with planks as shown or by stone or other masonry laid up without mortar. Round pits are best if masonry linings are used. Extending a plank cover beyond the walls as shown will reduce the danger of cave-ins.

may carry silt and thus reduce the disposal area.

Although any kind of garbage can be disposed of in this kind of a pit, it is best to use it only for wet garbage and such things as dead birds, dead farm animals, and refuse from dressed meat. Papers, tin cans, bottles, etc., which do not readily decompose will quickly fill the pit.

Figure 11-37 illustrates a new type of pit for disposal of both toilet waste and wet garbage. The designers claim that 90-95 percent of the waste is converted to odorless gas and water vapor which escape through the vent. The remaining solids collect in the storage chamber, can be removed through the clean-out hatch and can be used as fertilizer. No water, chemicals, or moving parts are involved. As the tank is made of fiberglass there is no leakage, therefore no danger of contaminating a water supply.

The system is a Sweedish invention and is called the "Clivus Multrum" system, meaning "Inclining Compost Room." It has been used in Scandinavia for a number of years, but was introduced into the

U.S. only recently, therefore, potential users should check on its acceptibility by local health departments before purchasing.

Containers

Convenient and sanitary containers for holding garbage until final disposal are important. In the kitchen two such containers, one for papers and the other for food scraps and other noncombustible materials, may save the chore of sorting at final disposal time. Step-on cans are good for this purpose.

Larger outdoor galvanized or plastic cans with tight lids make satisfactory depositories for daily emptying of the smaller cans. The outdoor cans should be watertight and should be stored where they cannot be disturbed by dogs or rodents.

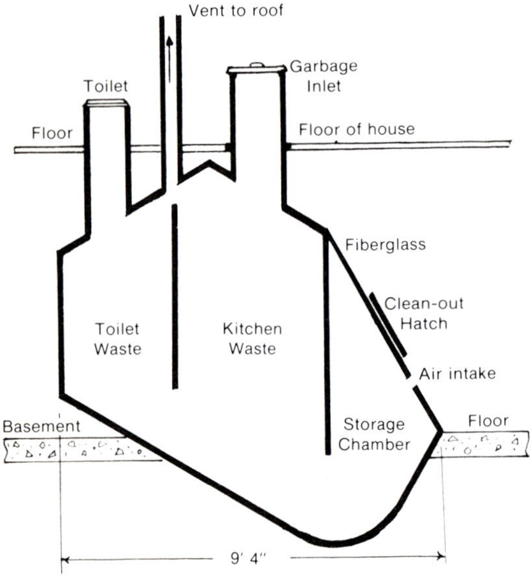

Fig. 11-37. A disposal system for both toilet waste and wet garbage. The tank is made of fiberglass and has a sloping bottom as shown. The wastes move slowly down the sloping bottom as they decompose.

Courtesy Mr. Stewart D. McBride and The Christian Science Monitor.

Figure 11-38 illustrates an enclosed storage built in the side of an outbuilding. It keeps dogs and flies away and tends to confine the odors. The cans should be emptied and cleaned at least once a week.

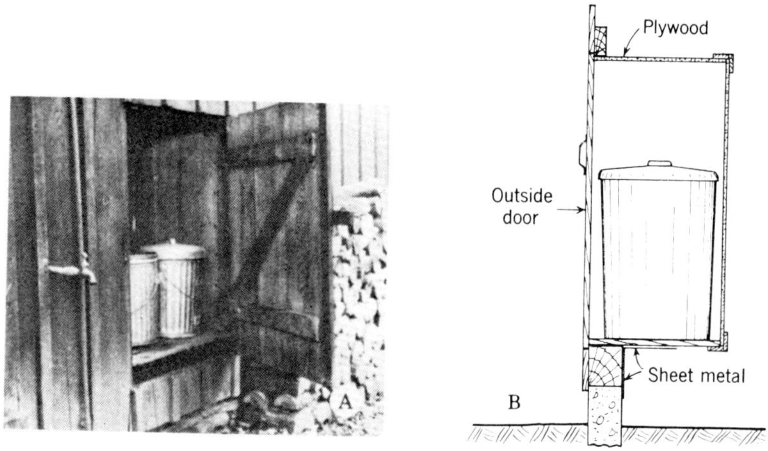

Fig. 11-38. A garbage can enclosure built in the side of an outbuilding. The enclosure can be made insect-tight and almost odorproof by use of plywood with boxed-in joints. A door to the outside gives easy access to the cans. Sheet metal shields should be placed at points where rodents might gnaw through the walls. A water outlet nearby, as shown in A, is convenient for washing the cans.

PART TWO

Cutting to Measure, Reaming, and Threading Steel Pipe

JOB 1

Steel pipe is normally connected to fittings by threaded joints. For lengths under 21 feet the pipe must be cut and threaded with standard pipe dies.

MEASURING PIPE LENGTHS

The length of pipe should equal the distance between the faces of the fittings plus the lengths of the threaded ends which will extend into the fittings as indicated at Y in Figs. J-1-1 and J-1-2. Three accepted methods of measuring are as follows:

1. Measure distance X between the faces of the fittings as in Fig. J-1-1. For pipe sizes up to 1 inch allow ½ inch per thread to get the total length Y of the pipe. For pipe sizes 1¼ inches to 2 inches allow ¾ inch per thread.

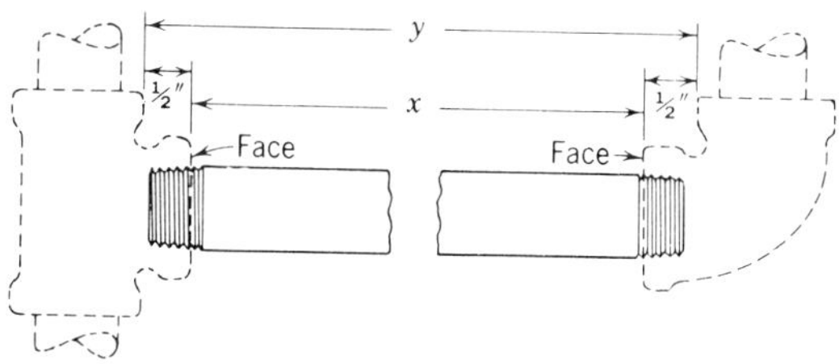

Fig. J-1-1. A method of measuring where exact dimensions are not important. Good for pipe up to 1 inch size.

2. A more accurate method for use when plumbing around fixtures or in close quarters is to measure distance X from center to center of the pipe as indicated in Fig. J-1-2, then subtract for each thread the nominal diameter of the pipe. For example, for ½-inch pipe subtract 2 × ½ inch or 1 inch from distance X to get length Y for the pipe. For ¾-inch pipe subtract 2 × ¾ inch or 1½ inch from distance X to get length Y, etc. This method is good for sizes up to 1 inch.

3. For pipe sizes of 1¼ inches and larger, measure distance X from center to center as shown in Fig. J-1-3. Mark two parallel lines on the

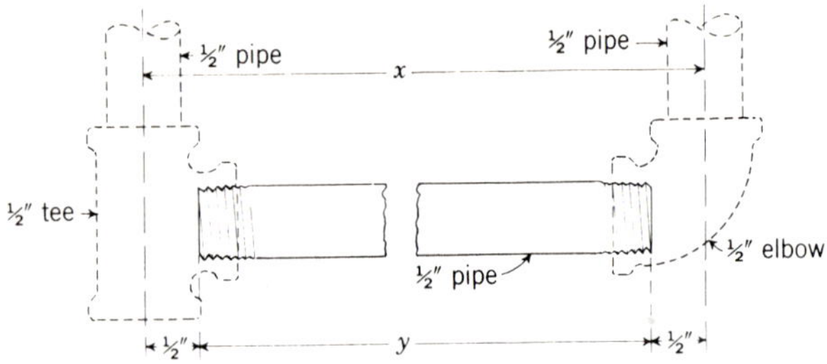

Fig. J-1-2. A more accurate method of measuring pipe lengths for sizes up to 1 inch. Measure distance x and subtract 2 × ½" to get distance y.

floor distance X apart. Lay the fittings on these center lines and measure distance Y between the back of the threads. Distance Y will be the length to cut the pipe.

The accuracy of these methods of measurement will be affected by the manner of cutting the thread. If the dies are not set accurately, or if the threads are not cut the right lengths, the pipe will not make up to the correct dimensions. The correct length of thread can be determined by measuring factory-cut threads.

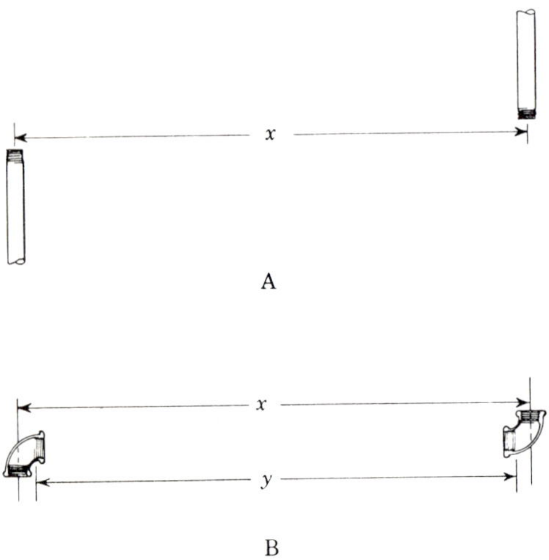

Fig. J-1-3. A method of measuring for large-diameter pipes.
1. Measure distance x as at A.
2. Lay out distance x on floor.
3. Place fittings centered on lines at ends of distance x as at B.
4. Measure distance y from back of threads of fittings.

CUTTING PIPE TO MEASUREMENT

When installing a plumbing system using steel pipe and fittings it is necessary to cut and thread pipe and to "make" the joints water tight. The following is a brief outline of the procedure.

1. With a ruler measure the length of pipe needed and mark with chalk. For exact measure, mark in the chalk with a pencil.

2. Place the pipe to be cut in a pipe vice as shown in Fig. J-1-5. Screw the jaws of the vice up tight so that the pipe will not turn and strip off the galvanizing.

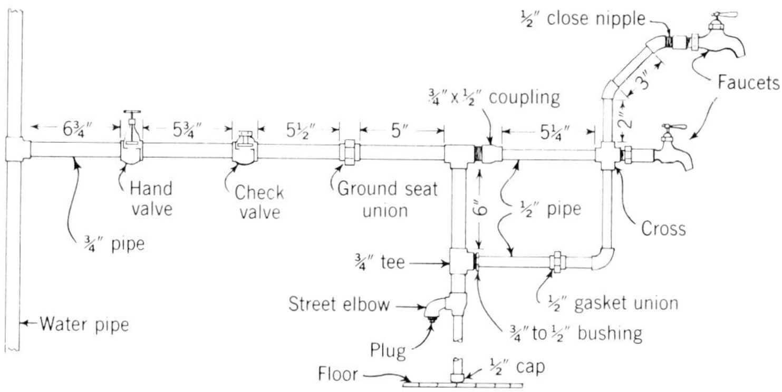

Fig. J-1-4. A piping assembly suitable for practice in cutting pipe and "making" joints. This assembly contains the most common pipe sizes and the most common valves and fittings used in farm plumbing. When the assembly is completed the water pressure can be turned on to test the joints, the valves, and the faucets. The faucets and valves may be used for practice in faucet and valve repair.

3. Cut the pipe at the pencil line.

Plumbers use a special pipe-cutting tool as shown in Fig. J-1-5. This tool is fast but expensive and has no other use than for cutting pipe. It also leaves a burr on the inside of the pipe, as shown in Fig. J-1-6A. This burr must be reamed out which means an additional investment in another expensive tool. For one who does only a limited amount of plumbing with the smaller sizes of pipe, a hacksaw is a very satisfactory tool for cutting pipe.

To cut pipe with the pipe-cutting tool:

1. Place the tool over the pipe as shown in Fig. J-1-5 with the cutter on the mark. Tighten the cutter by turning the handle to force the cutting wheel into the pipe. Swing tool around the pipe to make the initial cut, being sure that the cutting wheel "tracks." Continue swinging the tool around the pipe, tightening the cutter a little after each turn until the pipe is cut free.

2. Unless the burr is removed it will restrict the flow of water. The best way to remove the burr is with a pipe reamer as shown in Fig. J-1-7. Ream until the burr is all gone as indicated in Fig. J-1-6C.

To cut pipe with a hacksaw: Hold the saw at *right angles* to the pipe as indicated in Fig. J-1-8 or J-1-9. It is important to cut the pipe at right angles so that the thread cutter will start straight. Saw at no more than 60 strokes per minute. Sawing too fast heats the saw blade and softens the teeth. Use a full-length stroke. The teeth near the ends of the blade are just as good as those in the middle.

A hacksaw does not leave a burr on the inside of the pipe but may leave a rough edge. A few strokes with a round file in the end of the pipe will smooth the edges.

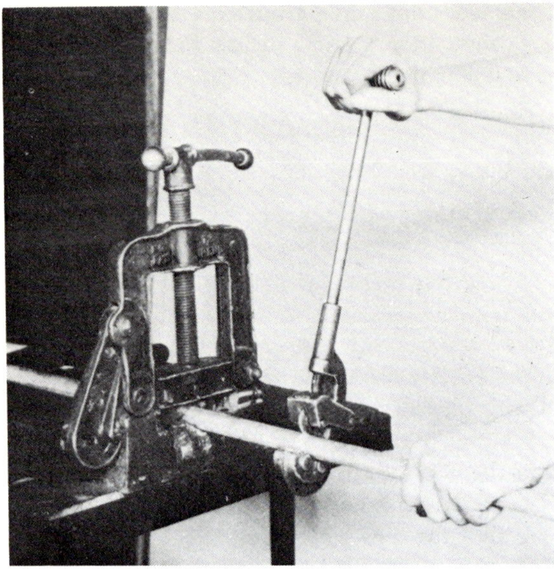

Fig. J-1-5. Cutting pipe with a wheeled pipe cutter.

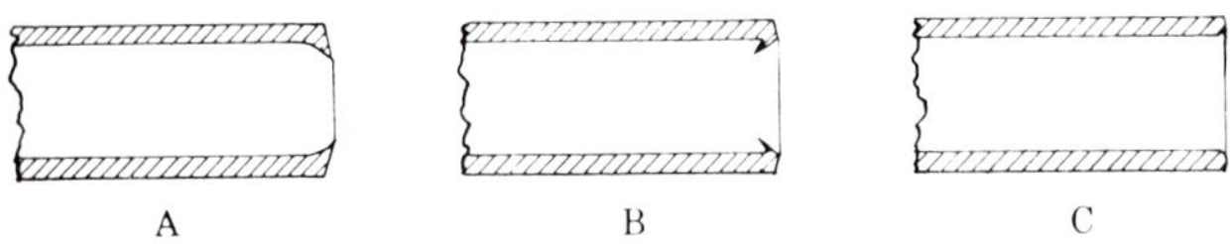

Fig. J-1-6. A — The burr made by a wheeled pipe cutter. B — Improper reaming. C — Pipe properly reamed.

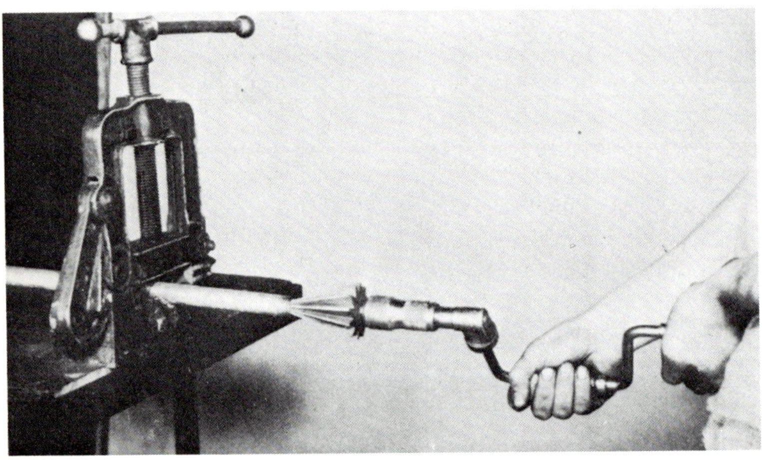

Fig. J-1-7. Reaming the end of a pipe.

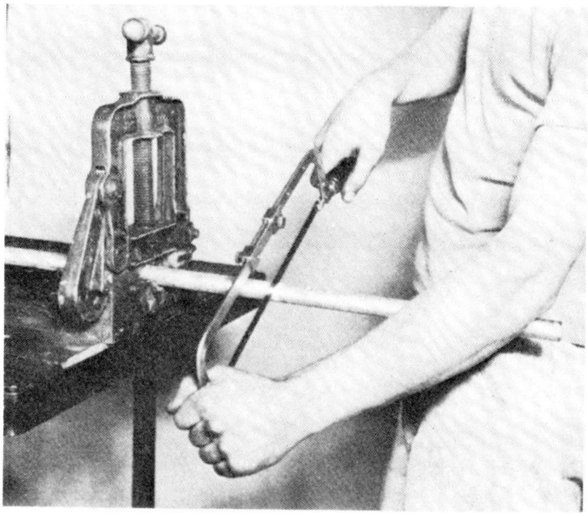

Fig. J-1-8. Cutting pipe with a hack saw.

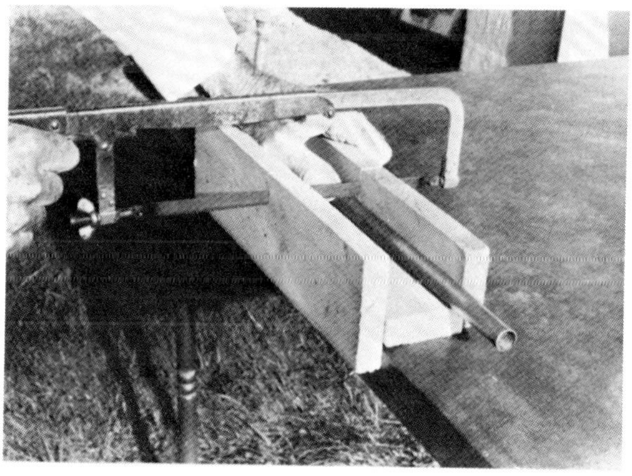

Fig J-1-9 A miter box can be used for cutting pipe and tubing square. The pipe can be held securely in place by means of "C" clamps if necessary.

THREADING PIPE

Tools Needed:

A pipe thread cutter with proper sized dies.
A pipe vise.
Thread-cutting oil.

Procedure:

Pipe thread cutters are made with two handles as shown in Fig. J-1-10 and with one handle and a ratchet as shown in Fig. J-1-11. The latter is easier to operate and is more accurate, but is more expensive than the two-handled type. Either will cut good threads if in good

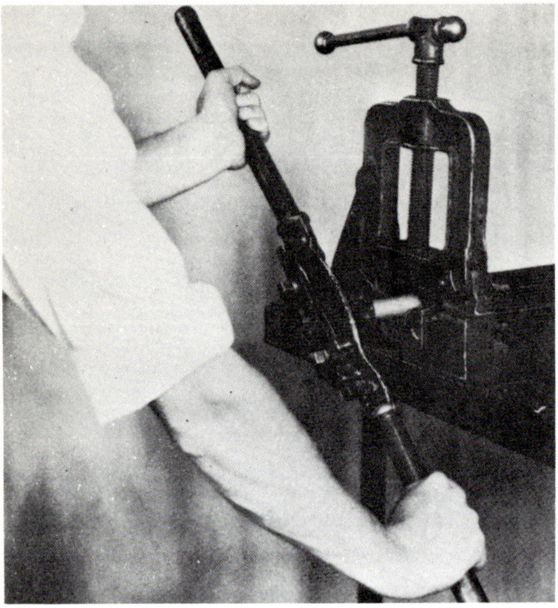

Fig. J-1-10. Cutting a thread with a two-handle non-ratchet stock and die.

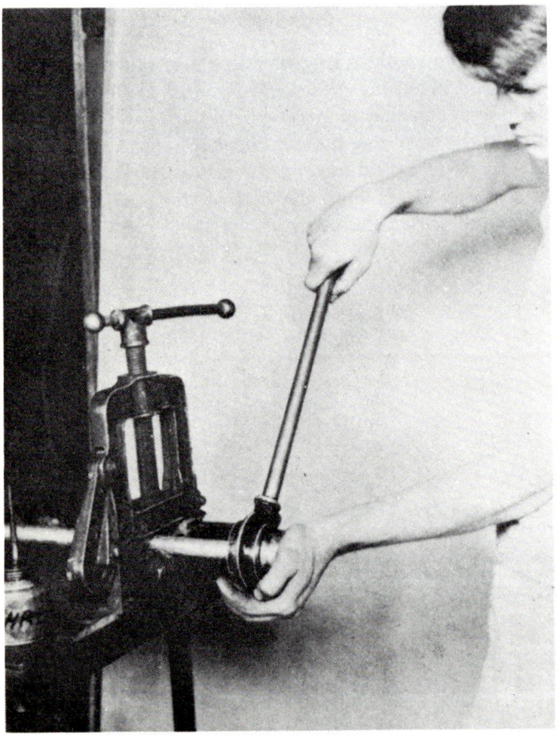

Fig. J-1-11. Cutting a pipe thread with a ratchet type of stock and die.

condition and properly used. Before using either type check it over to see that the dies are of the correct size, properly adjusted, and clean and sharp.

Place the tool on the end of the pipe, guide side first, as shown in Figs. J-1-10 and J-1-11. Press the dies firmly against the end of the pipe and turn the handle in a clockwise direction, at the same time keeping the handle at right angles to the pipe.

As soon as the threads are started, oil the dies and the end of the pipe with thread-cutting oil. This oil will aid in cutting a smooth thread and will make the dies easier to turn. It will also make the dies wear longer. After each two or three complete turns of the dies, re-oil.

Turn the dies until the end of the pipe is flush with the outside face of the dies. Remove the dies from the pipe, being careful that chips do not catch and spoil the threads. Turn the stock so that the dies are facing downward and strike the pipe a light blow with the handle of the stock. This will clean the die and the end of the pipe of chips.

Be sure to remove all metal chips from the inside of the pipe. If this is not done the chips may lodge under faucet washers and cause leaks.

Assemble the pipe and fittings as directed in Job 2.

"Making" a Threaded Joint in Steel Pipe

JOB 2

The plumber's term "making a joint" refers to the process of making a joint between a pipe and a fitting or valve watertight.

Tools Needed:

One pipe vise.
One Stilson wrench (pipe wrench).
One 12-inch flat jawed wrench.
One stiff-bristle paint brush (optional).

Supplies Needed:

One can of good quality pipe-joint compound.
One piece of threaded pipe.
Pipe fittings or valves of the same size as the pipe.

Procedure:

1. With the paint brush or swab cover the *entire pipe threads* with pipe-joint compound, brushing it well into the threads. This will help seal the joint and lubricate the thread.

2. Place the pipe tightly in the vise with the threaded end close to the vise.

NOTE: The pipe-joint compound should never be put in the fitting threads as it will be pushed ahead of the pipe and pile up, partially closing the pipe. Pipe-joint compound is better than paint because it makes a better seal and does not dry hard; therefore the joint can be more easily taken apart. Covering the entire thread with pipe-joint compound tends to prevent rusting where the galvanizing has been cut off by threading. See Fig. J-2-1.

3. Start the fitting on the pipe (or the pipe in the fitting) by hand and tighten with the pipe wrench until reasonably tight. If turned too tight the fitting may stretch or crack. Use a small wrench on small pipe.

NOTE: A pipe wrench will hold only when turned in one direction, as shown in Fig. J-2-2.

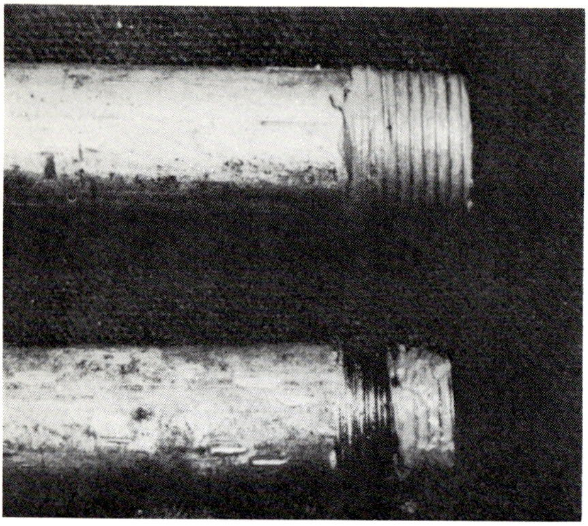

Fig. J-2-1. Top: correct application of pipe-joint compound. Bottom: incorrect application. The uncovered threads may rust badly.

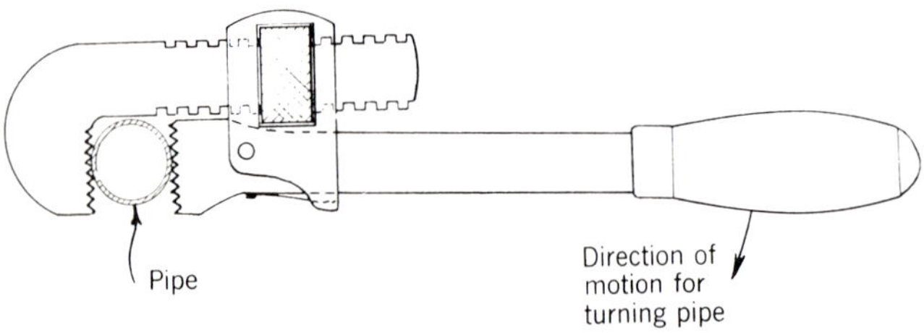

Fig. J-2-2. Method of using a pipe wrench.

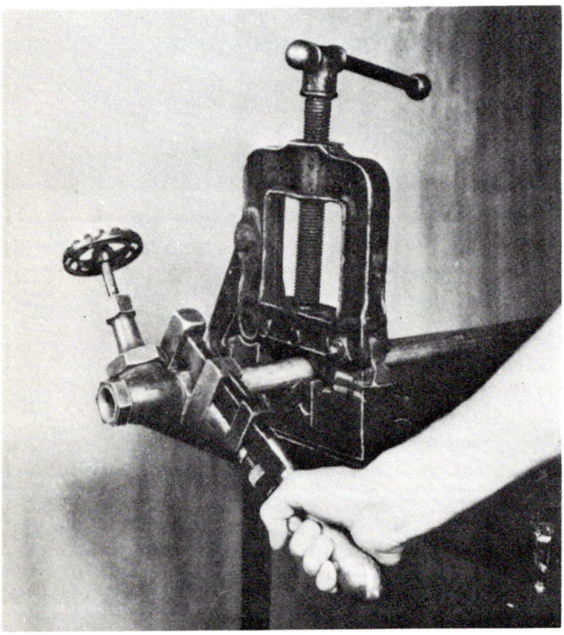

Fig. J-2-3. Proper method of screwing a brass valve on the end of a pipe.

Brass is a relatively soft metal; therefore, when screwing a brass valve onto pipe, place a flat-jawed wrench on the end of the valve next to the pipe, as shown in Fig. J-2-3. When screwing pipe into a brass valve, hold that end of the valve into which the pipe is to be screwed, as shown in Fig. J-2-4. This method will prevent twisting of the valve. Always tighten the bonnet and packing or gland nut on a new valve at the time of installation. A brass valve should not be placed in a vise as the pressure of the vise may squeeze the valve out of shape.

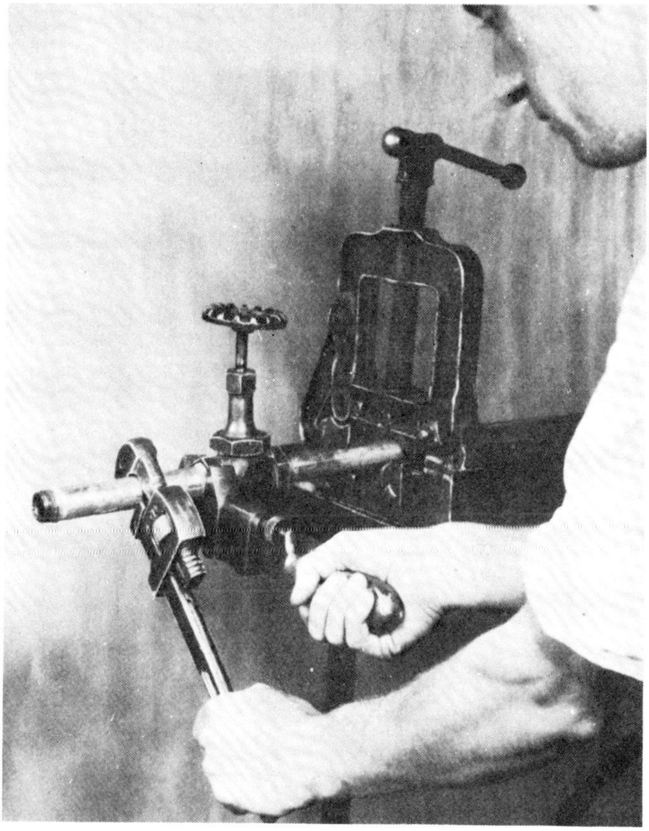

Fig. J-2-4. Proper method of screwing a piece of pipe into a brass valve.

Making Joints in Copper and Plastic Tubing

JOB 3

For joining copper to copper two types of fittings are used. They are the flared fittings shown in Fig. J-3-1 which are used on soft copper tubing only, and the solder fittings shown in Fig. J-3-2 which are used on both soft and hard tubing. Flared fittings are seldom used except where the tubing must be disconnected from time to time.

For joining copper to steel or to faucets and valves, various forms of flared or solder adapters are used. See Fig. J-3-3.

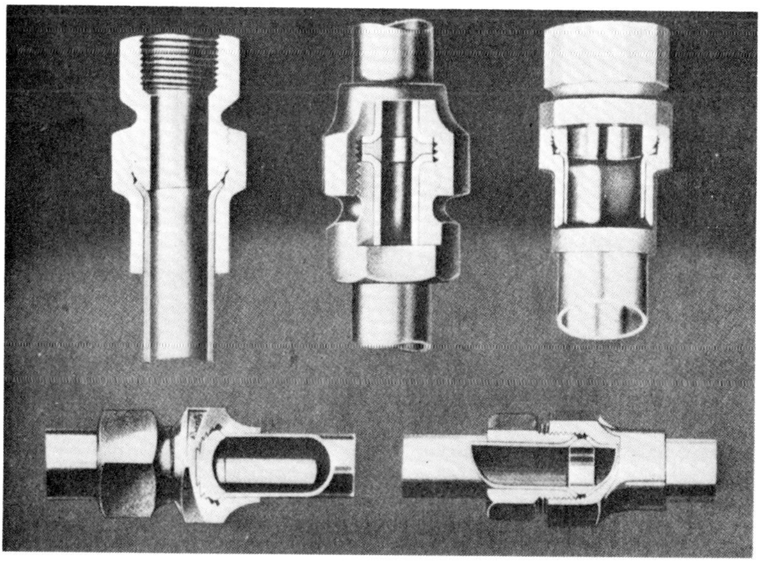

Courtesy Copper and Brass Research Association

Fig. J-3-1. A representative group of flared fittings cut away to show construction details.

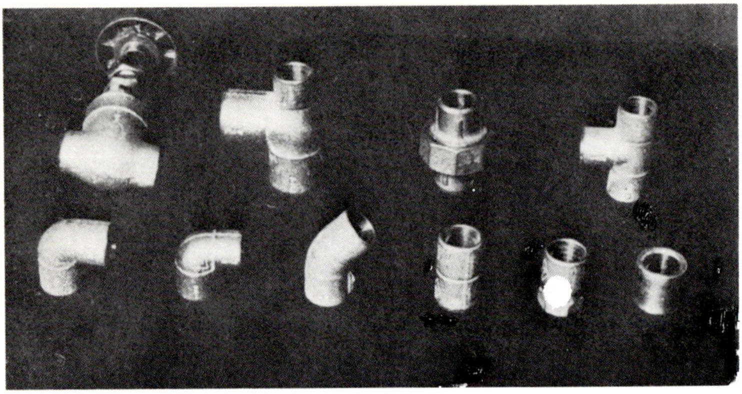

Fig. J-3-2. An assortment of solder fittings for use with copper tubing.

MAKING A JOINT WITH SOFT COPPER TUBING AND FLARED FITTINGS

Tools Needed:

Hacksaw or tubing wheel cutter. A tubing wheel cutter is shown in Fig. J-3-4. For a limited amount of plumbing a fine toothed hacksaw is adequate.

A miter box if hacksaw is used.

10-inch mill file or a reamer.

Flaring or flanging tool for the size of tubing to be used.

Hammer, if flanging tool is used.

Two wrenches large enough for the sleeve nuts on the fittings.

Materials Needed:

Tubing and fitting.

Light oil.

Procedure:

1. Cut the tubing to length with a hacksaw or a wheel cutter. Be sure to cut the tubing at right angles so the ends will be square. See Figs. J-3-4 and J-1-9.
2. With a file or reamer remove all rough edges on the cut end.
3. Slip the flange nut over the tube.
4. If a flaring tool is used, moisten the shank of the tool with oil and insert into the end of the tubing as shown in Fig. J-3-5A.
5. Hold the tubing firmly in one hand and strike the flaring tool with a hammer until the tubing is flared enough to cover the curved shoulder on the flaring tool as shown in Fig. J-3-5B.
6. If the flanging tool is used, place the tubing in the correct size

hole with the end flush with the tool surface, tighten tool on the tubing, and screw the flanger down into the end to form the flange.

7. Moisten the inside of the flange with a film of oil, pull the flange nut over the flange, and screw it hand tight onto the body of the fitting as shown at B in Fig. J-3-5.

8. With one wrench on the body of the fitting and another on the flange nut, draw the flange nut up tight. The soft copper flange serves as a gasket to make the joint watertight and as an anchor to hold the tubing in place.

9. If possible, test the joint under pressure to see if it leaks.

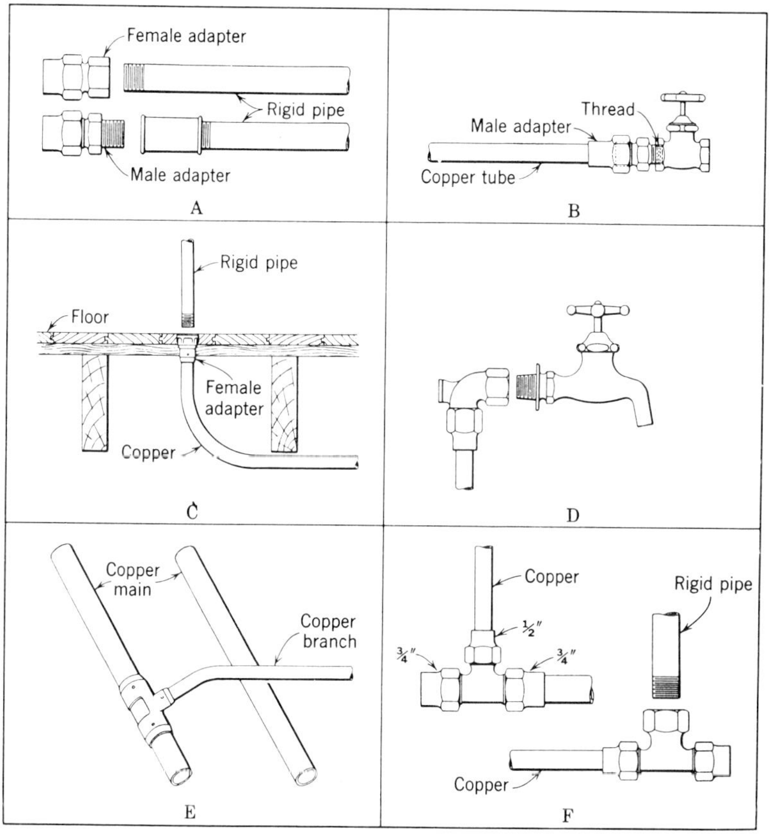

Fig. J-3-3. A — Male and female adapter connections to join copper tube to rigid pipe. B — Method of connecting copper tube to rigid female threaded valve. C — Female adapter used to connect copper tube under the floor to rigid pipe above the floor. D — Connection of a faucet to a bracketed elbow. E — Soldered fitting tee with bent branch line forming a "crossover." F — These and other forms of tees are used for copper water piping.

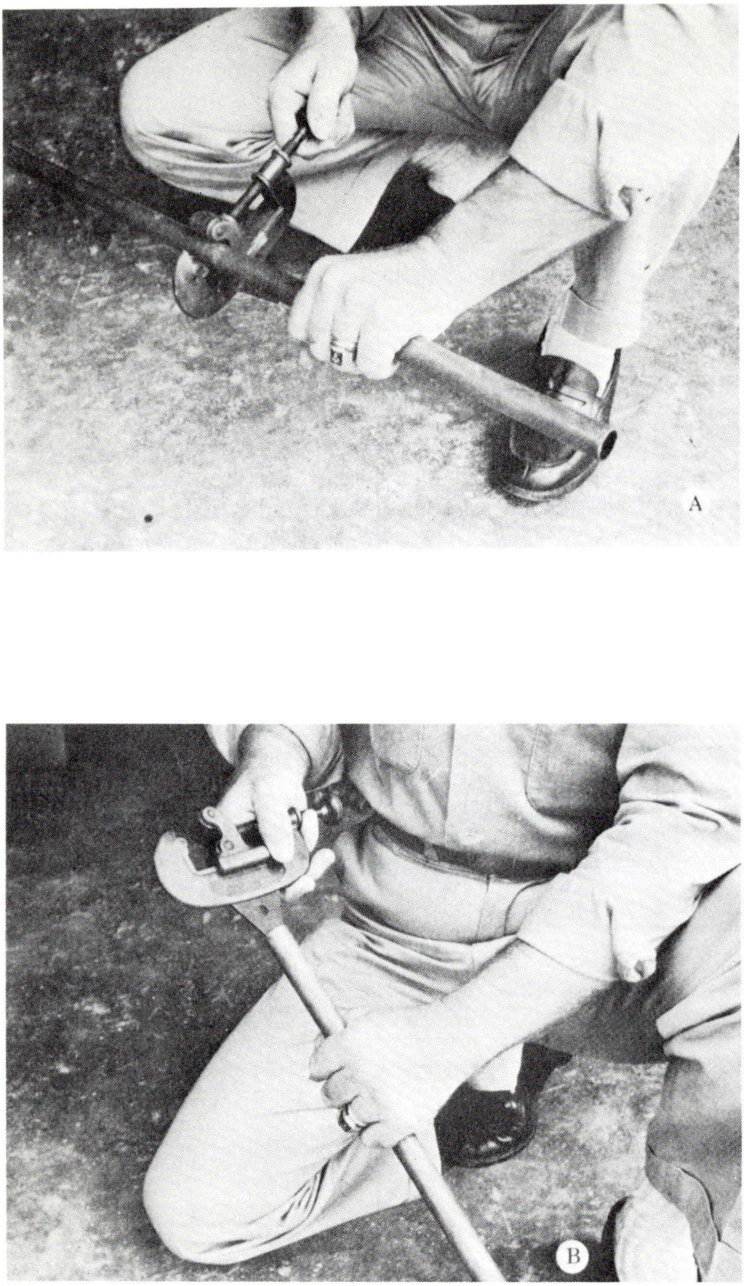

Fig. J-3-4. A — Cutting copper tubing with a wheel cutter. B — Reaming the end of the cut tubing.

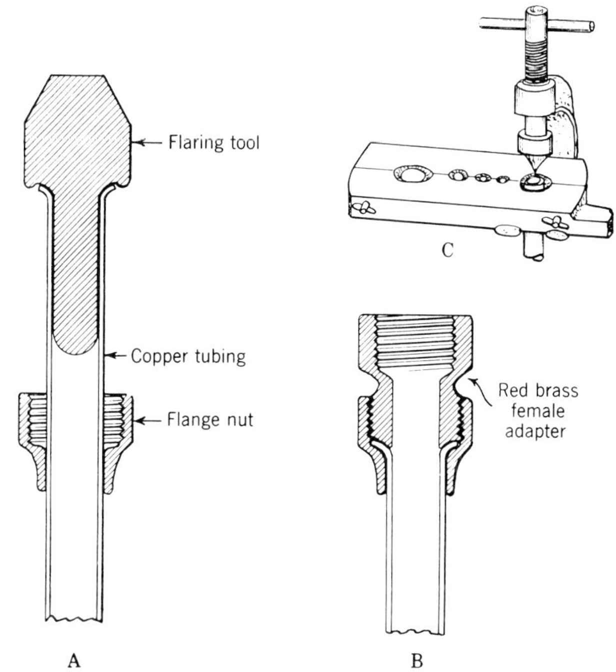

Fig. J-3-5. Flaring tool driven into end of tubing as shown at A turns a flange on the end of the tubing. This flange serves as an anchor to hold the pipe to the fitting and as a gasket to prevent leaking. B, the flanged tubing in place in a fitting. C, a flaring tool for five sizes of tubing.

MAKING A JOINT WITH SOLDER FITTINGS

Tools Needed:

Hacksaw or wheel cutter.

10-inch mill file.

00 steel wool or fine sand cloth made for this special purpose.

A steel wire brush made especially for polishing the inside of fittings. If not available use a strip of the fine sand cloth over a finger.

Heating torch.

Materials Needed:

Tubing and fittings.

Soldering flux suitable for the type of solder being used. Best results will be obtained by using both a flux and solder recommended by the tubing manufacturer. Wire solder, preferably of a grade recommended by the tubing manufacturer.

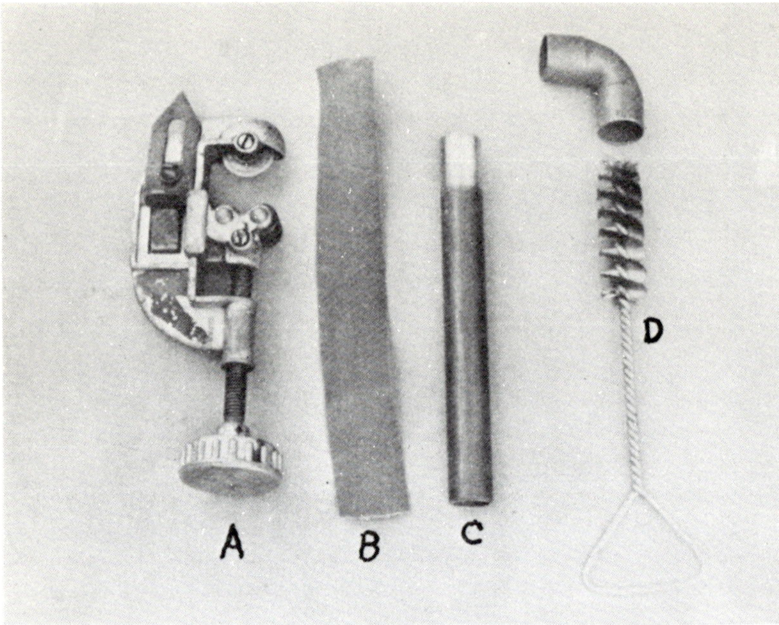

Fig. J-3-6. Tools needed in preparing copper tubing for soldering. At A, a wheeled tubing cutter. At B, a strip of fine emery cloth for polishing the ends of tubing. At C, a length of tubing, and at D, a wire brush for polishing the inside surface of fittings.

Important Steps in Successful Soldering:

The strength of a soldered joint does not depend upon the amount of solder showing on the outside but rather on the bond made by the solder *between* the two surfaces being joined. To make a strong bond the following four steps *must* be taken:

1. *The surfaces to be joined together must be clean.*
2. A suitable flux must be applied. The flux functions to prevent tarnishing of the metal while heating and makes the molten solder flow freely.
3. Heat must be applied in such a way that the entire joint is heated uniformly. Heat until the flux boils or until solder will melt when touched to the metal. Do not overheat.
4. As soon as the metal is hot enough solder is applied to the joint until the joint is filled.

Procedure:

1. Cut the tubing to length with a hacksaw or wheel cutter. See Fig. J-3-4. Be sure to cut the tubing off square.
2. With a file or a reamer remove any burrs or rough edges from both the inside and outside of the tube end.

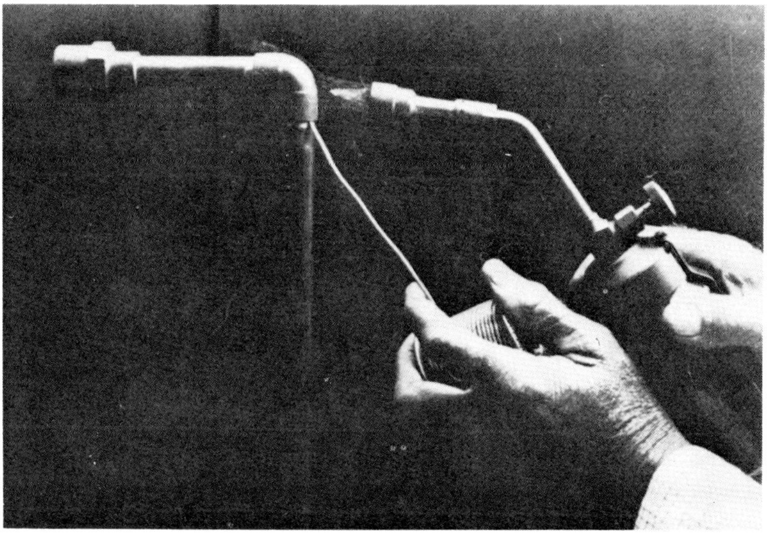

Fig. J-3-7. The tube and fitting, being properly cleaned and fluxed, are assembled and heated to the correct soldering temperature by playing the torch on the fitting and the tube adjacent thereto. Then solder is applied at the edge of the fitting and, melting, flows by capillary action into the space between the tube and fitting.

3. With steel wool or sand cloth burnish the end of the tubing until bright and shiny on the outside for the distance it will be covered by the fittings. This is of primary importance for making strong joints. Solder will not stick to tarnished or dirty surfaces.

4. Burnish the inside of the fitting as far back as the shoulder to remove any oxide. The special wire brush is best for this. See Fig. 3-6D.

5. Apply a thin coating of flux to the burnished outside surface of the tubing and to the inside of the fitting.

6. Push the tubing inside of the fitting *until the end butts against the shoulder of the fitting*. The tubing must remain in this position while soldering. When soldering a valve onto tubing be sure to remove barrel before applying heat. The heat will destroy the washer and stem packing of the valve.

7. Apply heat to the joint until the flux begins to boil or until the copper will melt the solder. See Fig. J-3-7. When soldering large-diameter tubing move the torch around the joint to apply heat on all sides. Apply heat to the fitting rather than the tubing.

8. With the heat still on apply solder to the joint as indicated in Fig. J-3-7 until the joint is filled all the way around. This can be determined by the appearance of solder at the edge of the fitting. Do not apply the flame directly on the solder. Because of the close fit between the tubing and the fitting the solder will flow by capillary ac-

tion throughout the joint, even upward, when the joint is correctly heated.

9. Remove the flame and solder wire as soon as the joint is filled. Excess heat may cause the solder to boil out of the joint. Excess solder is a waste and makes an unsightly job. If excess solder does appear, wipe it off quickly with a cloth.

10. Allow the joint to cool without being disturbed. The result should be a strong, watertight joint. If possible test the joint under pressure.

Making joints in plastic tubing.

For making joints in flexible plastic tubing:

1. Cut the tubing with a knife or a saw.
2. With a knife trim off any burrs and slightly bevel the inside edge of the tube.
3. For ease of inserting the fitting, place the end four or five inches of the tube in hot water for a minute or two. This will soften and lubricate the tube.
4. Place the clamp over the end of the tube and push the fitting in place.

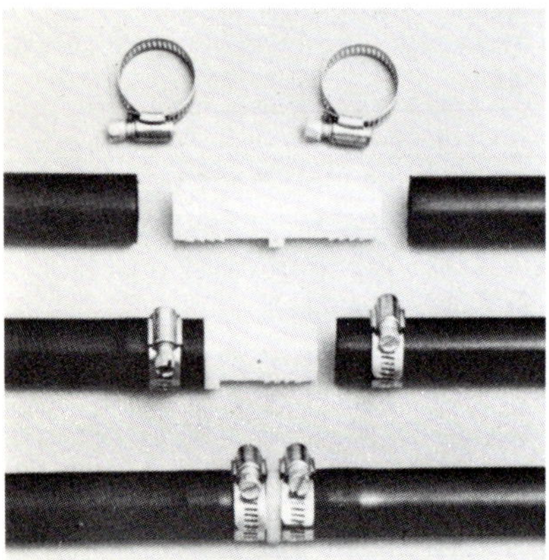

Courtesy ARMCO Chem. Corp.

Fig. J-3-8. Joining flexible plastic tubing.

5. Move the clamp over the tail of the fitting and tighten. See Fig. J-3-8.

For making joints in hard plastic tubing:

1. Cut the tubing square on the ends.
2. With a knife trim off any burrs left from sawing.
3. Clean the inside of the fitting socket and the outside of the end of the tubing.
4. If the fitting must be in a certain position when installed, position it on the tubing and mark both the fitting and the tubing as shown in Fig. J-3-9.

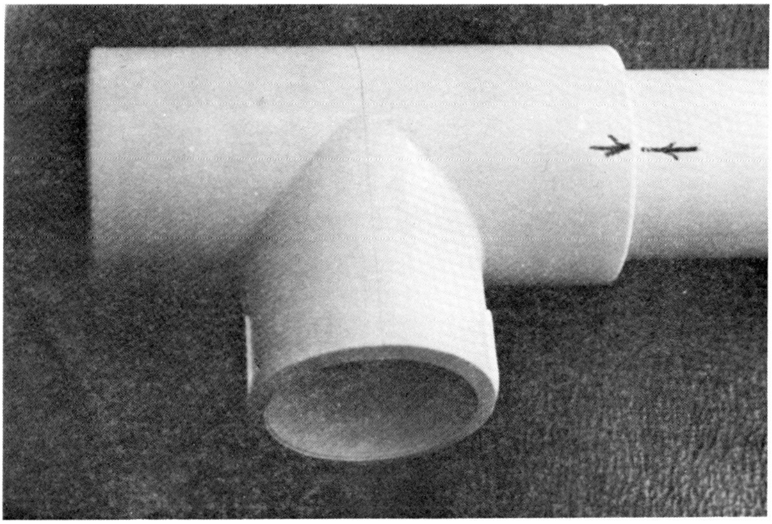

Fig. J-3-9. Mark the position of the fitting before cementing.

5. Remove the fitting and apply a liberal coating of the special cement made for that type of plastic. Be sure to cover the entire surface of the inside of the fitting socket and the outside of the end of the tubing. Read carefully the application instructions printed on the cement container before using.

6. Immediately push the fitting onto the tubing as far as it will go. Use a twisting motion and bring the fitting to rest with the marks lined up.

7. Hold the joint together firmly for a few seconds until the cement starts to set.

8. Wipe off excess cement.

9. Handle the joint carefully for a few minutes or until the cement has set firmly.

10. Do not subject the joint to water pressure for several hours.

Repairing Faucets

JOB 4

Reference: Chapter 10, pages 172–176

Investment in good quality faucets at the outset reduces the overall cost of repairs. However, any faucet will in time develop leaks resulting from wear or damage by scale, grit, or corrosive water.

Faucets develop leaks at two places: at the seat and at the stem. A leak at the seat is caused by wear of or damage to the seat, the washer, or to both. A leak at the seat is indicated by water dripping from the spout when the faucet is *closed.* A leak at the stem is caused by worn or loose stem packing. A stem leak is indicated by water flowing out around the stem at the top of the packing nut when the faucet is *open.* A seat leak is more serious because it wastes more water and sometimes causes staining of the fixtures.

Pipe threading chips, filings, or grit in the pipes is likely to ruin the seat and washer, even on a new faucet. For this reason a good plumber will always knock chips and dirt out of the pipes before they are installed.

Failure to close a faucet tightly may cause water to cut a washer or a seat, thus causing a leak. Faucets should always be closed tightly after use, especially the compression type. Some faucets, especially those which close with the pressure, can and should be closed with *very little pressure* on the handle.

A slow drip at a faucet may not seem important. However, the leak not only causes water to cut the washer or the seat but wastes a surprising amount of water. In the case of a leaking hot-water faucet there is also a considerable waste of heat energy.

Figure J-4-1 shows an average loss of water from commonly used types of faucets at five different rates of dripping. The figures shown will not necessarily apply to any particular faucet because the size of

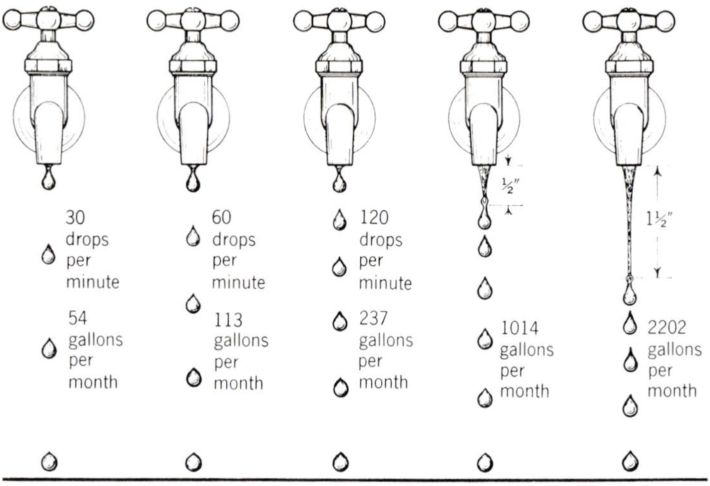

Fig. J-4-1. Showing average losses of water from leaking faucets for a period of 1 month.

drops varies widely with different faucets.

As already stated, in the case of a leaking hot-water faucet the loss of heat may be quite considerable. For example, with an automatic electric water heater set to heat the water to 140°F (60°C), an average of 1 kwhr is consumed for every 3½ to 4 U.S. gallons (1.94 to 3.33 Imp. gals.) of water heated. Assuming a heater with a high efficiency which will use 1 kwhr for every 4 gallons (3.33 Imp. gals.) of water, the additional energy required because of hot-water faucets leaking at the rates shown in Fig. J-4-1 would be as follows:

Faucet Leaking	Kwhr per Month
30 drops per minute	13.5
60 drops per minute	28.2
120 drops per minute	59.2
½-inch solid stream	253.5
1½-inch solid stream	550.5

If the electric rate for this heater were 1½ cents per kwhr, the additional cost for heat due to the leaking faucets would be as follows:

Faucet Leaking	Additional Cost per Month, Dollars	Additional Cost per Year, Dollars
30 drops per minute	0.20	2.43
60 drops per minute	0.42	5.04
120 drops per minute	0.89	10.68
½-inch solid stream	3.80	45.60
1½-inch solid stream	8.26	99.12

It is obvious from the figures just given that the little time and money spent repairing faucets yield good returns.

The following instructions are for repairing the types of faucets described in Chapter 10.

I. REPAIR PLAIN COMPRESSION FAUCETS

Tools Needed:

A flat jawed wrench large enough to fit the packing nut of the faucet. (Do not use a pipe wrench on faucets.)

A piece of soft cloth for the jaws of the wrench to protect the finish of the faucet.

A screw driver.

A faucet seat dresser.

Supplies Needed:

An assortment of faucet washers.

Stem packing material. (Graphite coated wicking is best. Lubricated candle wicking will do.)

Waterproof grease, if candle wicking is used.

An assortment of washer screws.

Procedure:

1. Examine the faucet to see where the leak is. If water is leaking at the spout the trouble is due to a damaged washer, a damaged seat, or both. If the faucet leaks around the stem when open, the trouble is with the stem packing.

2. Turn off the water. This may be done by closing a valve on the pipe under the fixture, if there is such a valve. Otherwise it is usually necessary to close the main valve on the supply line.

3. With the wrench remove the faucet packing nut. A piece of cloth over the wrench jaws will prevent marring the finish on the faucet.

4. Remove the stem from the faucet body.

5. If the leak is at the spout, examine the washer *and seat.* If there is evidence that the washer is damaged, it should be renewed as follows:

a. Remove the washer screw. Use a screw driver that fits snugly in the screw slot. If the screw is too tight to turn, try pounding it on a piece of wood or soak it with penetrating oil.

b. Remove the old washer.

c. Select a new washer of the correct size and quality. If the faucet is for hot water be sure to use a heat-resistant washer.

d. With the washer screw attach the new washer in place on the stem. If the old screw is damaged or badly corroded use a new one.

The seat can be examined by feeling for roughness with a finger or by use of a flashlight. If the seat is damaged it should be repaired, otherwise it will soon cut out the new washer. Nonrenewable seats

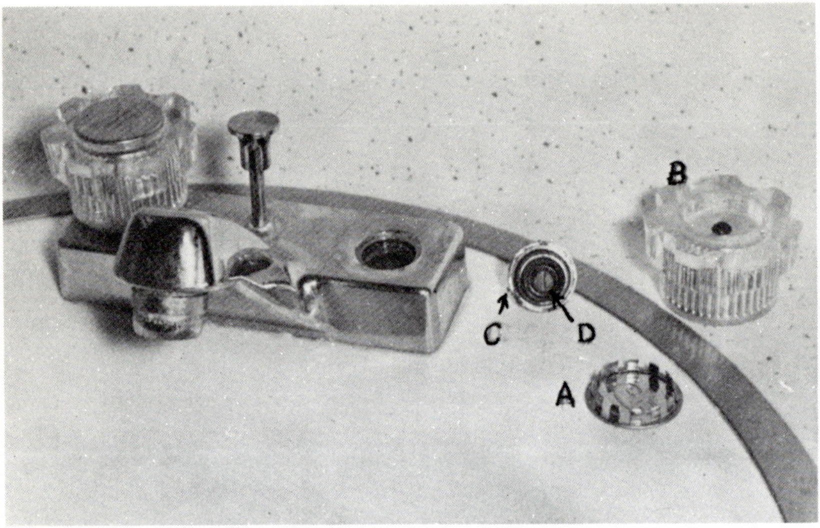

Fig. J-4-2. Procedure for repairing one type of compression mixing faucet.
(1) Turn off the water pressure.
(2) Pry off the metal cap A.
(3) Remove the handle B.
(4) With a flat jawed wrench remove the barrel C.
(5) Remove the old washer D, and replace with a new washer.
(6) Reassemble the faucet.
(7) Turn on the pressure and test for leaks.

can be recut with a seat dresser. There are a number of effective seat dressers on the market. One is illustrated in Fig. J-4-3. Follow the manufacturer's instructions for using the particular seat dresser at hand.

e. After repairs are made, reassemble the faucet and turn on the water.

If the leak was at the stem, examine the stem packing. This can be done by removing the handle and packing nut. It is not necessary to turn off the water or to remove the stem for this job. If the packing is not badly damaged it may be possible to repair it by the addition of a little wicking over the old packing. If candle wicking is used the wicking should be lubricated before winding it on the stem. Waterproof grease is good for this. Wind the wicking on the stem and in the direction the packing nut turns to tighten. If the old packing is badly damaged it should be removed and replaced with new packing. Use only enough wicking to make a snug fit when the packing nut is screwed in place on the faucet body. Some faucets will take prefabricated stem packings which can be purchased at plumbing supply houses.

6. Replace the handle. Set the handle in a convenient position on the stem before tightening the handle screw.

7. Test for leaks.

In lieu of the foregoing procedure for repairing compression faucets, patented "snap-in" repair washers and seats may be used. These are especially useful for repairing old faucets with badly damaged seats. They are easily installed by anyone handy with tools. Figure J-4-4 illustrates the washer and seat. Installation is as follows:

a. Take the faucet apart as directed in the foregoing.

b. Select the largest size snap-in seat that will enter the seat hole.

c. Place the seat on the holder tool as illustrated in Fig. J-4-5 and tap lightly with a hammer until the seat is firmly and evenly in place. The slanted grooves on the sleeve of the snap-in seat will bite into the faucet seat to hold the new seat. The neoprene gasket will make a tight seal on the old seat.

d. Remove the old washer from the stem.

e. With a pair of pliers break off the flange which holds the conventional washer in place.

f. Press the stem of a snap-in swivel washer into the screw hole in the faucet stem. See Fig. J-4-4.

g. Reassemble the faucet.

h. Turn on the water and test for leaks.

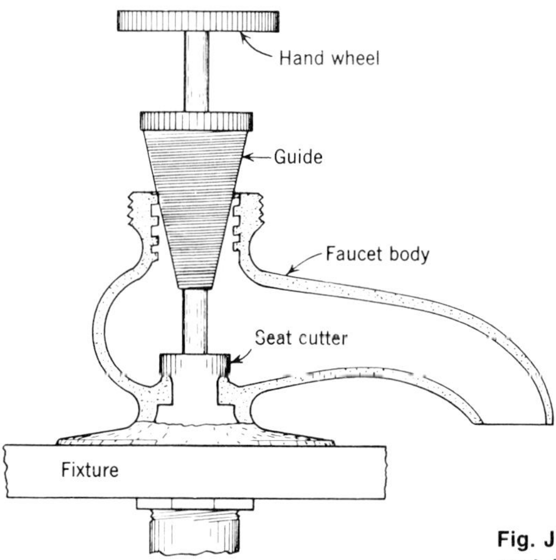

From Sears Roebuck and Co.

Fig. J-4-3. One type of faucet seat dresser. The guide serves to center the cutter and to hold it in position while being turned by means of the hand wheel.

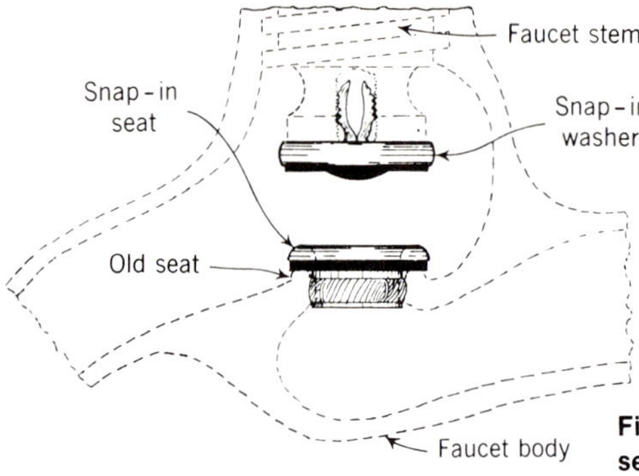

Fig. J-4-4. Snap-in washer and seat for repairing faucets.

II. REPAIR A RENEWABLE SEAT TYPE OF COMPRESSION FAUCET. See Fig. 10-15, page 174

Tools Needed:

Same as for I, plus a square or hexagonal rod which will fit the hole in the renewable seat.

Supplies Needed:

Same as for I, plus a renewable seat of the same size as the old one. Seats made of stainless steel or monel metal will last longer than brass ones.

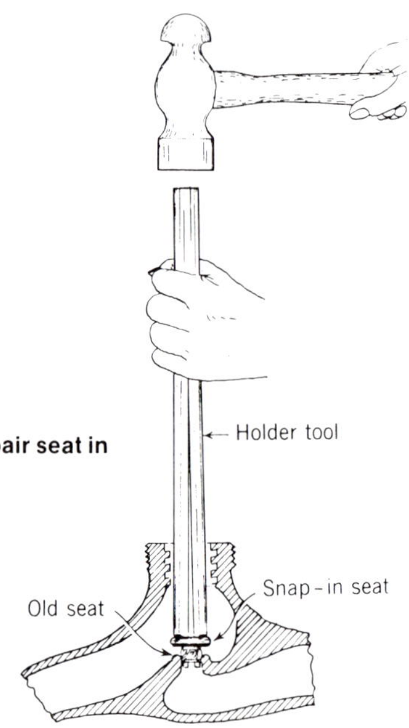

Fig. J-4-5. Driving a snap-in repair seat in place in a faucet.

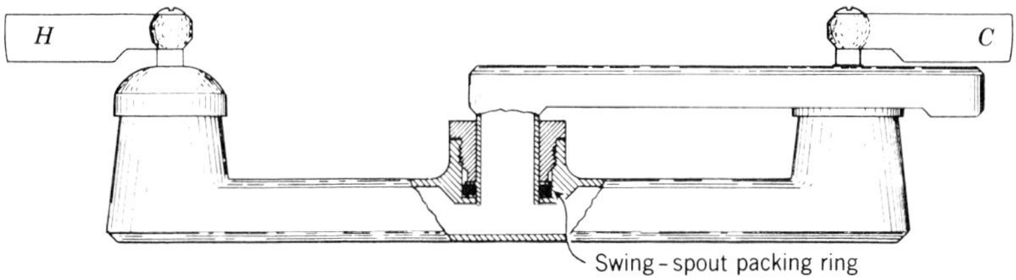

Fig. J-4-6. A swing-spout mixing faucet showing packing ring for spout.

Procedure:

The procedure is the same as for I except for seat repairs. In this case simply remove the old seat and screw the new one in place.

III. REPAIR LEAK AT SWING SPOUT ON MIXING FAUCET

Swing-spout mixing faucets sometimes leak at the base of the spout when either faucet is opened. This leak can be repaired by removing the spout and renewing the packing washer. Figure J-4-6 indicates the spout packing on one type of mixing faucet.

Repairing Toilet Tanks

JOB 5

Study Tank Operation: Refer to Fig. J-5-1

a) When the exterior handle is turned the flush value ball is lifted from its seat. This ball is hollow; therefore it floats upward.

b) The water in the tank flows rapidly through the wide flush valve to flush the toilet.

c) As the water level in the tank drops to approximately the level of the flush valve the flush valve ball drops back onto the valve seat to end the flushing period.

d) The ball-cock tank float also drops with the water level and in doing so opens the ball cock, allowing more water to flow into the tank for refill.

With elevated ball cocks of the type shown in Figs. J-5-1 the ball-cock discharge pipe leads downward so that the incoming refill water will be discharged below the residual water level in the tank. This arrangement prevents splashing and reduces the noise. On the submerged ball cock of Fig. J-5-2 this pipe is unnecessary.

As the tank refills, the ball-cock tank float rises and eventually closes the ball-cock valve to stop the flow of water.

Also, while the tank is refilling, a measured amount of water flows through the trap refill tube into the overflow pipe. This water runs down into the toilet to refill the trap. The trap is partially siphoned out during the flushing period. Figure 10-29F, page 191, shows a toilet trap with a normal water level.

Common Toilet Tank Troubles:

Toilet tank troubles are usually indicated by water leaking into the toilet bowl. The leaking water can reach the bowl either through the flush valve or through the overflow pipe.

If the water level in the tank is at or below normal the leak is at the

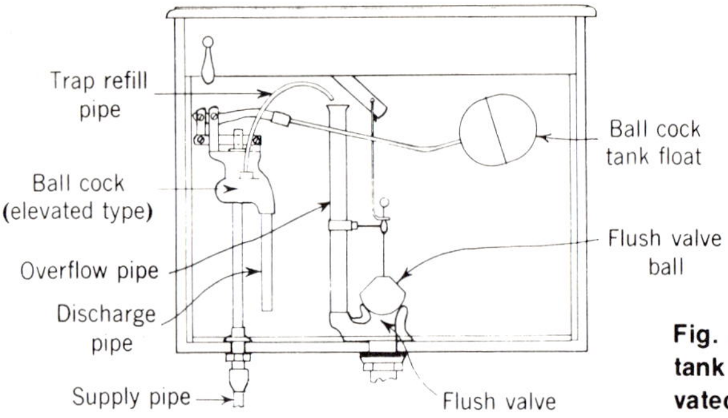

Fig. J-5-1. A toilet tank with an elevated ball cock.

flush valve. If the water level is at the top of the overflow pipe the leak is at the ball cock.

Flush valve leaks usually result from a worn or warped ball. The remedy is a new ball or a replacement with the hinged type shown in Fig. J-5-3. If the ball stem guide is worn, or not centered over the flush valve, the ball may fail to seat properly at the end of the flushing period. The remedy is a new guide or an adjustment of the old one.

A leak at the flush valve lets the ball-cock float drop enough to open the ball cock and water flows into the tank at the same rate that it leaks out. It is this flow of refill water through the ball-cock valve that makes the hissing noise which accompanies a leak.

Ball cock leaks may be due to:

1. A waterlogged ball-cock float.
2. Ball-cock float rod bent up too far.
3. A worn washer or seat.
4. Scale lodged between washer and seat.
5. Binding in the ball-cock mechanism or valve. Sometimes the valve packing swells because of the absorption of water and binds on the housing.

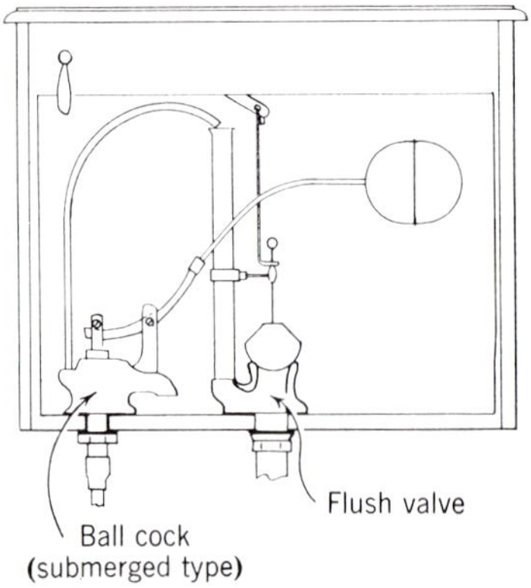

Fig. J-5-2. A toilet tank with submerged type of ball cock.

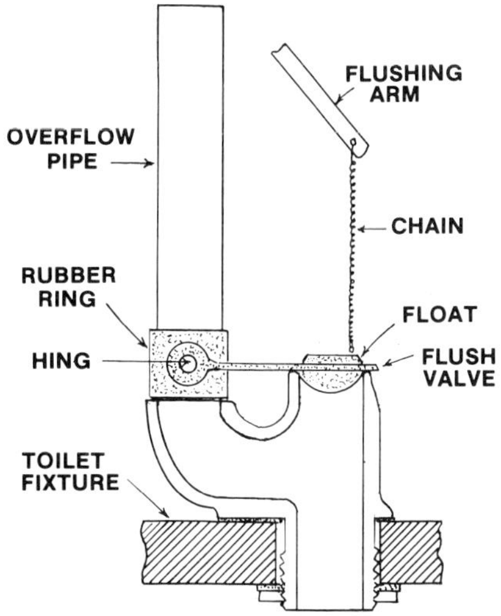

Fig. J-5-3. A relatively new type of flush valve. It can be used to replace the older ball type and is standard equipment on some of the new toilet tanks. To install, remove the old ball, the ball guide and the ball guide clamp on the overflow pipe. Press the rubber ring down over the overflow pipe until the rubber float rests firmly on the flush valve seat. Attach the chain, which is supplied with the float, to the flushing arm as shown.

This valve is long lasting and stays in place better than the ball type.

If there is a need to conserve water this valve can be used to flush only half a tank of water when flushing for urine only. This is accomplished by pushing the flushing handle down only far enough to obtain a good flow into the toilet, but not far enough to cause the float to float. Hold the handle in this position until the toilet trap starts to siphon. Release the handle and the float drops immediately saving about half a tank of water.

Waterlogged floats should be replaced. Glass or plastic floats are more corrosion resistant than copper floats. Bent float rods can usually be straightened.

Worn washers can be replaced as in a faucet after taking the valve stem out. Pliers and a screw driver are usually needed for this job.

If the ball cock seat is worn or damaged it can sometimes be repaired by recutting the seat with a faucet seat dresser. Otherwise a

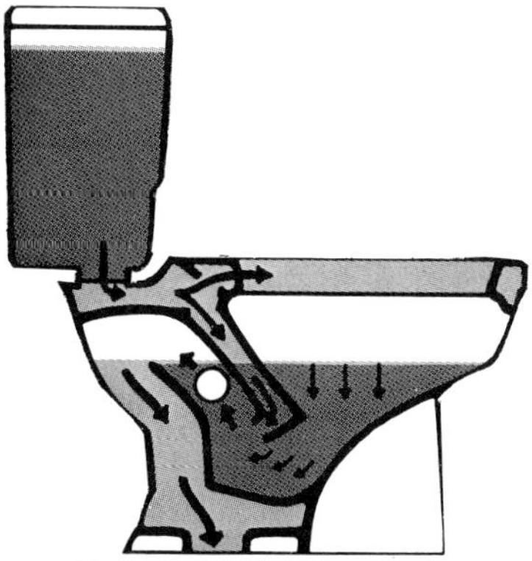

Siphon-Jet Flushing Action.

Courtesy Borg-Warner Corp.

Fig. J-5-4. A new type of flush toilet which the manufacturer claims will save 1½ gallons of water per flushing. It is quiet and easy to clean. Has hinged type of flush valve.

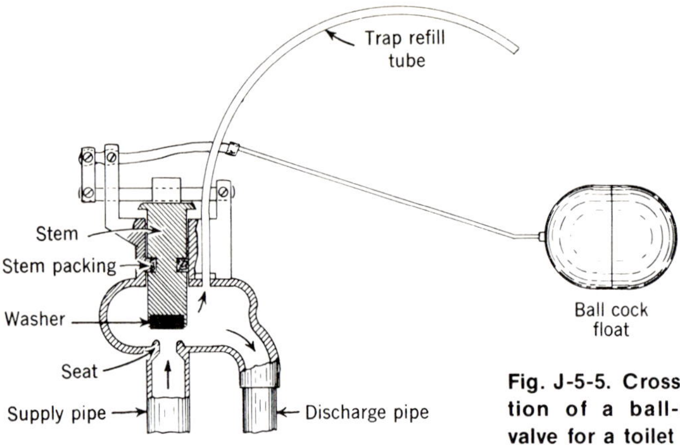

Fig. J-5-5. Cross section of a ball-cock valve for a toilet tank.

new seat or a whole new ball cock will have to be used.

Scale lodged in the valve can sometimes be flushed out by repeatedly pushing the ball-cock float completely down. If this fails the valve will have to be taken apart.

Binding may occur because of corrosion on the valve mechanism or a swelling of the packing. A good cleaning of the metal parts and light sanding on the packing will relieve this trouble.

If the valve packing is badly worn or deteriorated, the valve will leak at the top during the refill period. This makes a noticeable "run-

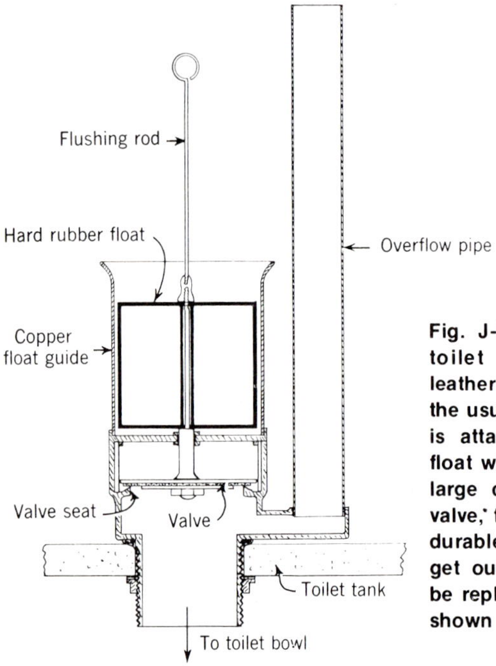

Fig. J-5-6. Cross section of a toilet flush valve having a leather-faced valve rather than the usual rubber ball. The valve is attached to a hard rubber float which float is housed in a large copper tube guide. The valve, float, and guide are very durable and the guide cannot get out of adjustment. Cannot be replaced by the hinged type shown in Fig. J-5-3.

ning-water" noise and sometimes causes a leak over the top of the tank. New packings can be purchased at plumbing supply stores and installed by removing the valve stem, breaking out the old packing, and pressing the new one in place.

If the water level in the toilet bowl stands too low, the trouble is with the trap refill tube. The tube may be plugged with scale, bent out of position from over the overflow pipe, or broken off. Cleaning, adjusting, or renewal of the refill pipe will remedy this trouble. It is important that the toilet trap be filled to its normal level (see Fig. 10-29F) in order to prevent sewer gases from escaping into the room.

Determining Pipe Sizes

JOB 6

Reference: Chapter 5, Pg. 69.

The loss of head on flowing water in pipes due to friction is a very important consideration in the proper installation of a plumbing system or a pump. This factor is often neglected entirely, with the result that the flow of water is not satisfactory.

Where long runs of pipe are used, as might be the case with a natural gravity water system or where a pump is located at some distance from the buildings, it is most necessary, for satisfactory operation of the system, to see that the pipes are large enough.

To determine the size of pipe to use in any case the following facts must be known:

1. The length of the pipe to be used.
2. The number of fittings, valves, faucets, etc., on the pipe-line.
3. The kind and condition of pipe used.
4. The rate of flow of water desired in gallons per minute.
5. The amount of head (gravity or pressure) available for forcing water through the pipe.
6. The altitude above sea level.

Length of Pipe

The actual length of the pipe should be measured from the source of water to the point of delivery; i.e., for a suction pipe to a pump, measure the entire length including that portion which is submerged in the water.

Number of Fittings, Valves, Faucets, etc.

Straight-through fittings such as couplings and unions offer a negligible amount of friction; therefore they may be neglected in calculating pipe sizes. On the other hand, elbows, T's, return bends, and reducing fittings do cause appreciable friction losses and when used in considerable numbers should be considered in determining pipe sizes. Ordinarily one or two such fittings in a long pipeline can safely be neglected.

The losses in valves and faucets vary widely with the type and design. Globe valves offer appreciably more resistance than do gate valves. The resistance of faucets, when wide open, can be considered the same as that of globe valves of the same size.

Space will not permit a presentation here of exact friction losses for every type of fitting, valve, and faucet. However, Table J-6-I indicates average losses in the most commonly used ones. The losses are expressed in terms of equivalent length of pipe of the same size.

TABLES J-6-I
FRICTION LOSSES IN FITTINGS, VALVES, FAUCETS, ETC. EQUIVALENT TO LENGTHS OF SAME SIZE PIPE*

	Type of Fittings, Valve, Faucet, Etc.								
Nominal Size,	90° Elbow	45° Elbow	Stand. T	Gate Valve Fully Open	Globe Valve Fully Open	Check Valve Fully Open	Faucet Fully Open	Foot Valve Fully Open	Strainer
Inches	Equivalent Length Straight Pipe, Feet								
½	1.80	0.78	3.40	0.35	16.00	3.80	16.00	4.00	10.00
¾	2.25	1.00	4.50	0.47	21.00	5.20	21.00	5.00	12.00
1	2.75	1.35	5.80	0.60	27.00	6.50		6.00	14.00
1¼	3.75	1.72	7.50	0.80	37.00	9.00		7.00	16.00
1½	4.45	2.00	9.00	0.95	45.00	11.00		8.00	18.00
2	5.30	2.50	12.00	1.25	55.00	14.00		9.00	20.00
2½	6.50	3.00	14.00	1.40	65.00	17.00		10.00	22.00
3	8.20	3.80	16.00	1.75	85.00	19.00		12.00	25.00

Nominal Size,	90° Elbow	45° Elbow	Stand. T	Gate Valve Fully Open	Globe Valve Fully Open	Check Valve Fully Open	Faucet Fully Open	Foot Valve Fully Open	Strainer
Inches	Equivalent Length Straight Pipe, Meters								
½	0.55	0.24	1.04	0.11	4.88	1.16	4.88	1.22	3.05
¾	0.69	0.30	1.37	0.14	6.40	1.58	6.40	1.52	3.66
1	0.84	0.41	1.77	0.18	8.23	1.98		1.83	4.27
1¼	1.14	0.52	2.29	0.24	11.28	2.74		2.13	4.88
1½	1.36	0.61	2.74	0.29	13.71	3.35		2.44	5.49
2	1.62	0.76	3.66	0.38	16.76	4.27		2.74	6.10
2½	1.98	0.91	4.27	0.43	19.81	5.18		3.05	6.71
3	2.50	1.16	4.88	0.53	25.90	5.79		3.66	7.62

*Compiled from "Flow of Fluid Through Valves, Fittings and Pipe," Technical Paper No. 409, May 1942, page 17, Crane Company Engineering and Research Division, Chicago, Ill.

Kind and Condition of Pipe

The kind and condition of pipe used affect materially the rate of flow of water. The smoother the inside of the pipe the less the friction losses. As steel pipe often corrodes and has scale deposits on the inside after a few years of use, the friction losses are increased. For this reason most friction tables for steel pipe are based upon the use of pipe which is 10 to 15 years old. Copper and plastic tubing seldom corrode and do not hold scale deposits to any appreciable extent; therefore, the friction losses remain fairly constant over a period of

TABLE J-6-11 A (U.S. UNITS)
FRICTION RESISTANCE TO FLOW OF WATER*
FIGURES IN BODY OF TABLE SHOW LOSS OF HEAD IN FEET PER 100 FEET OF PIPE FOR INDICATED RATES OF FLOW OF WATER

Rate of Flow, Gallons per Minute	Nominal Diameter of Pipe, Inches							
	½	¾	1	1¼	1½	2	2½	3
1	2.10	0.49						
2	7.40	1.90						
3	15.80	4.10	1.26					
4	27.00	7.00	2.14	0.57	0.26			
5	41.00	10.50	3.25	0.84	0.39	0.12		
6	54.86	14.15	4.39	1.15	0.52	0.17		
7		18.19	5.63	1.61	0.75	0.23		
8		24.05	7.50	1.93	0.89	0.32		
9		28.58	9.04	2.45	1.18	0.38		
10		38.00	11.70	3.05	1.43	0.50	0.17	0.07
12		53.00	15.76	4.13	1.93	0.66	0.27	0.10
15		80.00	24.05	6.50	3.00	1.00	0.36	0.15
18		108.20	35.00	9.10	4.24	1.49	0.50	0.21
20		236.00	42.00	11.10	5.20	1.82	0.61	0.25
25			64.00	16.60	7.80	2.73	0.92	0.38
30			89.00	23.50	11.00	3.84	1.29	0.54
35			119.00	31.20	14.70	5.10	1.73	0.71
40			152.00	40.00	18.80	6.60	2.20	0.91

**Courtesy Sears Roebuck and Company.*
Note: For new smooth pipe multiply the above values by 0.7

years. However, the actual inside diameter of copper tubing is less than that of steel pipe per nominal size.

Plastic tubing has the same inside diameter as steel pipe, but the small difference in friction losses, in sizes up to and including 1-inch,

TABLE J-6-II B (METRIC UNITS)
FRICTIONAL RESISTANCE TO FLOW OF WATER
FIGURES IN THE BODY OF TABLE SHOW LOSS OF HEAD IN METERS PER 30.48 METERS (100 FT.) OF PIPE FOR INDICATED RATES OF FLOW OF WATER

Rate of Flow, Imp. Gals. per Min.	Nominal diameter of Pipe, Inches — Friction Loss in Meters of Head per 30.48 M. (100 ft.) of 15 Year-Old Pipe							
	½"	¾"	1"	1¼"	1½"	2"	2½"	3"
0.93	0.64	0.15						
1.67	2.26	0.58						
2.50	4.82	1.25	0.38					
3.33	8.23	2.13	0.65	0.17	0.08			
4.17	12.50	3.20	0.99	0.26	0.12	0.04		
5.00	16.72	4.31	1.34	0.35	0.16	0.05		
5.83		5.54	1.72	0.49	0.23	0.07		
6.67		7.33	2.29	0.59	0.27	0.10		
7.50		8.71	2.76	0.75	0.36	0.12		
8.33		11.58	3.57	0.93	0.44	0.15	0.05	0.02
10.00		16.15	4.80	1.26	0.59	0.20	0.08	0.03
12.50		24.38	7.33	1.98	0.91	0.30	0.11	0.05
15.00		33.00	10.67	2.77	1.29	0.45	0.15	0.06
16.67		71.93	12.80	3.38	1.58	0.55	0.19	0.08
20.83			19.51	5.06	2.38	0.83	0.28	0.12
25.00			27.13	7.16	3.35	1.17	0.39	0.16
29.17			36.27	9.51	4.48	1.55	0.53	0.22
33.33			46.33	12.19	5.73	2.01	0.67	0.28

does not justify the use of one size smaller tubing than indicated by the friction table. It is therefore recommended that the same friction table (Table J-6-II) be used for all three types of piping materials, at least for sizes up to and including 1 inch. For sizes over 1 inch the next size smaller plastic tubing can be used and, where the friction table indicates a borderline choice, the next size smaller copper tubing can be used.

Rate of Discharge

A faucet discharges at the rate of 3 to 5 U.S. gallons (2½ to 4.2 Imp. gals.) per minute when wide open. If two or more faucets or other discharge units are to be supplied simultaneously through the same pipe, the discharge rate of all the units should be added to obtain the total rate of flow desired.

The Amount of Head Available

The amount of head available for forcing the water through the pipes is important because the more the head available the more we can afford to lose by friction, therefore the smaller the pipe necessary. Conversely, with very little head available we cannot afford to lose much of it by friction and must therefore use larger pipes.

The Elevation Above Sea Level

The elevation above sea level affects the suction lift of pumps; see Table 5-I, page 76.

The following examples will illustrate how to use friction Table J-6-II in determining pipe sizes. The solution of such problems is made easier if sketches are made, as illustrated in Figs. J-6-1, J-6-2, and J-6-3.

Example 1.

A 100-foot length of ¾-inch pipe carries water at the rate of 5 gallons (4.17 Imp. gals.) per minute. How much head would be lost due to friction?

Solution: using Table J-6-II-A

1. Referring to Table J-6-II-A locate a flow of 5 U.S. gallons per minute in column 1 on the left. Reading horizontally to the right from this figure to the figure in the column under ¾-inch pipe we find the figure 10.50, which is the loss of head in feet per 100 feet of pipe.

2. If the pipe were 300 feet long the loss of head would be 3 × 10.5 or 31.5 feet.

3. If the rate of flow were 8 U.S. gallons per minute, the loss of head would be found by reading to the right from 8 U.S. gallons per minute in the left-hand column to the figure 24.05 under ¾-inch pipe.

4. If the rate of flow were 8 U.S. gallons per minute through a 1-inch pipe, the loss of head would be 7.50 feet.

5. What would be the loss of head with a rate of flow of 10 U.S. gallons per minute through 200 feet of 1¼-inch pipe?

Example 1.

Solution, using metric Table J-6-II-B

1. Locate in column I a rate of flow of 4.17 Imp. gals. per minute (5 U.S. gals. per min.). Reading horizontally to the right from that figure to the column under ¾-inch pipe we find the figure 3.2 meters loss of head in 30.48 meters (100 ft.) of pipe.

2. If the pipe were 91.44 meters (300 ft.) long the loss of head would be 3 × 3.32 meters or 9.6 meters.

3. If the rate of flow were 6.67 Imperial gallons per minute the loss of head through ¾″ pipe would be 7.33 meters (100 ft.) of pipe.

4. If the rate of flow were 6.67 Imperial gallons per minute through 1″ pipe the loss of head would be 2.29 meters.

5. What would be the loss of head with a rate of flow of 10 Imperial gallons per minute through 61 meters (200 ft.) of 1¼″ pipe?

Example 2. Using U.S. Units

A 200-foot length of pipe is to be used to carry water downhill from a spring to a swimming pool. The elevation of the spring is 5 feet above the top of the pool; therefore the gravity head on the water is 5 feet. If the desired rate of flow is 4 U.S. gallons per minute what size pipe should be used?

Solution

Referring to Table J-6-II-A we locate 4 U.S. gallons per minute rate of flow, then read to the right until we find a figure which, when multiplied by 2, will not exceed 5 feet of head. We find that the figure 2.14 is the nearest (2 × 2.14 = 4.28) and that figure is in the column under 1-inch pipe; therefore a 1-inch pipe would be the size to use.

Example 2. Using Metric Units

A 61 meter (200 ft.) length of pipe is used to carry water down hill from a spring to a swimming pool. The elevation of the spring is 1.52 meters above the top of the pool; therefore the gravity head on the water is 1.52 meters. If the desired rate of flow is 3.33 Imperial gallons per minute what size pipe should be used?

Solution

Referring to Table J-II-B we locate 3.33 gallons per minute rate of flow. Reading to the right until we find a figure which, when multiplied by 2 will not exceed 1.52 meters of head, we find that figure to be 0.65 meters of head in the column under 1 inch pipe; therefore 1 inch pipe would be the size to use.

Example 3 *

If in the problem of Example 2 a ½-inch pipe were used what would be the rate of flow?

Solution

The only available head for making the water flow is the 5 feet of gravity head. Regardless of the size of pipe all of this head and only this head would be used up. Referring to the column under ½-inch pipe we locate a figure which, when multiplied by 2, would equal 5. the nearest figure is 2.10 which would give a loss of head of 4.2 feet. Reading to the left to column 1, we see that the rate of flow for that figure is only 1 gallon per minute. As we have 5 feet of head the actual rate of flow would be a little over 1 U.S. gallon per minute instead of the desired 4 U.S. gallons per minute.

Example 4. See Fig. J-6-1.

A gravity storage tank is located on a hill back of the house. The tank has an elevation of 58 feet above the faucet and requires 365 feet of pipe with a strainer, two 90° elbows, a gate valve, and a ½-inch faucet. The desired rate of flow at the faucet is 6 gallons per minute. What size pipe should be used?

Solution

1. Here we have, in addition to the pipe, some fittings, valves, and faucets which must be considered. The equivalent length of pipe is equal to the measured length of 365 feet plus the losses in the fittings. These losses are indicated in Table J-6-1, pg. 278.

If we used ¾-inch pipe the losses in the fittings, valve, faucet, and strainer would be equivalent to the following lengths of pipe:

Two ¾-inch, 90° elbows	4.50 feet	—	1.38 m.
One ¾-inch gate valve	.47 feet	—	0.14 m.
One ½-inch faucet	16.00 feet	—	4.88 m.
One ¾-inch strainer	12.00 feet	—	3.66 m.
Total	32.97 feet	—	10.06 m.

The equivalent length of pipe under these conditions would be 398 feet (365 plus 32.97). In using the friction table we will consider this as 400 (121.92 m.) feet of pipe.

If we used a 1-inch pipe the equivalent length of pipe for the fittings, etc., would be 36.10 feet as calculated from the Table J-6-I. This, added to the 365 feet, equals 401 feet. Again, in using the friction table we would consider this as 400 feet of pipe.

---

* 1 foot = 0.3048 meter
Imperial gallons = U.S. gallons ÷ 1.2

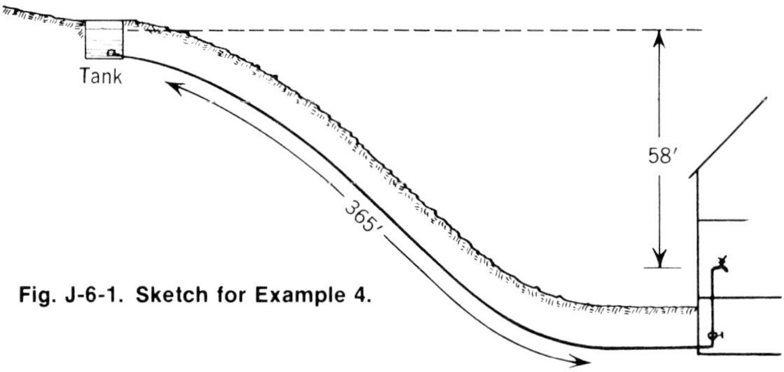

Fig. J-6-1. Sketch for Example 4.

2. The gravity head available is 58 feet; therefore the friction losses in the 400 feet of pipe should not exceed that value.

Referring to Table J-6-II-A, reading horizontally from 6 U.S. gallons per minute we find that even *one* 100-foot length of ½-inch pipe would require practically all of the head available; therefore ½-inch pipe is too small. The next larger size, ¾ inch, would require 14.15 feet of head per 100 feet of length. 14.15 × 4 = 56.60 feet total head required. As 58 feet of head is available a ¾-inch pipe would be adequate.

Example 5

Determine the size of suction pipe for a pump. In the case illustrated in Fig. J-6-2, we find:

1. The actual length of pipe from the strainer to the pump is 70 feet. There is one 90° elbow, one foot valve, one strainer, and a check valve, all of which add to the friction losses. For a pipe 70 feet long these losses should be considered.

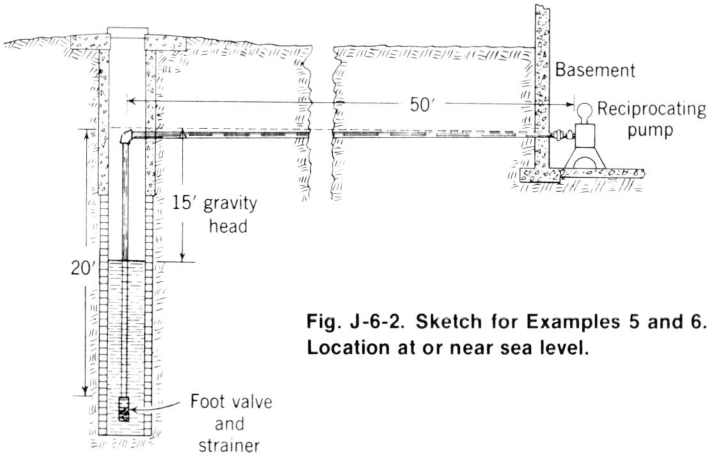

Fig. J-6-2. Sketch for Examples 5 and 6. Location at or near sea level.

2. The rate of flow is equal to the capacity of the pump, which we will assume to be 8 U.S. gallons per minute.

3. The gravity head is 15 feet. The pump has a rated suction lift of 25 feet at sea level. The pump must overcome the gravity head as well as friction head. The pump suction lift of 25 feet minus the 15 feet of gravity head leaves only 10 feet of suction head to overcome friction.

The intake opening on the pump is tapped for 1-inch pipe. Is 1-inch pipe large enough? As a general rule the suction pipe for a pump should never be smaller than the tapped intake opening on the pump.

Solution

1. Referring to Table J-6-I we find that the loss of head in the 1-inch fittings would be equivalent to that in the following lengths of 1-inch pipe.

One 90° elbow	2.75 feet
One foot valve	6.00 feet
One strainer	14.00 feet
One check valve	6.50 feet
Equivalent length of 1-inch pipe	29.25 feet

This equivalent length of 1-inch pipe added to the actual length of pipe gives us 99.25 feet of total equivalent length of pipe. Thus we see that the losses in the fittings and valves is equal to more than one-third the length of the pipe.

2. Referring to Table J-6-II in the column on the left we locate 8 gallons per minute. From this, reading to the right under 1-inch pipe, we find the loss of head due to friction is 7.50 feet per 100 feet of pipe.

The total suction head which the pump will have to work against will therefore be the 15 feet of gravity head plus the 7.50 feet of friction head, or a total of 22.50 feet. As the reciprocating pump has a rated suction lift of 25 feet the 1-inch pipe is adequate.

Example 6

If the foregoing installation were to be made at a higher elevation, say 5280 feet above sea level, what size suction pipe should be used?

Solution

1. Referring to Table 5-I on page 76 we find that the practical suction lift of a reciprocating plunger pump at that altitude is 17 feet instead of 25 feet as at sea level.

2. As the pump is 15 feet above the water the available suction head for friction would be 17 feet minus 15 feet, or 2 feet.

3. The loss of head in 1-inch pipe would be 7.50 feet. As only 2 feet of suction head is available the 1-inch pipe is too small.

4. If 1¼-inch pipe were used the loss of head would be 1.93 feet. Therefore 1¼ inches would be the correct size for stee pipe or copper tubing. One size smaller, or 1 inch, plastic tubing could be used.

Example 7

Determine the size of suction pipe for the shallow-well jet pump installation shown in Fig. J-6-3.

1. The actual length of pipe is 170 feet. There are two 90° elbows, one foot valve, one strainer, and one check valve at the pump.

2. The desired rate of pumping is 10 U.S. gallons per minute or 600 U.S. gallons per hour.

3. The discharge capacity of the pump is as follows:

TABLE J-6-III

With a Suction Lift in Feet, Including Pipe Friction, of	Capacity in U.S. Gallons per Minute at 20 Pounds Discharge Pressure
5	18
10	15
15	12
20	10
25	6

From these figures it is evident that the capacity of the pump falls off rapidly as the suction lift increases, and in order to obtain 10 U.S. gallons per minute the total suction head must not exceed 20 feet.

4. Elevation of pump above water level is 12 feet. This leaves 8 feet of head which can be lost in friction.

5. Pump intake opening is tapped for 1-inch pipe.

Will 1-inch pipe and fittings, with a rate of flow of 10 U.S. gallons per minute cause more than an 8 foot loss of head?

Solution

1. Referring to Table J-6-I we find the friction losses in the 1-inch fittings would be equal to those of the following lengths of 1-inch pipe:

Two 1-inch 90° elbows	(2 × 2.75) or 5.50 feet
One foot valve	6.00 feet
One strainer	14.00 feet
One check valve	6.50 feet
Total	32.00 feet

The total equivalent length of suction pipe would be 170 + 32 or 202 feet. Use 200 feet for the friction table.

2. Referring to Table J-6-II we find under 1-inch pipe at 10 U.S. gallons per minute the loss of head per 100 feet of pipe is 11.70 feet. This times two 100-foot lengths equals 23.40 feet loss of head, as only 20 ft. of suction head is available. It is evident that 1-inch pipe is too small.

3. Referring again to Table J-6-I we find that the 1¼-inch fittings would equal 39.5 feet of pipe. The equivalent length of pipe would therefore be 170 + 39.5 or 209.5 feet.

4. Referring to Table J-6-II we find the loss of head in 200 feet of

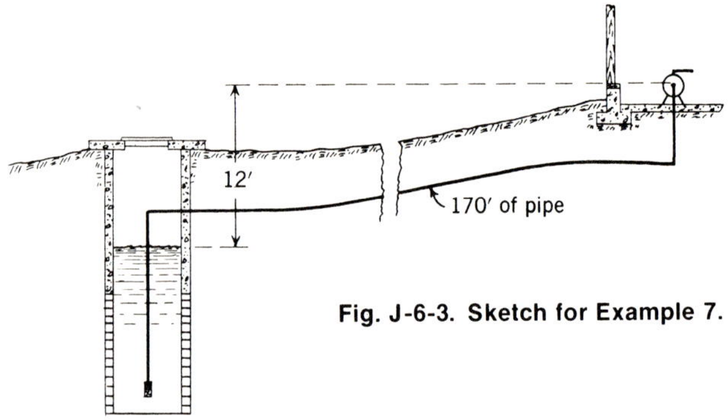

Fig. J-6-3. Sketch for Example 7.

1¼-inch pipe at 10 U.S. gallons per minute is 2 × 3.05 or 6.10 feet. As 8 feet of suction head is available this allows a little for the extra length of pipe; therefore, 1¼ inch would be the correct size for steel pipe and copper tubing. One size smaller, or 1 inch, plastic tubing could be used.

5. If the size of the suction pipe for this installation were chosen on the basis of the size of the intake opening on the pump, as is often done, the capacity of the pump would be reduced to about 7 U.S. gallons per minute instead of the desired 10.

Example 8: See Fig. J-6-4

From a pressure tank in the basement of a house it is desired to pipe water to drinking cups in a barn 250 feet away. There is only one elbow and two gate valves are used. The maximum rate of flow desired for the cows is 15 gallons per minute. The minimum pressure on the water in the tank at the house is 20 pounds per square inch. The outlets in the barn are 18 feet above the low-water level in the tank. What size pipe should be used to the barn?

Solution

1. The length of pipe = 250 feet.
2. Fittings are so few that they can be neglected, on a long run of pipe.
3. Rate of flow, 15 U.S. gallons per minute.
4. Minimum head available is 20 pounds' pressure per square inch × 2.3 feet per pound, or 46 feet.
5. Of the 46 feet of available pressure head, 18 feet must be used to lift the water through the 18-foot difference in elevation. This leaves 28 feet of head for overcoming friction.
6. Referring to Table J-6-II-A at 15 U.S. Gallons per minte through 1-inch pipe we find a 24.05-foot loss of head per 100 feet of pipe. 24.05 × 2.5 = 60.1 foot loss of head in the 250 feet of pipe. As we have only 28 feet of pressure head available, 1-inch pipe would not be

large enough.

Referring again to Table J-6-II-A we find that with 1¼-inch pipe the loss of head would be 6.50 feet per 100 feet of pipe. 6.5 × 2.5 = 16.25 feet total loss of head. As this is less than the 28 feet of available head, 1¼ inches would be the size for steel pipe, or a combination of 1-inch and 1¼-inch pipe such that the combined loss of head would not exceed 28 feet could be used.

7. If 1-inch pipe were used instead of 1¼-inch, what would be the rate of flow? This can be determined by reference to Table J-6-II-A. We have 28 feet of available head to force the water through the pipe. Reading upward under 1-inch pipe we look for a value which when multiplied by 2.5 will equal 28 feet. The nearest figure is 11.70 feet loss of head. 11.70 × 2.5 = 29.25. Reading horizontally to the left to the rate of flow column we find 10 U.S. gallons per minute. Therefore, the rate of flow with 1-inch pipe would be less than two-thirds of the desired 15 gallons per minute. As a major item is the labor of installing the pipe, the extra cost of the 1¼-inch pipe would be a good investment.

As the table indicates a considerable margin of head (11.75 feet) when using 1¼-inch steel pipe, it would be possible to use 1-inch plastic tubing.

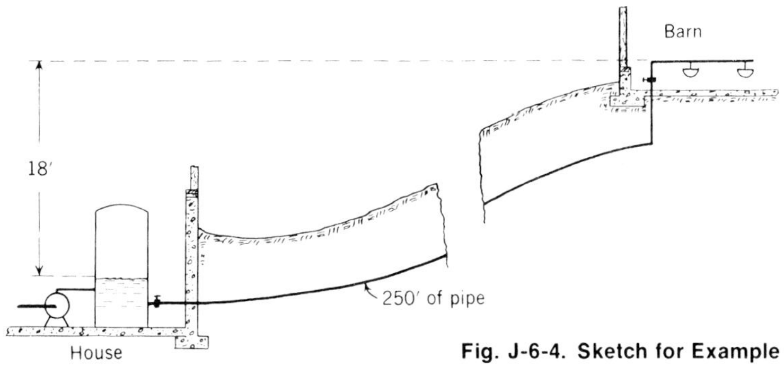

Fig. J-6-4. Sketch for Example 8.

Laying Sewer Tile and Drain Tile

JOB 7

References: Chapter 11

The sewer tile and the drain tile for the absorption field must be carefully laid to make the sewage system function properly. In some areas Health Departments have established regulations on the type of sewer pipe to use and its installation. Such regulations should be complied with wherever they exist. The refernce for this job gives general recommendations on location and installation.

Regardless of the kind of tile used, it should be laid in a straight line, if possible, and on a uniform grade, the inside should be smooth.

Stoppage in sewer lines is caused by (1) broken pipes, (2) poor grading, (3) solids of excessive size, such as newspapers, rags, children's toys, and large pieces of garbage, (4) excessive amounts of grease, and (5) poor joints which may offer obstructions of permit roots to enter the pipe in search of water.

LAYING SEWER TILE

The main job in laying sewer and drain tile is the digging of the trenches and the establishing of the grades. When this is done the rest of the job is comparatively easy.

The digging can be done by hand or by machinery. Two types of machines are used for this purpose. One is a trenching machine which digs a narrow trench suitable for sewer lines but usually is not wide enough for drain tile. The other machine is a back hoe, which can be used for both sewer lines and for drain tile lines. The trenching machine can dig almost exactly to grade. If a back hoe is used the trench should be roughed in then brought to the exact grade by hand. The grade of a sewer line should be ¼″ (0.64 cm.) per foot and the grade of the drain tile should be 1/16″ to ⅛″ (0.16 to 0.32 cm.) per foot.

A common method for determining a grade is by means of batter boards as illustrated in Fig. J-7-1. If machinery is used for the digging the batter boards can be set up after the trench is roughed in and before the hand leveling to grade is done.

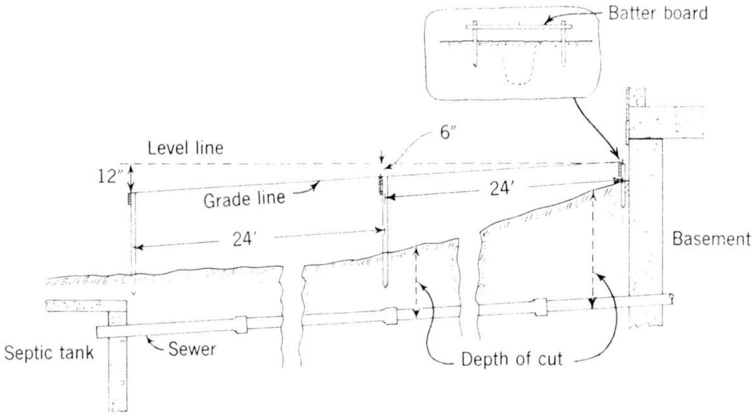

Fig. J-7-1. Method of establishing a grade line for sewer or absorption tile. Note that the pipe is parallel to the grade line regardless of the contour of the soil.

Procedure for erecting batter boards.

1. At the house where the sewer is to come through the foundation, drive two stakes 4 or 5 feet (1.22 or 1.52 m) apart, one on each side of the proposed trench, as shown in Fig. J-7-1.
2. Across these stakes nail a straight board called a "batter board" (see inset), being sure that the top edge is level. A carpenter's level may be used for leveling.
3. At a point 24 feet (7.3 m) away from the first stakes, drive two more stakes.
4. Across these stakes nail another batter board at a point 6 inches (15.24 cm) lower than the first board for a grade of ¼″ (0.64 cm) per foot.
5. At a point 24 feet (7.3 m) from the second set of stakes place another batter board and so continue with the line of stakes and batter boards to the septic tank location. When the batter boards are all up, sight over the top of them to determine if the top edges are in a straight line as they should be.
6. In the top edge of each board drive a nail directly over the center of the proposed trench. When finished these nails should be in a straight line. A string may be used to align the nails.
7. Stretch a stout string from nail to nail for the full length of the trench.

Assume that the inlet tile of the septic tank is in place and that the bottom edge is 4 feet (1.22 m) below the grade string at that point. The bottom of the trench should be 4 feet below the string at all points up to the foundation. This grade should be maintained regardless of the contour of the soil surface.

The width and depth of drain tile trenches should be determined by the requirements outlined in Chapter 11.

If cast-iron soil pipe is used for the sewer line the joints should be caulked with oakum and lead or an approved plastic joint sealer. If bituminous tile is used for the sewer line care should be taken to see that the joints are water tight. Bituminous tile and plastic tile for the drainage field have two rows of holes or a series of slots along the sides. These holes should be placed on the downward side of the tile. See Figs. 11-18 and 11-20.

After the tile is in place cover it with at least 2″ (5 cm) of gravel. Cover the gravel with two inches of straw or a layer of *porous* building paper to keep the dirt out of the gravel. Backfill the trench, or trenches, preferably with sandy or loam soil. Mound the backfill to allow for settling. Sod or seed the backfill.

Leveling to Determine Gravity Head on Water Systems

JOB 8

Often in the development of a water system, particularly the gravity types of systems, it is desirable to know the difference in elevation between the source of water and the point where the water is to be used.

As a preliminary step in determining whether careful differential leveling would be worth while, a rough measurement can be made with a carpenter's level as shown in Fig. J-8-1. A set of sights for the level is desirable but not essential. See Fig. J-8-2.

Set the level on a support at the high point. Aim the level towards the low point and bring it to an exact level position. Sighting across the level toward the low point will indicate roughly the difference in elevation. This is much more accurate than judging the elevation by eye. If the measurement indicates that the elevation is likely to be satisfactory, then it would be worth while to proceed with differential leveling.

Leveling to determine differences in elevation is known as "differential leveling." When very careful work must be done, as in laying

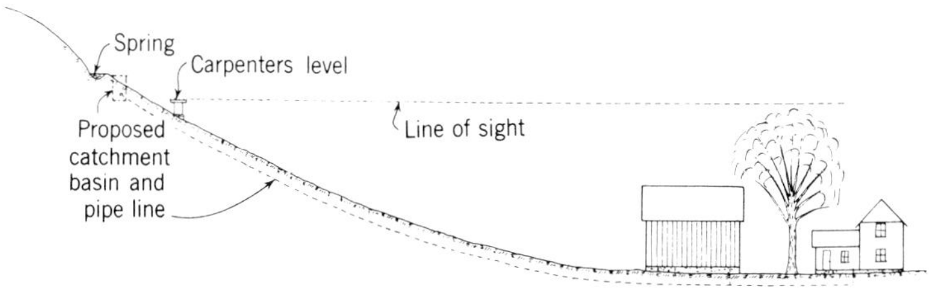

Fig. J-8-1. A method of making a rough check of differences in elevation.

out a building foundation, a good leveling instrument should be used. When leveling for a water system a satisfactory job may be done by means of a carpenter's level, as follows:

Equipment Needed:

Carpenter's level, preferably one equipped with sights. See Fig. J-8-2.

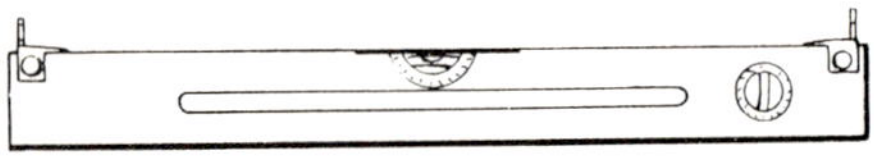

Fig. J-8-2. A carpenter's level equipped with clamp-on sights.

Stick or rod 10 or 12 feet (3 or 4 m) long, marked off in tenths of a foot (or cm) from the bottom up, as shown in Fig. J-8-3.

. A wooden box or a barrel to support the level.

Paper and pencil.

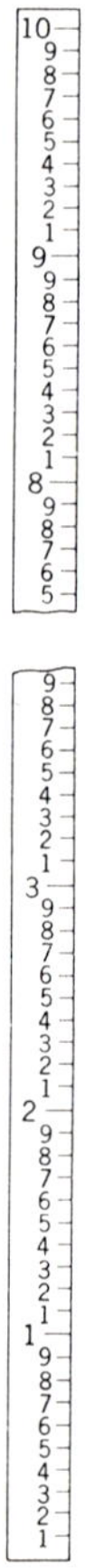

Fig. J-8-3. A rod marked off for use in leveling.

Procedure:

If the difference in elevation between the two points in question is not too great and if the distance between them is not so far that readings cannot be taken on a rod, the procedure may be as follows:

1. Set the level up between the two points, as shown in Fig. J-8-4. Point the level toward one of the points in question, as shown, and wedge or block it up until the bubble shows that it is level.
2. Ask a helper to set the rod on point A, toward which the level is sighted. If this point is the source of water, the rod should be supported on a stone or stake at the surface of the water as shown.
3. Look through the sights and take a reading on the rod. If the rod is too far away to read the figures, it may be necessary to ask the helper to hold a pencil or a stick across the rod in line with the cross hair of the sights to get the reading.
4. Record the reading. In Fig. J-8-4, the reading is 1 foot.
5. Ask the helper to move the rod to the other point B.
6. Turn the level around with the sights pointing toward point B, being sure that the level is leveled.
7. Take the reading on the rod. In Fig. J-8-4 the reading is 9 feet. We now know that the line of sights on the level is 1 foot above the first point A and 9 feet above the second point B. Therefore, the difference between the two readings, 9 feet and 1 foot, or 8 feet.

In Fig. J-8-4 the faucet is 5 feet above point B. Therefore, to obtain the height of the spring above the faucet, subtract 5 feet from 8 feet. The spring therefore has an elevation of 3 feet (0.914 m) above the faucet.*

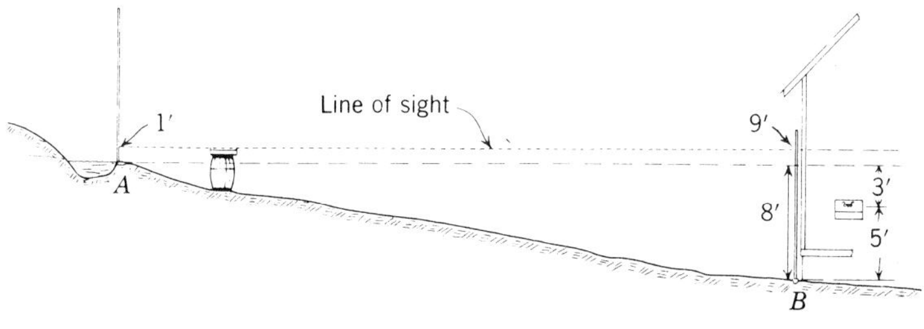

Fig. J-8-4. A method of measuring differences in elevation between two points which are close together.

If the difference in elevation between two points is obviously more than the length of the rod, of if the distance between them is too great to take readings, it will be necessary to set the level up at two or more

*If the rod is marked in metric units the readings will of course be different, but the results will be the same.

Field Notes for Fig. J-8-5.

Station	Backsights, Feet	Foresights, Feet
1	0.5	9.8
2	1.5	8.2
	2.0	18.0

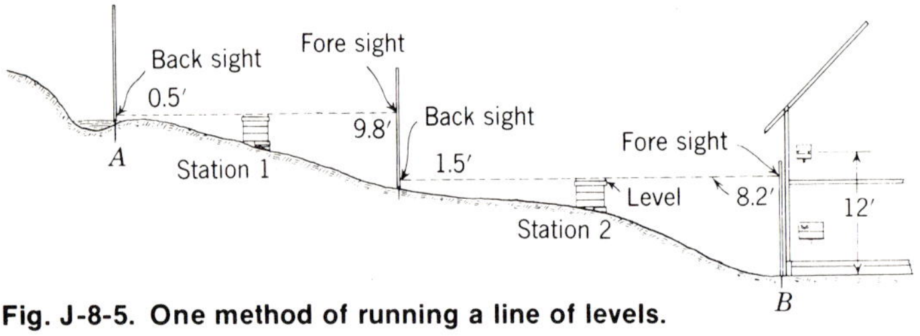

Fig. J-8-5. One method of running a line of levels.

stations and take a series of readings. Such a series of readings is called a "line of levels." The procedure is essentially the same as outlined in the foregoing but is duplicated successively toward point B as shown in Figs. J-8-5 and J-8-6, until the entire distance between the two points has been covered.

At each location or station of the level a sight is taken backward on the rod at its last location and then one forward on the rod at a new location. The sights taken backward are called *backsights* and those taken forward are called *foresights.* For most accurate results the rod should be an equal distance from the level on the backsight and the foresight at each station.

The readings on the rod should be set down on paper, with all the backsights in one column and all the foresights in another column. See field notes for Fig. J-8-5 above. When the leveling is finished the difference in elevation between the two points in question may be obtained by finding the difference between the *sum* of the foresights and the *sum* of the backsights. In the case illustrated in Fig. J-8-5 the sum of the foresights is 18 feet and the sum of the backsights is 2 feet. The difference in elevation between points A and B is therefore 16 feet.

If the sum of the foresights is *greater* than the sum of the backsights, then point B is below point A, as is the case in Fig. J-8-5. If the

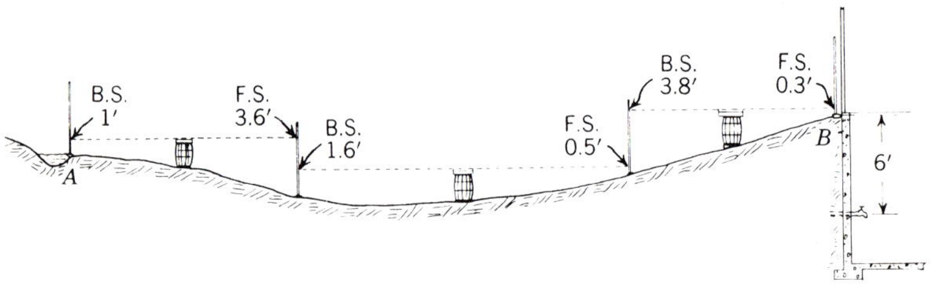

Fig. J-8-6. A line of levels showing the difference in elevation between points A and B.

sum of the foresights is *less* than the sum of the backsights, as would be the case if the levels of Fig. J-8-5 were run from the house to the spring, or as is shown in Fig. J-8-6, then the last point is above the first point.

In any event, the difference in elevation between the last point B and the highest faucet must be taken into consideration in order to determine the difference in elevation between the source of water and the faucet. In Fig. J-8-4 the difference in elevation is 3 feet, as has been shown. In Fig. J-8-5 the highest faucet is 12 feet above point B. The difference in elevation between A and B is 16 feet; therefore, the spring at point A is 4 feet above the highest faucet. In Fig. J-8-6 the faucet is 6 feet below point B. Point B is 2 feet above point A at the spring; therefore, the spring is 4 feet above the faucet.

NOTE: The difference in elevation between points A and B in Fig. J-8-5 is sufficient for satisfactory flow at the faucet if the distance is not too great and if the pipe is large enough. The difference in elevation shown in Fig. J-8-6 is not enough for satisfactory flow, therefore the water would have to be pumped, either directly from the pipe or from a catchment basin as shown in Figs. 3-3 and 3-4, page 24.

MEASUREMENT CONVERSIONS

Linear measure
1 inch = 2.54 cemtimeters (cm)
1 foot = 30.48 cm. = 0.3048 meters (m)
1 cm. = 0.39 inches
1 meter = 39.37 inches
1 mile = 5,280 feet = 1.61 km
1 km = 0.621 mile = 3.281 ft.

Area measure
1 square inch (sq. in.) = 6.45 square centimeters (sq. cm.)
1 square foot (sq. ft.) = 144 sq. in. = 929 cm^2 = 0.09 m^2
1 cm^2 = 0.155 sq. in.
1 m^2 = 10.76 sq. ft. = 1549 sq. in.
1 acre = 43,560 sq. ft. = 0.41 hectare
1 hectare = 2.47 acres

Cubic measure
1 cu. in. = 16.39 cu. cm.
1 cu. ft. = 1728 cu. in. = 28322 cu. cm. = 0.02832 cu. m.
1 cu. cm. = 0.06 cu. in.
1 cu. m = 35.3 cu. ft.

Volume measure
1 liquid quart = 0.946 liters
1 liter = 1.057 liquid quarts
1 U.S. gallon = 0.833 Imperial gallons = 3.79 liters
1 Imperial gallon = 1.2 U.S. gallons

Weight measure
1 pound = 453.6 grams
1 ounce = 28.35 grams
1 gram = 0.035 ounce
1 kilogram = 2.2 pounds
1 U.S. ton = 0.91 metric ton
1 metric ton = 1.1 U.S. ton

$$\text{Grams head per sq. cm.} = \frac{\text{head in feet} \times 453.6}{6.45}$$

Temperature measure
Degrees Fahrenheit (F°) = degrees Centigrade (C°) × 1.8 + 32

$$\text{Degrees centigrade (C°)} = \frac{\text{degrees F} - 32}{1.8}$$

USEFUL INFORMATION

1 U.S. gallons = Imperial gallons ÷0.833

1 Imperial gallons = U.S. gallons ÷1.2

One U.S. gallon of pure water weighs 8.33 lbs. (3.778 kg.) and contains 231 cu. in. (3786 cu. cm.).

One Imperial gallon of pure water weighs 10.26 lbs. (4.65 kg.) and contains 277.2 cu. in. (4543.3 cu. cm.).

One cubic foot of pure water weighs 62.5 pounds (28.35 kg.) and contains 7.48 U.S. gallons. (6.23 Imp. gals.)

The capacity of round tanks and cisterns in U.S. gallons equals the inside diameter in feet squared × 0.7854 × inside height in feet (to overflow pipe) × 7.48. For Imperial gallons divide U.S. gallons by 1.2.

The capacity of square or rectangular tanks or cisterns in U.S. gallons equals the inside length in feet × the inside width in feet × the inside height in feet (to overflow pipe) × 7.48. For Imperial gallons divide U.S. gallons by 1.2.

Atmospheric pressure at sea level 14.7 pounds per sq. in. (6.68 kg. per 6.45 sq. cm.) and will support a column of water 33.9 feet (10.34 m/) high under a vacuum.

One pound (453.6 grams) of pressure on water = 2.3 ft. of head (70.1 cm.).

Head in meters = head in feet × 0.3048

Doubling the diameter of a pipe line increases its capacity four times.

One acre-inch of water = 27,154 U.S. gallons (22,628 Imp. gals.).

Index